T0286274

Thoracic Surgery: Advanced Concepts

Thoracic Surgery: Advanced Concepts

Edited by **Charles Heim**

New Jersey

Published by Foster Academics,
61 Van Reypen Street,
Jersey City, NJ 07306, USA
www.fosteracademics.com

Thoracic Surgery: Advanced Concepts
Edited by Charles Heim

International Standard Book Number: 978-1-63242-401-3 (Hardback)

The publisher's policy is to use permanent paper from mills that operate a sustainable forestry policy. Furthermore, the publisher ensures that the text paper and cover boards used have met acceptable environmental accreditation standards.

Trademark Notice: Registered trademark of products or corporate names are used only for explanation and identification without intent to infringe.

Printed in the United States of America.

Contents

Preface

This book has been a concerted effort by a group of academicians, researchers and scientists, who have contributed their research works for the realization of the book. This book has materialized in the wake of emerging advancements and innovations in this field. Therefore, the need of the hour was to compile all the required researches and disseminate the knowledge to a broad spectrum of people comprising of students, researchers and specialists of the field.

This book on thoracic surgery has been contributed by many famous specialists from across the globe elucidating numerous distinct topics. This book is a compilation of distinct conventional topics elucidating Pancoast Tumors and Repetition Patterns of Stage-I Lung Disorder, Lung Transplantation, Hyperhidrosis, Bronchiectasis, Vena Cava Syndrome, etc. The book provides new techniques in thoracic surgery for students, researchers and surgeons.

At the end of the preface, I would like to thank the authors for their brilliant chapters and the publisher for guiding us all-through the making of the book till its final stage. Also, I would like to thank my family for providing the support and encouragement throughout my academic career and research projects.

Editor

Pancoast Tumors: Surgical Approaches and Techniques

N. Barbetakis

Consultant Thoracic Surgeon, Thoracic Surgery Department, Theagenio Cancer Hospital, Greece

1. Introduction

1.1 History

Tumors of the superior sulcus represent less than 5% of lung malignancies. The distinctive symptomatology was first described by Edwin Hare in 1838 [1], and it has been nearly 80 years since clinical and radiographic features of this tumor were described by Dr Henry Pancoast, a radiologist, in 1924 [2]. As a radiologist, he noted the difficulty in detecting the tumor on a plain chest radiograph. He initially thought that these tumors arose from epithelial crest cells from the fifth brachial cleft. These tumors have been named Pancoast tumors or Pancoast-Tobias tumors after further descriptions of their features by these authors in 1932 [3, 4]. This was the first time that bronchogenic carcinoma was recognised as the primary cause of this syndrome.

Prior to the 1950s, superior sulcus tumors were uniformly fatal. Chardack and McCallum reported a long-term survival after surgical resection and postoperative irradiation therapy [5]. Paulson, using preoperative irradiation followed by surgical resection, published the first series, which included 18 patients, in 1966 [6]. Shaw and Paulson identified that preoperative irradiation and a well-defined resection were associated with a 5-year survival of 34% [7]. Based upon these studies, preoperative irradiation and an extended posterolateral paravertebral thoracotomy (Shaw Paulson approach) has been the "standard of care" over the last 5 decades. However surgical resection remained limited to tumors invading the ribs only, and any further involvement of vascular or neural structures was still considered to remain a contraindication for an operation. This was changed by Dartevelle who was the first to develop an anterior transcervical approach for the resection of tumors involving subclavian vessels. Later on several other modifications of this technique were reported but with no remarkable improvement on overall survival.

In the last century, the management of the superior sulcus tumor changed from inoperability and incurability to the current regimen of preoperative chemoradiation therapy, with an attempt at complete resection. Interest in trimodality treatment led to the South-West Oncology Group (SWOG) 8805 study of induction chemoradiotherapy (cisplatin, etoposide, 45Gy) followed by surgery that resulted in a complete response rate of 22% and encouraging results [8]. A recent prospective phase II study (SWOG 9416) suggests that preoperative concurrent chemoradiation (cisplatin, etoposide, 45Gy) improves the rate of complete resection, intermediate survival and decreases the rate of local or distal recurrence [9]. The 2-year survival was 55% for all eligible patients and 70% for patients who had a complete resection.

The superior sulcus tumor is a rare tumor posing a unique challenge to thoracic surgeons. The current regimen of preoperative chemoradiation with complete surgical resection leads to reasonable long term survival. Progress is being made in the understanding of the anatomy and biology of this disease. A choice of incisions provides options that have the potential to increase the rate of complete resection. New techniques allow resection of structures that were previously considered unresectable. Future efforts to improve the results will entail not only multidisciplinary approach to en bloc extended resection of adjacent structures but also preoperative therapy (chemotherapy or biologic agents) that yields greater tumor regression, thereby improving complete resection rates that are so critical to long-term survival in this form of non-small cell lung cancer (NSCLC).

2. Definition and surgical anatomy

Pancoast tumor is a cancer of the apex of the lung with no intervening lung tissue between tumor and chest wall. Subsequently, there is involvement of structures of the apical chest wall above the level of the second rib. The chest wall involvement may be limited to invasion of parietal pleura or may extend deeper to involve the periosteum or the bone of the first rib or apical vertebral bodies, or it may include invasion of subclavian vessels, the nerve roots of the brachial plexus or the stellate ganglion. Involvement of the chest wall only at the level of the second rib or lower should not be considered to meet the criteria for Pancoast tumor [10]. An apical tumor involving only the visceral pleura and not the chest wall by clinical staging should not be classified as a Pancoast tumor. However, it seems reasonable to include tumors that are thought to involve chest wall by clinical criteria.

Superior sulcus tumors may occur in the three compartments of the thoracic inlet and symptoms are related to the location. The anterior compartment lies anterior to the insertion of the anterior scalene muscle onto the first rib, the middle compartment extends from there to the posterior border of the middle scalene muscle, whereas the posterior compartment lies behind the middle scalene muscle [11]. Tumors located in the anterior component may invade the subclavian vessels, whereas those in the middle mainly invade the brachial plexus (Figures 1, 2). Posterior Pancoast tumors usually invade the stellate ganglion or vertebral bodies (Figure 3).

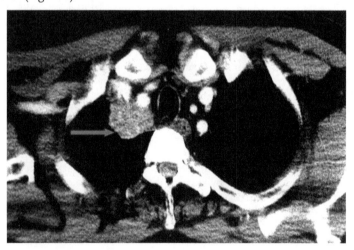

Fig. 1. Pancoast tumor located in the anterior component (anterior Pancoast tumor).

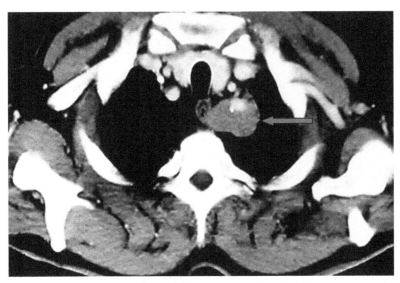

Fig. 2. Pancoast tumor occupying the middle component (median Pancoast tumor).

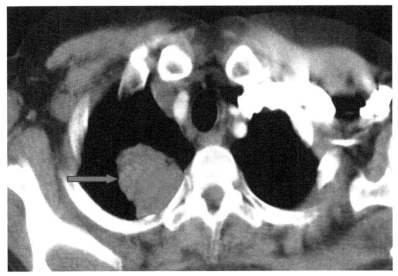

Fig. 3. Pancoast tumor located in the posterior component (posterior Pancoast tumor).

In case of invasion of the brachial plexus, patients often present with intense pain that begins in the shoulder and scapular region and extends down to the ulnar aspect of the arm (T1 dermatome) onto the small and ring fingers (C8 dermatome). Due to increasing pressure on the nerve roots, muscle atrophy of the ulnar aspect of the hand and loss of the triceps reflux can occur. In about 20-30% of patients, tumor invasion of the sympathetic chain and the stellate ganglion causes Horner's syndrome (ipsilateral ptosis, miosis and anhydrosis) [12].

COMPARTMENT	BOUNDARIES	included STRUCTURES	SIGNS AND SYMPTOMS
Anterior	Between sternum and anterior edge of anterior scalene muscle.	Platysma, sternocleidomastoid and omohyoid muscles, jugular and subclavian veins, scalene fat pad.	Pain radiating to the upper anterior chest wall, venous thrombosis.
Middle	Between anterior and posterior border of middle scalene muscle	Anterior and middle scalene muscles, subclavian artery and primary branches, phrenic nerve, trunks of brachial plexus	Pain and parasthesia radiating to the shoulder and upper limb, arterial thrombosis, diaphragmatic paralysis
Posterior	Behind middle scalene muscle	Posterior scalene muscle, posterior scapular artery, posterior aspect of subclavian and vertebral artery, paravertebral sympathetic chain, stellate ganglion, nerve roots of brachial plexus, long thoracic and spinal accessory nerves, neural foramina, vertebral bodies and prevertebral muscles.	Pain in the axilla and in the medial part of the upper arm, Horner's syndrome.

Table 1. Anatomical definition of the thoracic inlet and main clinical features in case of superior sulcus tumor invasion [13].

3. Biological behaviour

Advanced molecular biology techniques have accelerated the understanding of cancer biology. It is well established that the application of such technology has led to the recognition of lung cancer as a molecularly diverse set of tumor types whose only commonality is their origination in the lung [14]. Lung cancer classification is far more complex than the simplistic grouping into small cell and non-small cell variants with a comparable outcome when treated in a similar fashion [15]. Histologic subdivision of lung cancer uses only one of many phenotypic manifestations of the genetic changes that underlie lung cancer development.

Lung cancer development is a result of a stepwise progression of malignant transformation of normal respiratory epithelium. This transformation is driven by the cumulative effect of genetic alterations induced predominantly by inhaled carcinogens from tobacco smoke [16]. The Noguchi classification of lung adenocarcinoma is a pioneering effort to relate tumor histology with clinical and radiologic characteristics. This has resulted in the identification of atypical adenomatous hyperplasia and adenocarcinoma in situ as preinvasive neoplastic lung lesions that serve as precursors to invasive lung adenocarcinoma through a progressive transformation into the type A, B, and C adenocarcinomas with lepidic growth (referring to growth along alveolar structures) characterized by an increasing component of invasive carcinoma but showing excellent survival outcome, and the type D, E, and F solid-type adenocarcinomas with a well-recognized poor prognosis [17]. The most frequently described acquired genetic aberrations within the tumor involve the tumor protein p53 (TP53), KRAS, fragile histidine triad (FHIT), epidermal growth factor receptor (EGFR), cyclin-dependent kinase 2a (CDKN2), LKB1, retinoblastoma (RB), and Myc genes. Larger genomic mishaps such as chromosomal deletions involving the short arms of chromosomes 1, 3, and 9 (del 1p36, del 3p, and del 9p, respectively) are also frequently observed in different lung cancer histologic subtypes and stages. More recently, inversion translocation of the echinoderm microtubule-associated protein-like 4 (EML4) and anaplastic lymphoma kinase (ALK) genes on chromosome 2 (2p21 and 2p23) was shown to characterize a small subset of NSCLC with a characteristic clinical and histologic profile. The discovery of other molecularly defined lung cancer subsets is likely to be hastened by this finding [18].

The treatment options for patients with lung cancer have improved considerably in recent years. Improvements in survival have been noted for patients with every stage of the disease with the integration of new systemic therapy options, improvements to local therapy, and supportive care measures. A number of molecularly targeted agents that modulate a wide array of cell signaling pathways are currently under development. The remarkable success achieved with the use of EGFR tyrosine kinase inhibitors and the ALK inhibitors are the initial steps toward an era of individualized treatment options for patients with NSCLC. Several groups are now involved in screening tumor specimens for dominant oncogenic drivers in individual patients to guide treatment selection. A total of 13 known molecular abnormalities including 8 mutations are evaluated in the tumor specimens. By developing novel clinical trials across institutions to target each of these molecular events, the oncologist is evaluating a variety of individualized treatment approaches for patients with NSCLC. Because these molecular changes are noted in much smaller subsets of patients, such clinical trials are unlikely to complete accrual within a single institution in a reasonable time and therefore require such collaborative efforts to accelerate research.

The tremendous increase in the knowledge of lung cancer biology notwithstanding, a number of important questions remain unanswered. With lung cancer in never-smokers having been recognized as a unique entity, insights into the underlying mechanism and etiological factors will help in the development of novel therapies for this group of patients. The differences in lung cancer biology based on gender are another important area of research that will hopefully lead to the development of gender-driven therapeutic approaches. As newer therapeutic options are developed, participation of patients in clinical trials must be encouraged and supported by health care delivery systems. Currently, fewer than 5% of the patients diagnosed with cancer participate in therapeutic clinical trials [19]

Concerning Pancoast tumors it was traditionally believed that the biology was different from that of other non–small cell lung cancers and in that these tumors had a strong propensity to local invasion and a diminished incidence of spread through lymphatic or hematogenous routes. However, recent data does not support this belief [20]. Additionally the incidence of pathologic N2 disease, is similar to that of other peripheral stage I or II lung tumors and survival is better following a formal lobectomy rather than a wedge resection alone. The unique feature of Pancoast tumors appears not to lie in the tumor biology but rather in the anatomy of the region in which these tumors occur.

Ipsilateral supraclavicular nodal involvement is classified as N3 disease. However, there is some evidence that such involvement in patients with a Pancoast tumor may not preclude long-term survival. Ipsilateral supraclavicular node involvement in these patients may have a prognostic importance more akin to that of N1 disease [21].

4. Surgical approaches

4.1 Posterior approach

The ideal tumor for the posterolateral approach is situated posteriorly in the superior sulcus and does not invade the anterior structures of the thoracic inlet. It may however invade the vertebral bodies or the brachial plexus. The C8 and T1 nerve roots are most commonly invaded. It is important to assess the patient's neurologic function preoperatively and to inform him properly concerning postoperative neurological morbidity [22].

The patient is placed in the lateral decubitus position. The incision starts anteriorly, allowing exploration of the chest cavity (usually through the fourth/fifth interspace) to assess resectability. The extension of the tumor onto the thoracic chest wall, thoracic inlet, lung, and mediastinum should be assessed. The incision is then extended posteriorly around the tip of the scapula and vertically upward between the spinous processes and posterior edge of the scapula, up to C7 (Figure 4). The division of muscle layers starts from the latissimus dorsi and trapezius to expose and subsequently divide the serratus anterior, rhomboidius major and minor, and levator scapulae muscles. The dorsal scapular nerve and scapular artery branches should be avoided when dividing the rhomboids at their insertion into the medial border of the scapula. These muscles will all be meticulously reapproximated at the end of the case. The chest wall resection is carried out first, in order to release the involved chest wall into the pleural cavity allowing for a safer lobectomy. En bloc resection of the chest wall and lung is preferred to extrapleural dissection without rib sacrifice, which often leads to incomplete resection. In most cases, the first two or three ribs are removed, although more ribs may be resected if required. The resection should guarantee large free margins, resecting 3-4 cm of uninvolved rib anteriorly and one rib and the intercostal muscle below the tumor inferiorly.

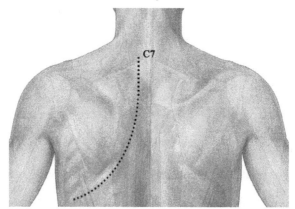

Fig. 4. Posterior approach for Pancoast tumors (Shaw Paulson thoracotomy). The incision extends up to the 7th cervical vertebrae.

First, the anterior and inferior dissection is started along the established resection margins beginning with the healthy rib. The invaded ribs and intercostal muscles are divided using rib shears and electrocautery, in succession from below to above, and the intercostal neurovascular pedicles are ligated. When the first rib is reached, the anterior and middle scalenus insertions to the second and first rib are divided with cautery, exposing the structures of the thoracic inlet crossing above the first rib. It is very important to note the insertions of the anterior and middle scalene on the first rib. Also of note is the phrenic nerve lying on the anterior surface of the anterior scalene. This, as well as the subclavian vein and artery should be identified before dividing the anterior scalene.

The posterior phase of the dissection starts by incising the erector spinae muscle along its anterior border from T1 to T5 and retracting it outward to expose the costotransverse joint. If the tumor involves the parietal pleura only, with no rib or vertebral erosion, the ribs may be disarticulated from the transverse processes, preserving the latter structures. The intercostal nerve and vessel originating from the intervertebral foramen are identified and divided between clips or sutured with 3-0 Prolene. This manoeuvre is repeated for each rib, until the first rib is reached. If the tumor involves the ribs posteriorly, the transverse processes are removed along with the adjacent lateral cortex of the vertebrae using an osteotome.

The lower trunk of the brachial plexus is identified by retracting the first rib downward and can be dissected posteriorly until it splits into the C8 (above the neck of the first rib) and T1 (below the neck of the first rib) nerve roots. Most commonly, the neoplastic invasion is limited to the first thoracic nerve root, which may be divided medial to its entry into the lower trunk and lateral to tumor involvement, keeping the C8 nerve root intact. This is very important in order to avoid the morbidity of loss of function of the intrinsic muscles of the hand [23]. When the tumor involves the C8 nerve, the lower trunk of the brachial plexus should be divided medially, at its origin from the spine. When the T1 nerve root is divided there is usually only a sensory deficit along the medial aspect of the hand.

With a hand inside the chest, the first rib is cut either at its neck if the head is not involved with tumor or beyond the attachment of its tubercle to the transverse process. The chest wall is then released from the apex of the chest en bloc by sequentially dividing the lower portion of the stellate ganglion and first intercostal artery.

Then a formal upper lobectomy with systematic lymph node dissection is the final step. The tumor attached to the chest wall is removed as one specimen. At this time a routine evaluation of the margins is done, obtaining biopsies and placing clips for helping postoperative irradiation.

It is not usually necessary to reconstitute the posterior defect in the chest wall, as it is covered by the scapula. A defect of three or more ribs or over the tip of the scapula should be closed with synthetic mesh. It is well established that meticulous reapproximation and closure with mesh prevents major morbidity in respiratory chest wall motion.

The posterior approach allows excellent exposure of the posterior chest wall including the transverse processes and thoracic nerve roots. It also allows standard exposure of the pulmonary hilum. However, surgical manipulation of the subclavian vessels is very difficult. Furthermore, visualization of the apex is poor making assessment of the appropriate extent of resection problematic.

4.2 Anterior approach
The anterior surgical approach to Pancoast tumors is modified to optimize exposure. Depending on location and size of the tumor there are two basic incisions: 1) a transclavicular incision and 2) a hemi-clamshell incision with supraclavicular extension.

The transclavicular incision (Dartevelle approach) is used with the patient in the supine position with the neck hyperextended and the head turned toward the uninvolved side [24]. The skin is prepared from the mastoid process to the xyphoid process and from the midaxillary line to the contralateral midclavicular line. The cervicotomy uses an L-shaped incision that follows the anterior border of sternocleidomastoid muscle and the inferior border of the clavicle to the deltopectoral groove (Figure 5). In first reports, a standard clavicular resection was included but this was associated with functional disability and suboptimal cosmetic results. An alternative approach involves bisecting the manubrium to preserve the claviculomanubrial junction (Grunenwald approach) (Figure 6) [25].

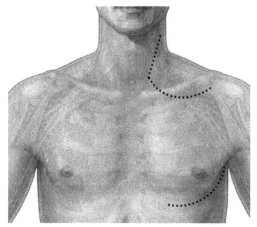

Fig. 5. Anterior transclavicular approach for Pancoast tumors (Dartevelle approach).

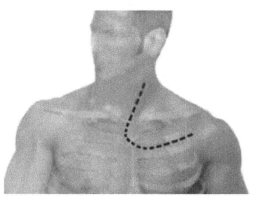

Fig. 6. Anterior approach for Pancoast tumors (Grunenwald approach).

The hemi-clamshell incision is a clavicular-sparing approach [23]. The patient is in full lateral position with slight posterior rotation. The skin is prepared in the same manner as described for the transclavicular approach. In patients requiring a supraclavicular extension, the ipsilateral arm is incorporated in the skin preparation.

The sternocleidomastoid muscle is divided and the medial half of the clavicle is resected. Variations of this approach include simple division of the mid-portion of the clavicle and subsequent reconstruction with plates and screws, or disarticulation of the sternoclavicular joint and lateral retraction of the clavicle.

The sequential steps involve dissection of the jugular veins, dissection of the arteries and exposure of the brachial plexus. Dissection of the jugular veins is important for adequate exposure. Ligation of the internal jugular vein is well tolerated. Especially on the left side, the thoracic duct is ligated with care.

The anterior scalene muscle is divided either at its insertion on the scalene tubercle of the first rib, or as close as it gets to its origin at the transverse processes of C3-C5. The anterior scalene muscle is well defined in 2/3 of patients and may be located behind the subclavian artery or split into two with the artery passing between the bundles [26]. The subclavian artery is mobilized by dividing most of its branches. Care is taken to preserve the vertebral artery and resection of the vessel is done only if it is involved with the tumor. A preoperative Doppler ultrasound is important to detect any extracranial occlusive disease. If the subclavian artery is invaded by the tumor, the affected portion is resected and reconstructed with a PTFE vascular graft. A small dose of heparin is administered during vascular clamping. Following anterior traction of the subclavian artery, the middle scalene muscle comes into good view.

The middle scalene muscle originates from the transverse processes of C2-C7and inserts onto the first rib between the subclavian groove and the posterior tubercle of the transverse process. In tumors invading the middle compartment of the thoracic inlet, the middle scalene muscle may be extensively involved. In these cases resection of the middle scalene muscle requires mobilization along its origin from the lower cervical vertebrae.

At this stage the cords of the brachial plexus are identified laterally. The anterior surface of vertebral bodies C7 and T1 are in view. The sympathetic chain and the stellate ganglion are lying in front of the vertebral bodies of C7 and T1. C8 and T1 nerve roots are visualized and dissected medially up to the lower trunk of the brachial plexus. The C8 nerve component of the plexus is preserved for better functional outcome of the upper limb. For carcinomas affecting the spine a multilevel unilateral laminectomy, nerve root division inside the spinal canal and vertebral body division can be performed by neurosurgeons.

The chest wall resection is performed with progressive resection of the first, second and third ribs. The ribs are resected from the costochondral junction anteriorly to the articulation with the transverse process. To facilitate mobility of the en bloc mass, resection of a short segment of rib (1-2 cm), may create a "mobile" chest wall. Resection of lower ribs is difficult and pulmonary resection by means of a conventional lobectomy is difficult. It may sometimes be necessary to perform a separate posterior thoracotomy to complete the resection and lymph node dissection.

The anterior approach facilitates direct visualization of vascular structures and provides excellent exposure of brachial plexus, sympathetic chain and stellate ganglion. There is freedom for hemi-vertebrectomy for tumors invading anterior parts of the vertebrae. Oncological clearance seems to be optimal due to the fact that the tumor is the last structure to be encountered. Finally the anterior approach seems to offer less morbidity than the posterior one.

A relative disadvantage of the anterior approach is the difficulty in removing the transverse processes and the head of the ribs in order to disarticulate them. The need to perform an additional posterior thoracotomy for the lobectomy and systematic mediastinal lymph node dissection could be seen as a factor that negates the routine use of anterior approach.

4.3 Future perspectives

Although the understanding of the biology and treatment of Pancoast tumors has evolved significantly, it is clear that more progress is needed. When considering that a large randomized trial may not be performed due to the relative rarity of the disease, the present clinical evidence from several phase II studies suggests that induction chemoradiotherapy and surgery be recommended as modern standard of care for Pancoast tumors. However, there are many issues still remaining for debate or are under discussion [27].

1. Recruitment of patients with N2 disease for surgery.
2. Ipsilateral supraclavicular lymph node disease should be considered as N1 disease.
3. The role of high dose preoperative radiotherapy (6000 cGy).
4. The role of prophylactic cranial irradiation.
5. The role of adjuvant postoperative chemotherapy.
6. The role of more aggressive surgery in cases of extensive involvement of the brachial plexus.

5. Acknowledgements

Sincere thanks to:
*   Dr Francess Gillespie-Tsilikas (Consultant Anesthesiologist) for her valuable help in language editing.
*   Dr Christos Asteriou and Dr Athanassios Kleontas (Residents in Cardiothoracic Surgery) for the photos and figures.
*   Dr Christodoulos Tsilikas (Chief Thoracic Surgeon) for his mentoring and endless support.

6. References

[1] Hare ES. Tumor involving certain nerves [Letter]. London Med Gaz 1838;1:16-18.
[2] Pancoast H. Importance of careful roentgen-ray investigation of apical chest tumors. JAMA 1924;83:1407.
[3] Pancoast HK. Superior pulmonary sulcus tumor: tumor characterized by pain, Horner's syndrome, destruction of bone and atrophy of hand muscles. JAMA 1932;99:1391-1396.
[4] Tobias J. Sindrome apico-costo-vertebral doloroso por tumor apexiano: su valor diagnostico en el cancer promitivo pulmonary (Spanish) Rev Med Lat Am 1932;19:1552-1556.
[5] Chardack WM, Mc Callum JD. Pancoast tumor: five-year survival without recurrence or metastases following radical resection and postoperative irradiation. J Thorac Surg 1956;31:532-534.
[6] Paulson DL. The survival rate in superior sulcus tumors treated by presurgical irradiation. JAMA 1966;196:342.
[7] Shaw RR, Paulson DL Kee JL Jr. Treatment of superior sulcus tumor by irradiation followed by resection. Ann Surg 1961;154:29-40.
[8] Albain KS, Rusch VW, Crowley JJ. Concurrent cisplatin/etoposide plus chest radiotherapy followed by surgery for stages IIIA (N2) and IIIB non small cell lung

cancer: mature results of South West Oncology Group phase II study 8805. J Clin Oncol 1995;13:1880-1892.

[9] Rusch VW, Giroux DJ, Kraut MJ. Induction chemoradiation and surgical resection for non-small cell lung carcinomas of the superior sulcus: Initial results of South West Oncology Group Trial 9416 (Intergroup Trial 0160). J Thorac Cardiovasc Surg 2001;121:472-483.

[10] Detterbeck FC. Changes in the treatment of Pancoast tumors. Ann Thorac Surg 2003;75:1990-1997.

[11] Dartevelle P, Macchiarini P. Resection of superior sulcus tumors. In Kaiser LR, Kron IL, Spray TL, eds. Mastery of cardiothoracic surgery. Philadelphia: Lippincott-Raven 1998:257-265.

[12] Komaki R, Putnam JB, Walsh G, Lee JS, Cox JD. The management of superior sulcus tumors. Semin Surg Oncol 2000;18:152-164.

[13] Rea F, Marulli G, Sartori F. Posterolateral (Shaw-Paulson) approach to Pancoast tumor. http://www.ctsnet.org/sections/clinicalresources/thoracic/expert_tech-38.html

[14] Fujii T, Dracheva T, Player A et al. A preliminary transcriptome map of non-small cell lung cancer. Cancer Res 2002;62:3340-3346.

[15] Brambilla E, Travis WD, Colby TW, Corrin B, Shimoshato Y. The new World Health Organization classification of lung tumors. Eur Respir J 2001;18 :1059-1068.

[16] Boyle P. Cancer, cigarette smoking and premature death in Europe: a review including The Recommendations of European Cancer Experts Consensus Meeting. Lung Cancer 1997;17:1-60.

[17] Noguchi M. Stepwise progression of pulmonary adenocarcinoma–clinical and molecular implications. Cancer Metastasis Rev. 2010; 29: 15-21.

[18] Soda M, Choi YL, Enomoto M, et al. Identification of the transforming EML4-ALK fusion gene in non-small-cell lung cancer. Nature. 2007; 448: 561-566.

[19] Ramalingam SS, Owonikoko TK, Khuri FR. Lung cancer: New biological insights and recent therapeutic advances.CA Cancer Journal for Clinicians 2011;61:91-112.

[20] Detterbeck F.C., Jones D.R., Rosenman J.G. Pancoast tumors. In: Detterbeck F.C., Rivera M.P., Socinski M.A., Rosenman J.G., eds. Diagnosis and treatment of lung cancer: an evidence-based guide for the practicing clinician. Philadelphia: WB Saunders, 2001:233-243.

[21] Ginsberg R.J., Martini N., Zaman M., et al. Influence of surgical resection and brachytherapy in the management of superior sulcus tumor. Ann Thorac Surg 1994;57:1440-1445.

[22] Nicastri GD, Swanson JS. Pros and Cons of anterior and posterior approaches to Pancoast tumors: posterolateral superior sulcus tumors resections. Operative Techniques in Thoracic and Cardiovascular Surgery 2006;6:141-153.

[23] Nesbit JC, Wind GG, Rusch VW (Consulting Ed), Walsh GL (Consulting Ed). Superior Sulcus Tumor resection in Nesbit JC, Wind GG (Eds): Thoracic Surgical Oncology: Exposures and Techniques, Philadelphia, Lippincott Williams and Wilkins, 2003.

[24] Dartevelle P, Macchiarini P. Surgical management of superior sulcus tumors. Oncologist 1999;4:398-407.

[25] Grunenwald D, Spaggiari L. Transmanubrial osteomuscular sparing approach for apical chest tumors. Ann Thorac Surg 1997;63:563-566.

[26] Dartevelle P, Mentzer SJ. Anterior approach to superior sulcus tumors. Operative Techniques in Thoracic and Cardiovascular Surgery 2006;6:154-163.

[27] Parissis H, Young V. Treatment of Pancoast tumors from the surgeon's prospective: reappraisal of the anterior-manubrial sternal approach. J Cardiothorac Surg 2010;5:102.

2

Surgical Treatment of Bronchiectasis

Hidir Esme and Sevval Eren
Konya Education and Researc Hospital,
Dicle University, School of Medicine,
Turkey

1. Introduction

Bronchiectasis is pathologically defined as a condition in which there are abnormal and permanent dilatations of proximal bronchi with predominance at the level of the second to the sixth bronchial division. This definition differentiates true bronchiectasis from functional bronchiectasis or pseudobronchiectasis, which is expected to return to normal once control of infection has been achieved (Deslauriers et al., 1998). Bronchiectasis was first described by Laenec in 1819 and, before the antibiotic era, was considered a morbid disease with a high mortality rate from respiratory failure and cor pulmonale (Balkanli et al., 2003). With the development of antibiotics in the 1940s, this entity began to be seen less frequently, but, with the emergence of drug-resistant microorganisms and the increasing frequency of drug-resistant tuberculosis, an increased incidence of postinfectious bronchiectasis is being noted (Miller, 2000). The current increase in tuberculosis rates is directly related to insufficient and irregular medication. Additionally, irregular and inadequate treatment, the cessation of medication shortly after symptom improvement, and a lack of check-ups after treatment are factors accelerating recurrent pulmonary infection in developing countries. As the disease progresses, physical activities become increasingly limited, patients fail to thrive, and ultimately they suffer from social deprivation, intrinsic depression, and respiratory failure (Al-Kattan et al., 2005). Therefore, bronchiectasis is still a major cause of morbidity and mortality in developing countries.

2. Pathophysiology

Reid categorized bronchiectasis as having three main phenotypes: 1) tubular characterized by smooth dilation of the bronchi; 2) varicose in which the bronchi are dilated with multiple indentations; and 3) cystic in which dilated bronchi terminate in blind ending sacs (Reid, 1950). The current major form seen on High resolution computed tomography scanning (HRCT) is the tubular form of bronchiectasis. The most definitive study of the pathology of bronchiectasis was performed by Whitwell (Whitwell, 1952). Whitwell suggested that bronchiectasis should be divided into (1) follicular bronchiectasis, characterized by excessive formation of lymphoid tissue both in the walls of dilated bronchi and in enlarged lymph nodes and thought to be sequelae of whooping cough, measles, or bronchopneumonia, (2) saccular bronchiectasis, characterized by loss of bronchial structures in the sacculi and of alveoli around them, and (3) atelectatic bronchiectasis, in which lung collapse leads to bronchiectasis. Follicular bronchiectasis was the dominant form and this corresponded to tubular bronchiectasis. In his study, he demonstrated marked inflammation of the bronchial wall, principally in the smaller airways. Bronchial dilation was characterized by deficiency/loss of elastin and more advance disease by destruction of muscle and cartilage. There was variable bronchial wall fibrosis, atelectasis and peribronchial pneumonic change (King, 2009).

Follicular bronchiectasis was characterized by the presence of lymphoid follicles in the bronchial wall. The inflammatory process commenced in the small airway. This small airway inflammation caused the release of mediators such as proteases which damaged the large airways causing loss of elastin and other components such as muscle and cartilage which resulted in bronchial dilation. With progression of the disease lymphoid follicles enlarged in size and caused airflow obstruction to the small airways. The final event was spread of the inflammation beyond the airways to cause interstitial pneumonia (King, 2009). The dominant cell types involved in the inflammatory process in bronchiectasis are neutrophils, lymphocytes, and macrophages. Neutrophils are the most prominent cell type in the bronchial lumen (Loukide et al., 2002; Khair et al., 1996) and release mediators, particularly proteases/elastase which cause bronchial dilation (Khair et al., 1996; Zheng et al., 2000). The infiltrate in the cell wall is predominantly composed of macrophages and lymphocytes (Loukide et al., 2002; Lapa a Silva et al., 1989)

Bronchiectasis can occur as focal or localized disease, or in a diffuse manner. Localized bronchiectasis is usually the result of childhood pneumonia and often has a benign course characterized by recurrent pulmonary infections always in the same anatomic territory. By contrast, diffuse bronchiectasis is often related to immune deficiencies, is bilateral, and may lead to death from respiratory failure (Deslauriers et al., 1998). Karadag et al. found that bronchiectasis most commonly involved the lower lobes. Only one lobe was found to be diseased in 46%, bilobar involvement in 28.1%, and multilobar involvement in 31.9% (Karadag et al., 2005). Karakoc et al. found bronchiectasis affecting the left lower lobe in 30.4%, and multilobar involvement in 56.5% (Karakoc et al., 2001). Dogru et al. found the most common lobe affected by bronchiectasis was the left-lower lobe in the 204 children they evaluated (Dogru et al., 2005). Isolated upper lobe bronchiectasis generally relates to prior tuberculosis, bronchopulmonary aspergillosis, or bronchial obstruction. Overall, one-third of cases of bronchiectasis are unilateral and affect a single lobe, one-third are unilateral but affect more than one lobe, and one-third are bilateral (Figure 1) (Deslauriers et al., 1998).

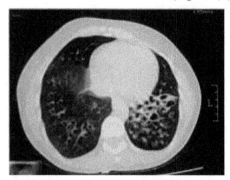

Fig. 1. Chest CT scan showing bilateral cystic bronchiectasis in the lower lobes.

The middle lobe syndrome consists of a small atelectatic lobe, often owing to extrinsic bronchial compression secondary to enlarged peribronchial nodes (Deslauriers et al., 1998). The right middle lobe bronchus is long, often bends sharply at its bifurcation and is of relatively small caliber. A collar of lymph nodes also surrounds the proximal bronchus and any condition that causes a prolonged enlargement of these nodes may lead to obstruction and secondary bronchiectasis. This may also occur in malignancy and in nontuberculous mycobacterial infection (Figure 2) (Bertelsen et al., 1980; Levin, 2002).

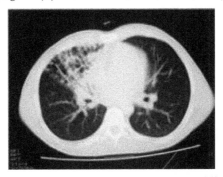

Fig. 2. Chest CT scan showing the bronchiectasis in the right middle lobe

3. Etiology

There have been a large number of factors that have been described as causative for bronchiectasis. A list of etiologic factors in different studies is given in Table 1. Recurrent pulmonary infection during childhood is an important factor in the etiology. Most of patients had recurrent infections in their histories and insufficient medication for pulmonary infection (Prieto et al., 2001; Agasthian et al., 1996; Fujimoto et al., 2001). The insufficient and inadequate use of medications for pulmonary infections and tuberculosis in patients, and the lack of follow-up over time, create a background for lung destruction (Figure 3). Bronchiectasis should not be mistaken with pseudo-bronchiectasis, temporary (up to 6 months) cylindrical dilatation of the bronchi accompanying lung infection in children (Sirmali et al., 2006). In developing countries, tuberculosis is still one of the most important causes of bronchiectasis. Bronchiectasis commonly develops between 1 and 3 months after the initial infection and usually in the same pulmonary region (Karakoc et al., 2001; Haciibrahimoglu et al., 2004).

Deficiencies in immune function, especially in humoral immunity, cause children to be at risk for recurrent sinopulmonary infections, which can lead to the development of bronchiectasis. This includes both primary immunodeficiency and secondary, or acquired, disease states (Boren et al., 2008). Cystic fibrosis is the most common cause of bronchiectasis among Caucasians of North America and Europe. Muco-ciliary clearance is a key defence mechanism against pulmonary infection. Its compromise is important in the development of the vicious cycle of bronchiectasis. The most prominent cilial disorder is primary ciliary dyskinesia which combines upper and lower respiratory tract infection, male infertility and in approximately 50%, situs inversus (King, 2009). Bronchial obstruction from either endobronchial pathology or external compression can also be an acquired factor predisposing to the development of bronchiectasis. Aspirated foreign bodies or gastric contents, slow-growing neoplasms, and mucous impaction can all cause local retention of secretions, secondary infection, and bronchiectasis (Deslauriers et al., 1998).

Etiolgic factor	Balkanli n, %	Eren n; %	Sırmali n, %	Cobanoglu n, %	Giovannetti n, %
Pneumonia	86 (36.1)	22 (15.3)	109 (61.9)	18 (29.0)	10 (22.2)
Childhood infection	63 (26.4)	19 (13.2)	-	7 (11.3)	-
Obstruction due to foreign body	1 (0.4)	4 (2.7)	23 (13)	1 (1.6)	-
Pulmonary sequestration	4 (1.6)	2 (1.4)	-	4 (6.4)	-
Postobstructive pneumonitis	-	34 (23.7)	-	2 (3.2)	-
Measles	-	-	-	4 (6.4)	-
Pertussis	-	-	-	3 (4.8)	4 (8.8)
Tuberculosis	-	22 (15.3)	44 (25)	11 (17.7)	6 (13.3)
Immunodeficiency (IgG, IgA)	-	-	-	1 (1.6)	-
Cystic fibrosis	-	-	-	2 (3.2)	-
Unknown etiology	84 (35.2)	40 (27.9)	-	4 (6.4)	25 (55%)

Table 1. Etiologic factors of bronchiectasis

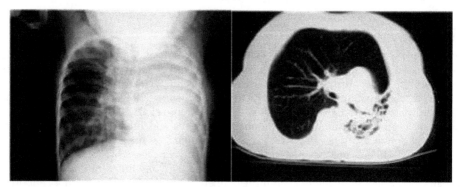

Fig. 3. Standart PA chest radigraph and Chest CT scan of a 4-year-old boy shows a destroyed left lung.

4. Clinical presentation

The clinical presentation of patients with bronchiectasis is variable and depends on the etiology of bronchiectasis and on whether the condition is localized of diffuse. Semptoms of the patients in different studies were presented in Table 2. The primary clinical symptom of bronchiectasis is a recurrent or permanent cough with ample sputum production. The sputum is frequently purulent and is often accompanied by hemoptysis in advanced stages of the disease (Nicotra et al., 1995). In the past, some bronchiectasis has been described as being nonproductive or "dry", although in retrospect these were mostly cases of post-tuberculous bronchiectasis located in the upper lobes (Deslauriers et al., 1998). Severe and life-threatening bleeding may result from erosions of the hypertrophic bronchial arteries or lesions in abnormal anastomoses between the pulmonary and bronchial arterial circulations.

Symptoms may be mild (eg, unproductive cough) or even absent if the disease is restricted to the upper lobes. Patients may also present with symptoms of the underlying disease that has led to the development of bronchiectasis (Zhang et al., 2010). Acute exacerbations of bronchiectasis are defined by symptomatic changes, including increased thick sputum production with change in color, shortness of breath, pleuritic chest pain, and generalized malaise. Chest roentgenograph (CXR) rarely shows new infiltrates, and the patient may lack fever and chills (Boren et al., 2008).

Symptoms	Balkanli n, %	Eren n, %	Zhang n, %	Sirmali n, %	Cobanoglu n, %	Haciibrahimoglu n, %
Productive cough	133 (55.8)	94 (65.7)	671 (85)	167 (94.9)	48 (77.4)	32 (91.4)
Recurrence of pulmonary infection	84 (35.2)	69 (48.2)	-	-	41 (66.1)	33 (94.2)
Fetid sputum	116 (48.7)	72 (50.3)	277 (35)	139 (79)	27 (43.5)	28 (80)
Hemoptysis	39 (12.1)	21 (14.6)	411 (52)	78 (44.3)	7 (11.3)	4 (11.4)
Chest pain	-	12 (8.3)	56 (7.1)	-	7 (11.3)	-
Fatigue	-	-	-	-	17 (27.4)	-
Dyspnea	-	-	-	-	34 (54.8)	-
Growth retardation	-	-	-	34 (19.3)	-	-
Asymptomatic	10 (4.2)	2 (2.0)	25 (3.2)	-	10 (16.1)	-

Table 2. Semptoms of the patients

Physical examination is often nonspecific. Crepitation, wheezing, and coarse expiratory rhonchi may be heard over the lung bases, whereas clinical signs of cor pulmonale and denutrition are uncommon and indicate advanced disease. Routine clinical assessment should include a careful recording of personal and familial history, which may indicate an inherited disorder (Deslauriers et al., 1998).

Pulmonary function testing can help determine the degree of lung damage because of bronchiectasis. Bronchiectasis typically results in obstructive lung function changes as the disease progresses. Typical obstructive changes on lung function testing include a reduced forced vital capacity (FVC), reduced forced expiratory volume in 1 s (FEV1), and reduced FEV1 to FVC ratio. Airway hyperresponsiveness with reversibility after the administration of inhaled bronchodilator should also be evaluated (Boren et al., 2008).

5. Imaging

Diagnosis of bronchiectasis is based on clinical history and imaging. CXR findings that are suggestive but nondiagnostic of bronchiectasis include stranding, cystic lesions, volume loss with crowding of vessels, air-fluid levels and honeycombing, and areas of infiltrates and atelectasis (Agasthian et al., 1996). Computed tomography scanning is currently the best technique to establish the presence, severity, and distribution of bronchiectasis, replacing Lipiodol bronchography, which is considered more invasive and more unpleasant to the patient as well as being occasionally associated with complications such as alveolitis or allergy to the local anesthetic agent or contrast medium. HRCT has replaced this procedure in the diagnosis of bronchiectasis, with only a 2% false negative and a 1% false positive rate (Young et al., 1991). The detailed images demonstrate bronchial dilatation, peribronchial inflammation, and parenchymal disease.

Perfusion isotopic lung scans using 99m Tc albumin particles in microspheres are considered important in the preoperative evaluation of patients with bronchiectasis because they may demonstrate abnormal territories considered normal on CT scans but representing potential areas of bronchial dilatations. This is explained by bronchial artery hyperplasia creating flow reversal through systemic to pulmonary artery shunting, thus causing areas of defective perfusion on the isotopic scan. Bronchial arteriography may be done to document the origin of hemoptysis. Esophageal studies if gastroesophageal reflux is suspected and ultrastructural examination of cilia from biopsy of the nasal respiratory epithelium if ciliary dyskinesia is suspected may be done (Deslauriers et al., 1998).

6. Therapy for bronchiectasis

Treatment options for the management of bronchiectasis include pharmacologic agents such as antibiotics, nonpharmacologic measures such as chest physiotherapy, and surgical procedures involving removal of the affected portion or portions of the lung. In general, treatment goals are to control infections and improve bronchial hygiene. General measures include avoidance of smoking and second-hand smoke, proper nutrition, and ensuring proper immunizations, including yearly influenza vaccinations. Depending on the specific cause of bronchiectasis, additional medical therapies may be warranted. This is especially true in patients with immunoglobulin deficiency, who could benefit from administration of intravenous or subcutaneous immunoglobulin for passive protection (Boren et al., 2008).

The goals of surgical therapy for bronchiectasis are to improve the quality of life for those patients in which medical treatment has failed and to resolve complications such as empyema, severe or recurrent hemoptysis, and lung abscess (Agasthian et al., 1996; Annest et al., 1982). There is a broad consensus concerning the indications for surgical removal. The surgical treatment is based on two physiopathologic hypotheses. First, the resection involves removal of lung tissue with destroyed bronchi that are no longer functional. Second, it permits the removal of a localized area of bronchiectasis, which could otherwise be involved in the infectious contamination of adjacent territories (Mazieres et al., 2003).

Mazierez and colleagues bring some arguments to help in the selection of patients who should be considered for operation (Mazieres et al., 2003). First, respiratory function and performance status must be compatible with the anesthetic risk. Second, the resection should be done quite early in the evolution of the disease because of the risk of contamination of healthy bronchi by an "active" territory and because of the low morbidity when the pulmonary function is good (Etienne et al., 1996). Third, operation is recommended for patients exhibiting disabling bronchiectasis with hemoptysis or a recurring infection that becomes resistant to medical treatment. Fourth, the etiology of bronchiectasis should not be considered in the decision for operation. Some studies showed the benefit of operation in primary ciliary dyskinesia (Simit et al., 1996), Kartagener's syndrome (Figure 4) (Mazieres et al., 2003), and in hypogammaglobulinemia (Cohen et al., 1994). Lastly, the ideal candidate has a nonhomogenous disease. Some territories are more severely involved and constitute real targets. The removal of an active infectious territory may protect the healthy bronchi from infectious contamination. Removal of diseased segments can break the vicious circle as described by Cole and colleagues, and stop the progression of the disease (Cole et al., 1985). In children growth retardation due to bronchiectasis and drop in school attendance secondary to the illness should be included in the indications for surgery as well (Sirmali et al., 2006).

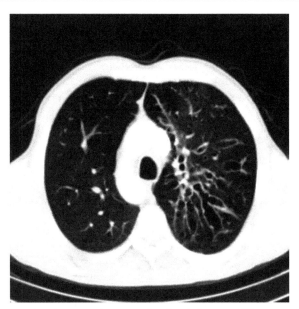

Fig. 4. Computed tomography scan showing the classic image of Kartagener's syndrome caharacterized by dextrocardia and cylindrical bronchiectasis in the right upper lobe (patient's left side).

7. Preoperative preparation

Careful preoperative preparations are of the utmost importance to reduce operation-related morbidity and mortality. The preoperative treatment should include reducing airway obstruction and elimination of microorganisms from the lower respiratory tract, which consists of antimicrobial therapy, postural physiotherapy, bronchodilators, and corticosteroids (Agasthian et al., 1996). Patients should be well prepared during the preoperative period with regard to infection to minimize postoperative complications. Bacterial infections, particularly those involving potentially necrotizing agents such as Staphylococcus aureus, Pseudomonas aeruginosa, Streptococcus pneumonia, and various anaerobes, remain important causes of bronchiectasis, particularly when there is a delay in treatment or other factors that prevent eradication of the infection (Deslauriers et al., 1998). Antimicrobial therapy is particularly true in the setting of mycobacterial disease, such as M. tuberculosis and various environmental mycobacterial species. Patients with focal bronchiectasis and M. avium complex infection typically are started on a three-or four-drug regimen for 2-3 months before surgery based on in vitro susceptibility testing of the isolated organism. The regimen is continued through the hospital stay and for several months thereafter, often to a total of 24 months (Kim et al., 2005).

Preoperative bronchoscopy should be routinely done to rule out benign or malignant cause of obstruction. Preoperative bronchoscopic examinations were performed in 117 (81.8%) of our patients as an adjuvant diagnostic method, to rule out benign or malignant bronchial obstruction, and for localization, collection of samples for microbiology, and bronchial toilet. We consider it essential in the preoperative evaluation and tracheobronchial cleaning of all patients. In our study, patients in whom bronchoscopy was not performed had a significantly higher rate of postoperative complications (Eren et al., 2007). Patients should be preoperatively monitored until they produced less than 20 mL/day of sputum with little purulence. Operation should be not conducted until bronchofibroscopy showed no engorgement or edema in the tunica mucosa bronchiorum (Zhang et al., 2010).

Most patients with chronic suppurative disease of the lungs are malnourished, often to a considerable degree, as a result of the long-standing catabolic state these patients experience. If malnutrition is present, an aggressive preoperative regimen of nutritional supplementation is advised (Sherwood et al., 2005). Pulmonary function studies should be preoperatively performed in all patients. The patients with bronchiectasis are showed a mixed or obstructive ventilatory pattern. In patients with low FEV1 (<60% of the predicted value) the postoperative complication rate was significantly high. This indicated that surgery should be delayed in cases of severe inflammation until adequate control has been achieved (Eren et al., 2007).

In all patients undergoing pulmonary resection, it is imperative to clearly determine preoperatively the extent of resection to be done because at surgery it may be difficult to judge with great accuracy the segments that are involved.

Balloon tamponade of the bleeding bronchus, which can be performed under emergency conditions is an effective method to manage massive hemoptysis in bronchiectasis patients. Embolization of the bronchial artery is a good alternative, capable of stopping the hemorrhage in 75−90% of the cases (Freitag et al., 1994). On the other hand, once the first episode of hemorrhage is stopped, preoperative assessment should be promptly undertaken because recurrence in the first month after the embolization is frequent and fatal (Fujimoto et al., 2001; Mal et al., 1999). Planning surgical operation in patients with hemoptysis should involve bronchoscopic as well as radiological assessments. Yielding 2% false negative and 1% false positive results, HRCT is a fairly reliable method for the diagnosis of bronchiectasis (Young et al., 1991). In such cases the most appropriate approach is to excise the pathological regions both depicted by HRCT and identified by bronchoscopy.

8. Surgical technique

A left-sided double-lumen endotracheal tube is used to avoid contralateral contamination of secretions. In children under 13 years old, in whom the double-lumen endotracheal tube is not used, bronchoscopy should be performed, and the bronchus of the side ready for resection should be cleaned by aspiration before the introduction of an endotracheal tube. A Fogarty embolectomy catheter may be used as a bronchus blocker in children (Eren et al., 2007). A thoracic epidural catheter is employed when an open approach is planned based on the extent of resection. In patients in whom a thoracoscopic lobectomy or segmentectomy is performed, the epidural is omitted. An arterial line and urinary catheter are placed.

Posterolateral thoracotomy or video-assisted thoracoscopic surgery (VATS) were performed for lung resection. Thoracotomy is performed so as to conserve as much muscle as possible. The resection type is selected according to the affected sides and cardiopulmonary reserve (Balkanli et al., 2003). Excessive bronchial dissection is avoided, and peribronchial tissues are preserved. The bronchial stump may manually be sutured with nonabsorbable materials or closed with a mechanical stapler. The bronchial stump is kept short. Stump covering with mediastinal pleura or tissue is performed. Complete resection is defined as an anatomic resection of all affected segments assessed preoperatively by either HRCT. Two silicon drains are placed into the thoracic cavity before the thorax is closed. All resected specimens are examined histopathologically in order to confirm the diagnosis. At the end of the procedure, the bronchial suture is bronchoscopically checked, and secretions are removed from the airways. Patients are extubated in the operating room. When postoperative mechanical ventilation was necessary, a standard endotracheal tube is substituted for the double-lumen tube (Zhang et al., 20101).

9. Complete resection and preserved segments

Complete and anatomic resection should be done with preservation of as much lung function as possible to avoid cardiorespiratory limitation (Laros et al., 1988). It was reported that the symptoms persisted when incomplete resection was carried out (Campbell & Lilly, 1982). We performed complete resection in 82.5% of our patients and preoperative symptoms resolved completely in 75.9% and improved in 15.7%, i.e. 92.8% benefited from the surgery. In the light of these findings, we suggest that complete resection should be performed for the surgical treatment of bronchiectasis and that incomplete resection should only be used for the palliative treatment of certain life-threatening symptoms. In our study, postoperative complications were observed in 11% of patients that underwent complete resection and in 80% of those that underwent incomplete resection (Eren et al., 2007). When suspicious lung regions are not excised with the aim of sparing as much lung tissue as possible, a second operation that carries a higher morbidity and mortality might be required to remove the residual diseased tissues (Sirmali et al., 2007). Therefore, we suggest that, during intraoperative examinations, if suspected areas that could not be determined by radiological examination are present, these parenchymal areas should be resected to perform complete resection and to decrease relapse rates. Bronchopulmonary development continues during childhood and the space occupied by the resected segments would be filled by the healthy lung segments. Therefore, surgeons should not refrain from wide resection of the lung to achieve complete resection of the diseased area (Sirmali et al., 2007). Incomplete resection should not be preferred in children except for palliative treatment of life threatening complications.

The goal of surgery is to excise all diseased lung areas whenever possible and to preserve as much healthy lung parenchyma as possible. It is known that even 2 or 3 preserved segments can fill the hemithorax (Campbell & Lilly, 1982). As recommended, we suggested to protect the anatomic structure of the superior segment in cases of bronchiectasis of the lower lobe when the superior segment of this lobe was normal (Fujimoto et al., 2001). In such patients, the superior segment had undergone a compensatory increase in volume and the affected basal segments had become small. Thus, the functional value of the superior segment was similar to that of the lower lobe (Yuncu et al., 2006). Patients with an uninvolved apical segment were found to have better spirometric values than those with more extensive disease (Ashour et al., 1996).

10. Resection for multisegmental bilateral bronchiectasis

Surgical treatment is usually offered only when the diseased area is well localized and restricted to one or several segments within the same lobe. Multiple or bilateral bronchiectasis is generally regarded as a contraindication to operation. From the end of the 1970s onward, some thoracic surgeons have suggested that bilateral bronchiectasis is not a contraindication to resection (George et al., 1979; Fujimoto et al., 2001). Nevertheless, the patients reported in the literature remained quite rare. The therapeutic options in nonfocal bronchiectasis are limited. Most of the time patients are treated with antibiotics and physiotherapy. Recently, progress has been made with the use of new antibiotics and inhalation of tobramycin solution in cases of Pseudomonas aeruginosa colonization (Barker et al., 2000). These therapies allow a good quality of life and symptomatic improvement for several years, but the usual evolution is a progression toward chronic respiratory failure with a poor prognosis and selection of resistant strains (Annest et al., 1982; Keistinen et al., 1997). Transplantation remains indicated for homogenous disease and for patients with advanced disease with seriously compromised pulmonary function and chronic respiratory failure (Hasan et al., 1995). The 3-year survival rate is 75% for patients undergoing double-lung transplantation (Barlow et al., 2000). Some investigators have proposed a radical operation for bilateral bronchiectasis (Kittle et al., 1985; Laros et al., 1988) but others report a higher mortality with pneumonectomy (McGovern et al., 1988). Considering the limited and palliative effect of medical treatment and the risk of transplantation or radical operation, it seems that a limited operation should be offered to some patients with diffuse bronchiectasis.

Mazierez and collegues suggested that surgical indications were offered to patients with multisegmental and severe bronchiectasis if (1) optimal medical treatment and physiotherapy were no longer efficient, (2) bleeding and sputum production were recurrent and abundant, (3) severely damaged territories could be identified, and (4) performance status and pulmonary function were compatible with the anesthetic risk (Mazierez et al., 2003).

Surgery in multiple segments on different lobes is technically more difficult, resulting in higher morbidity and mortality.[21] However, pulmonary resection is indicated early in patients with multisegmentar bronchiectasis, before other portions of the lung become grossly diseased. Our purpose in these patients was to protect as much pulmonary function as possible, with the aim of removing only the affected areas of different lobes. The types of procedures in different studies were presented in Table 3.

Operation type	Balkanli n, %	Eren n; %	Zhang n, %	Sırmali n, %	Haciibrahimoglu n, %	Giovannetti n, %
Pneumonectomy	13 (5.4)	12 (8.3)	90 (11.3)	40 (19.9)	7 (20)	1 (1.7)
Lobectomy	189 (79.4)	82 (55.4)	497 (62.9)	90 (44.7)	17 (48.5)	33 (56.8)
Bilobectomy		7 (4.7)	56 (7.1)	21 (10.4)	2 (5.7)	2 (3.4)
Lobectomy & segmentectomy	31 (13.0)	-	110 (14)	-	5 (14.2)	11 (18.9)
Lobectomy & lingulectomy		-		34 (16.9)	-	
Segmentectomy	10 (4.2)	17 (11.4)	37 (4.7)	16 (7.9)	4 (11.4)	11 (18.9)
Basal segmentectomy	-	16 (10.8)	-	-	-	-
Basal segmentectomy & lingulectomy	-	5 (3.3)	-	-	-	-
Basal segmentectomy & middle lobectomy	-	4 (2.7)	-	-	-	-

Table 3. Type of operation

11. Video-assisted thoracoscopic surgery

VATS for major lung resection has become a more frequent procedure in recent years with promising outcome. VATS represents a new approach; the indications for VATS major resection remain the same as for conventional resection. But not all the patients with bronchiectasis who needed operations were suitable for VATS lobectomy; severe scarring and adhesions on computed tomographic scan should be considered . The severity of adhesions to the chest wall, the hilum, and especially in the fissure, typically seen in inflammatory disease, was the key limiting factor for a safe VATS lobectomy (Weber et al., 2001). Adhesions need to be dissected to explore the relevant anatomy. If there were dense adhesions (such as destroyed lobes mainly after tuberculosis with or without aspergillosis) or enlarged lymph nodes, especially calcified, open operations were required (Zhang et al., 2011).

Bronchiectasis was considered the best lung benign disease suitable for VATS lobectomy (Yim, 2002). The VATS major resection has demonstrated to be a safe procedure when performed by experienced physicians. Postoperative pain after VATS is uncommon as compared with open surgery. Other documented advantages include better preservation of pulmonary function in the early postoperative period, earlier return to full activities, and better quality of life after recovery. One major advantage of VATS resection is that it allows recruitment of older and sicker patients with multiple comorbidities who would otherwise not be candidates for resection through a conventional thoracotomy approach (Farjah et al., 2009; Gonzales-Aragoneses et al., 2009). In study of Zhang and collegeus, the patients with VATS had a shorter length of stay in the hospital, fewer complications, and less pain in the postoperative period than those with thoracotomies (Zhang et al., 2011).

12. Postoperative complication

Bronchiectasis is an inflammatory disease of the lungs and the risk of developing postoperative empyema is higher than in other cases. Empyema, on the other hand, is a risk factor for bronchopleural fistula (Sirmali et al., 2006). Therefore, we suggest reinforcement of the bronchial stump in all patients. Bronchopleural fistula can be observed in as many as 9.1% of the cases (Fujimoto et al., 2001). Fujimoto and colleagues argued that the bronchial stump should be reinforced when the inflammation in the lung of bronchiectasis patients could not be effectively controlled (Fujimoto et al., 2001). We, however, suggest reinforcement the bronchial stump in all cases. Additionally, to avoid empyema, we recommend postoperative bacterial culture of thoracic effusion if the remaining lung shows signs of persisting inflammation. Sputum retention is common because patients with this disease might have problems with ciliary motion and postoperative expectoration, which would be easily disrupted (Fujimoto et al., 2001). In our series, respiratory physiotherapy was re-initiated on the first post-operative day, and continued for 2 weeks after discharge. We used bronchoscopy for sputum aspiration during the early postoperative period if physiotherapy was not effective. Virtually all patients had specific or large-spectrum intravenous antibiotic therapy for 1 week (Eren et al., 2007).

In bronchopleural fistula, drainage of the infected space is a key initial step to limit damage to the remaining lung. Bronchopleural fistula noted very early after the initial resection may be treated with primary reclosure and rebuttressing of the stump; later bronchopleural fistula usually require rib resection and creation of an Eloesser flap, followed by bronchopleural fistula closure and subsequent Clagett procedure, for successful treatment (Sugarbaker et al., 2009). The presence of a significant intrathoracic "space" appears to be more common after major lung resection for infectious lung disease such as bronchiectasis compared with other indications for surgery. The use of transposed muscle such as latissimus dorsi minimizes the potential complications in this setting, including postresection empyema or prolonged air leak (Sugarbaker et al., 2009). The rate of complications in the current literature varies between 9.4% and 24.6%. Mortality ranges from 0% to 8.3% in the literature (Fujimoto et al., 2001). Postoperative complications in different studies were presented in Table 4.

Complication	Balkanli n, %	Eren n, %	Zhang n, %	Sırmali n, %	Cobanoglu n, %	Haciibrahimoglu n, %	Giovannetti n, %
Postoperative Pneumonia	-	3 (2.0)	24 (3)	3 (1.7)	-	3 (8.8)	2 (4.4)
Atelectasis	7 (2.9)	11 (7.6)	16 (2)	8 (4.5)	4 (6.4)	-	
Prolonged air-leak	6 (2.5)	7 (4.8)	21 (2.7)	3 (1.7)	2 (3.2)	1 (2.9)	1 (2.2)
Residual air-space	-	-	-	-	-	-	1 (2.2)
Sputum retention	-	-	-	-	-	-	1 (2.2)
Bronchial infection	-	-	-	-	-	-	1(2.2)
Bronchopleural fistula	2 (0.8)	-	3 (0.4)	-	2 (3.2)	-	-
Postoperative hemorrhage	4 (1.6)	2 (1.3)	9 (1.1)	2 (1.1)	1 (1.6)	-	-
Empyema	2 (0.8)	5 (3.4)	5 (0.6)	5 (2.8)	2 (3.2)	2 (5.8)	-
Severe supraventricular arrhythmias	-	3 (2.0)	32 (4)	-	1 (1.6)	-	-
Respiratory insufficiency	-	2 (1.3)	10 (1.3)	-	-	-	-
Total	21 (8.8)	33 (23)	128 (16.2)	-	-	6 (17.6)	6 (13.2)

Table 4. Postoperative complications

13. Conclusion

Bronchiectasis is pathologically defined as a condition in which there are abnormal and permanent dilatations of proximal bronchi. Bronchiectasis can occur as focal or localized disease, or in a diffuse manner. Overall, one-third of cases of bronchiectasis are unilateral and affect a single lobe, one-third are unilateral but affect more than one lobe, and one-third are bilateral. Recurrent pulmonary infection during childhood is an important factor in the etiology. In developing countries, tuberculosis is still one of the most important causes of bronchiectasis. Bronchial obstruction from either endobronchial pathology or external compression can also be an acquired factor predisposing to the development of bronchiectasis.

Treatment options for the management of bronchiectasis include pharmacologic agents such as antibiotics, nonpharmacologic measures such as chest physiotherapy, and surgical procedures involving removal of the affected portion or portions of the lung. The goals of surgical therapy for bronchiectasis are to improve the quality of life for those patients in which medical treatment has failed and to resolve complications such as empyema, severe or recurrent hemoptysis, and lung abscess. The preoperative treatment should include reducing airway obstruction and elimination of microorganisms from the lower respiratory tract, which consists of antimicrobial therapy, postural physiotherapy, bronchodilators, and corticosteroids. Preoperative bronchoscopy should be routinely done to rule out benign or malignant cause of obstruction.

Complete and anatomic resection should be done with preservation of as much lung function as possible to avoid cardiorespiratory limitation. It was reported that the symptoms persisted when incomplete resection was carried out. When suspicious lung regions are not excised with the aim of sparing as much lung tissue as possible, a second operation that carries a higher morbidity and mortality might be required to remove the residual diseased tissues. Therefore, we suggest that, during intraoperative examinations, if suspected areas that could not be determined by radiological examination are present, these parenchymal areas should be resected to perform complete resection and to decrease relapse rates.

Surgery in multiple segments on different lobes is technically more difficult, resulting in higher morbidity and mortality. However, pulmonary resection is indicated early in patients with multisegmentar bronchiectasis, before other portions of the lung become grossly diseased. Our purpose in these patients was to protect as much pulmonary function as possible, with the aim of removing only the affected areas of different lobes. VATS represents a new approach; the indications for VATS major resection remain the same as for conventional resection. But not all the patients with bronchiectasis who needed operations were suitable for VATS lobectomy; severe scarring and adhesions on computed tomographic scan should be considered. When necessary, surgical treatment of bronchiectasis can be performed with acceptable morbidity and low mortality.

14. References

Agasthian, T.; Deschamps, C., Trastek, VF., Allen, MS. & Pairolero, PC. (1996). Surgical management of bronchiectasis. *Ann Thorac Surg*, Vol.62, No.4 , pp. 976-978

Al-Kattan, KM.; Essa, MA., Hajjar, WM., Ashour, MH., Saleh, WN. & Rafay, MA. (2005). Surgical results for bronchiectasis based on hemodynamic (functional and morphologic) classification *J Thorac Cardiovasc Surg* , Vol.130, No.5, pp. 1385-1390

Annest, LS.; Kratz, JM. & Crawford, FA Jr. (1982). Current results of treatment of bronchiectasis. *J Thorac Cardiovasc Surg*, Vol.83, No.4, pp. 546-550

Ashour, M.; Al-Kattan, KM., Jain, SK., Al-Majed, S., Al-Kassimi, F., Mobaireek, A., Al-Hajjaj, M. & Al-Zear, A. (1996). Surgery for unilateral bronchiectasis: results and prognostic factors. *Tuber Lung Dis*, Vol.77, No.2, pp. 168-72

Balkanli, K.; Genc, O., Dakak, M., Gurkok, S., Gozubuyuk, A., Caylak, H. & Yucel, O. (2003). Surgical management of bronchiectasis: analysis and short-term results in 238 patients. *Eur J Cardiothorac Surg*, Vol.24, No.5, pp. 699-702

Barker, AF.; Couch, L., Fiel, SB., Gotfried, MH., Ilowite, J., Meyer, KC., O'Donnell, A., Sahn, SA., Smith, LJ., Stewart, JO., Abuan, T., Tully, H., Van, Dalfsen J., Wells, CD. & Quan, J. (2000). Tobramycin solution for inhalation reduces sputum Pseudomonas aeruginoa density in bronchiectasis. *Am J Respir Crit Care Med* , Vol.162, No.2 Pt 1, pp. 481–485

Barlow, CW.; Robbins, RC., Moon, MR., Akindipe, O., Theodore, J. & Reitz, BA. (2000). Heart-lung versus double-lung transplantation for suppurative lung disease. *J Thorac Cardiovas Surg*,Vol.119, No.3, pp. 466–476

Bertelsen, S.; Struve-Christensen, E., Aasted, A. & Sparup, J. (1980). Isolated middle lobe atelectasis: aetiology, pathogenesis, and treatment of the so-called middle lobe syndrome. *Thorax*, Vol.35, No.6, pp. 449–452

Campbell, DN. & Lilly, JR. (1982). The changing spectrum of pulmonary operations in infants and children. *J Thorac Cardiovasc Surg*, Vol.83, No5. , pp. 680-685.

Cobanoglu, U.; Yalcinkaya, İ., Er, M., Isik, AF., Sayir, F. & Mergan, D. (2011). Surgery for bronchiectasis: The effect of morphological types to prognosis. *Ann Thorac Med*, *Vol.6*, No.1, pp. 25–32

Cohen, AJ.; Roifman, C., Brendan, J., Mullen, M., Reid, B., Weisbrod, G. & Downey, GP. (1994). Localised pulmonary resection for bronchiectasis in hypogammaglobulinaemic patients. *Thorax*, Vol.49, No.5, pp. 509–510

Cole, PJ.; Roberts, DE., Higgs, E. & Prior, C. (1985). Colonising microbial load a cardinal concept in the pathogenesis and treatment of progressive bronchiectasis due to "vicious circle" host mediated damage. *Thorax*, Vol.40, pp. 227

Deslauries, J.; Goulet, S. & Francois, B. (1998). Surgical treatment of bronchiectasis and broncholithiasis. In: *Advanced therapy in thoracic surgery*, Franco, LF., Putnam, JB, (ed.), pp. 300–309, ON: Decker, Hamilton

Dogru, D.; Nik-Ain, A., Kiper, N., Gocmen, A., Ozcelik, U., Yalcin, E. & Aslan, AT. (2005). Bronchiectasis: the consequence of late diagnosis in chronic respiratory symptoms. *J Trop Pediatr*, Vol.51, No.6; pp. 362–365

Eller, J.; Lapa, e Silva JR., Poulter, LW., Lode H. & Cole, PJ. (1994). Cells and cytokines in chronic bronchial infection. *Ann N Y Acad Sci*, Vol.725, pp. 331–345

Eren, S.; Esme, H. & Avci, A. (2007). Risk factors affecting outcome and morbidity in the surgical management of bronchiectasis. *J Thorac Cardiovasc Surg*, Vol.134, No.2, pp. 392-398

Boren, EJ.; Teuber, SS. & Gershwin, ME. (2008). A Review of Non-Cystic Fibrosis Pediatric Bronchiectasis. *Clinic Rev Allerg Immunol*, Vol.34, pp. 260–273

Etienne, T.; Spiliopoulos, A. & Megevand, R. (1993). Bronchiectasis: indication and timing for surgery. *Ann Chir*, Vol.47, No.8, pp. 729–735

Farjah, F.; Wood, DE., Mulligan, MS., Krishnadasan, B., Heagerty, PJ., Symons, RG. & Flum, DR. (2009). Safety and efficacy of video-assisted versus conventional lung resection for lung cancer. *J Thorac Cardiovasc Surg*, Vol.137, No.6, pp. 1415–1421

Freitag, L.; Tekolf, E., Stamatis, G., Montag, M. & Greschuchna, D. (1994). Three years experience with a new balloon catheter for the management of haemoptysis. *Eur Respir J*, Vol.7, No.11, pp. 2033−2037

Fujimoto, T.; Hillejan, L. & Stamatis, G. (2001). Current strategy for surgical management of bronchiectasis. *Ann Thorac Surg*, Vol.72, No.5, pp. 1711-1715

George, SA.; Leonardi, HK. & Overholt, RH. (1979). Bilateral pulmonary resection for bronchiectasis: a 40-year experience. *Ann Thorac Surg*, Vol.28, No.1, pp. 48–53

Giovannetti, R.; Alifano, M., Stefani, A., Legras, A., Grigoroiu, M., Collet, JY., Magdelenat, P. & Regnard, JF. (2008). Surgical treatment of bronchiectasis: early and long-term results Interactive. *CardioVascular and Thoracic Surgery*, Vol.7,No.4 ,pp. 609–612

Gonzalez-Aragoneses, F,; Moreno-Mata, N., Simon-Adiego, C., Peñalver-Pascual, R., Gonzalez-Casaurran, G. & Perea, LA. (2009). Lung cancer surgery in the elderly. *Crit Rev Oncol Hematol*, Vol.71, No.3, pp. 266 –271

Haciibrahimoglu, G.; Fazlioglu, M., Olcmen, A., Gurses, A. & Bedirhan, MA. (2004). Surgical management of childhood bronchiectasis due to infectious disease. *J Thorac Cardiovasc Surg*, Vol.127, No.5, pp. 1361-1365

Hasan, A.; Corris, PA., Healy, M., Wrightson, N., Gascoigne, AD., Waller, DA., Wilson, I., Hilton, CJ., Gould, FK. & Forty, J. (1995). Bilateral sequential lung transplantation for end-stage septic lung disease. *Thorax*, Vol.50, No.5, pp. 565–566

Karadag, B.; Karakoc, F., Ersu, R., Kut, A., Bakac, S. & Dagli, E. (2005). Non-cystic fibrosis bronchiectasis in children: a persisting problem in developing countries. *Respiration*, Vol.72, No.3, pp. 233–238

Karakoc, GB.; Yilmaz, M., Altintas, DU. & Kendirli, SG. (2001). Bronchiectasis: still a problem. *Pediatr Pulmonol*, Vol.32, pp. 175–178

Keistinen, T.; Saynajakangas, O., Tuuponen, T. & Kivela, SL. (1997). Bronchiectasis: an orphan disease with a poorly understood prognosis. *Eur Respir J*, Vol.10, No.12, pp. 2784–2787

Khair, OA.; Davies, RJ. & Devalia, JL. (1996). Bacterial-induced release of inflammatory mediators by bronchial epithelial cells. *Eur Respir J*, Vol.9, pp. 1913–1922

Kim, JS.; Tanaka, N., Newell, JD., Degroote, MA., Fulton, K., Huitt, G. & Lynch, DA. (2005). Nontuberculous mycobacterial infection: CT scan findings, genotype, and treatment responsiveness. *Chest* Vol.128, No.6, pp. 3863–3869

King, PT. (2009). The pathophysiology of bronchiectasis. *International Journal of COPD*, Vol.4, pp. 411–419

Kittle, CF.; Faber, LP., Jensik, RJ. & Warren, WH. (1985). Pulmonary resection in patients after pneumonectomy. *Ann Thorac Surg*, Vol.40, pp 294–299

Lapa e Silva, JR.; Guerreiro, D., Noble, B., Poulter, LW. & Cole, PJ. (1989). Immunopathology of experimental bronchiectasis. *Am J Respir Cell Mol Biol*, Vol.1, pp. 297–304

Laros, CD.; Van den Bosch, JM., Westermann, CJ., Bergstein, PG., Vanderschueren, RG. & Knaepen, PJ. (1988). Resection of more than 10 lung segments. A 30-year survey of 30 bronchiectatic patients. *J Thorac Cardiovasc Surg*, Vol.95, pp. 119-123

Levin, DL. (2002). Radiology of pulmonary Mycobacterium avium-intracellulare complex. *Clin Chest Med*, Vol.23, pp. 603–612

Loukides, S.; Bouros, D., Papatheodorou, G., Lachanis, S., Panagou, P. & Siafakas, NM. (2002). Exhaled H2O2 in steady-state bronchiectasis: relationship with cellular composition in induced sputum, spirometry, and extent and severity of disease. *Chest*, Vol.121, pp. 81–87

Mal, H.; Rulon, I., Mellot, F., Brugiere, O., Sleiman, C., Menu, Y. & Fournier, M. (1999). Immediate and long-term results of bronchial artery embolization for life-threatening hemoptysis. *Chest*, Vol.115, pp. 996–1001

Mazie`res, J.; Murris, M., Didier, A., Giron, J., Dahan, M., Berjaud, J. & Le´ophonte, P. (2003). Limited Operation for Severe Multisegmental Bilateral Bronchiectasis *Ann Thorac Surg*, Vol.75, pp.382-387

McGovern, EM.; Trastek, VF., Pairolero, PC. & Payne, WS. (1988). Completion pneumonectomy: indications, complications and results. *Ann Thorac Surg*, Vol.46, pp. 141–146

Miller, JI. (2000). Bacterial infections of the lungs and bronchial compressive disorders. In: Shields TW, editor. *General thoracic surgery*. 5th ed. Pp. 1048-1051, Lippincott Williams & Wilkins, Philadelphia

Nicotra, MB.; Rivera, M., Dale, AM., Shepherd, R. & Carter, R. (1995). Clinical, pathophysiologic, and microbiologic characterization of bronchiectasis in an aging cohort. *Chest*, Vol.108, pp. 955–961

Prieto, D.; Bernardo, J., Matos, MJ., Eugenio, L. & Antunes, M. (2001). Surgery for bronchiectasis. *Eur J Cardiothorac Surg*, Vol.20, pp. 19-23

Reid, L. (1950). Reduction in bronchial subdivisions in bronchiectasis. *Thorax*, Vol.5, pp. 223–247

Sherwood, JT.; Mitchell, JD. & Pomerantz, M. (2005). Completion pneumonectomy for chronic mycobacterial disease. *J Thorac Cardiovasc Surg*, Vol.129, pp. 1258–1265

Sirmali, M.; Karasu, S., Turut, H., Gezer, S., Kaya, S., Tastepe, I. & Karaoğlanoğlu, N. (2006). Surgical management of bronchiectasis in childhood. *Eur J Cardiothorac Surg*, Vol.31, No.1, pp. 120-123

Smit, HJ.; Schreurs, AJ., Van den Bosch, JM. & Westermann, CJ. (1996). Is resection of bronchiectasis beneficial in patients with primary ciliary dyskinesia? *Chest*, Vol.109, pp. 1541-1544

Sugarbaker DJ.; Bueno R, Krasna MJ, Mentzer ZJ & Zellos L. (2009). *Adult Chest Surgery*, The McGraw-Hill Companies, ISBN 978-0-07-145912-9, China

Weber, A.; Stammberger, U., Inci, I., Schmid, RA., Dutly, A. & Weder, W. (2001). Thoracoscopic lobectomy for benign disease–a single centre study on 64 cases. *Eur J Cardiothorac Surg*, Vol.20, pp. 443– 844

Whitwell, F. (1952). A study of the pathology and pathogenesis of bronchiectasis. *Thorax*, Vol.7, pp. 213-219

Yim, AP. (2002). VATS major pulmonary resection revisited– controversies, techniques, and results. *Ann Thorac Surg*, Vol.74, pp. 615-623

Young, K.; Aspestrand, F. & Kolbenstvedt, A. (1991). High resolution CT and bronchography in the assessment of bronchiectasis. *Acta Radiol*, Vol.32, pp. 439-441

Yuncu, G.; Ceylan, KC., Sevinc, S., Ucvet, A., Kaya, SO., Kiter, G., Unsal, S. & Ozsinan, F. (2006). Functional results of surgical treatment of bronchiectasis in a developing country. *Arch Bronconeumol*, Vol.42, No.4, pp. 183-188

Zhang, P.; Zhang, P., Jiang, S., Jiang, G., Zhou, X., Ding, J. & Gao, W. (2011). Video-Assisted Thoracic Surgery for Bronchiectasis. *Ann Thorac Surg*, Vol.91, pp. 239-243

Zheng, L.; Tipoe, G., Lam, WK., Leung, RY., Ho, JC., Shum, IH., Ooi, GC., Ip, MS. & Tsang, KW. (2000). Up-regulation of circulating adhesion molecules in bronchiectasis. *Eur Respir J*, Vol.16, No.4, pp. 691–696

3

Stage I Non-Small Cell Lung Cancer: Recurrence Patterns, Prognostic Factors and Survival

Jung-Jyh Hung and Yu-Chung Wu
*Division of Thoracic Surgery, Department of Surgery,
Taipei Veterans General Hospital and School of Medicine,
National Yang-Ming University, Taipei,
Taiwan*

1. Introduction

Lung cancer is the leading cause of cancer-related death worldwide. Surgical resection is the treatment of choice for early-stage non-small cell lung cancer (NSCLC).[1,2] Five-year survival in patients with resected stage I NSCLC ranges between 55% and 80%.[3-6] Tumor recurrence is the most common cause of death, and thus the main obstacle for long-term survival after resection.[4-10] The postoperative recurrence rates in stage I NSCLC range between 22% to 38%.[4-8] The incidence of local or regional recurrence in stage I NSCLC after surgical resection has been reported between 7% to 15%,[4-6] while distant metastasis been reported between 14% and 23%.[4-8] Post-recurrence survival in resected stage I NSCLC is poor.[7,10-12]

The fifth edition of the TNM staging system for lung cancer was published in 1997, and stage I NSCLC was subdivided into IA (T1N0M0, tumor size ≤ 3 cm) and IB (T2N0M0, tumor size > 3 cm).[3] In addition to tumor size greater than 3 cm, the T2 descriptor also includes tumors that invade the visceral pleura regardless of size, tumors that involve the main bronchus ≥ 2 cm distal to the carina, and tumors that result in associated atelectasis and obstructive pneumonitis that extends to the hilar region but does not involve the entire lung radiographically.[3] In the sixth edition of the TNM classification (TNM 6)[13] for lung cancer published in 2002, no change was made to the previous edition.[3] The seventh edition of the TNM classification (TNM 7) for lung cancer has been published in 2009.[14,15] The changes to the TNM 6 for lung cancer were based upon the proposals from the International Association for the Study of Lung Cancer (IASLC). In the seventh edition, T1 descriptor has been classified into T1a (≤ 2 cm) and T1b (> 2 to ≤ 3 cm), while size-based T2 descriptor has been classified into T2a (> 3 to ≤ 5 cm), T2b (> 5 to ≤ 7 cm), and T3 (> 7 cm).[16] Stage I NSCLC was subdivided into IA (T1aN0M0, T1bN0M0) and IB (T2aN0M0).[17] T2bN0M0 was reclassified as stage IIA.[17]

This review focuses on recurrence patterns of stage I NSCLC after surgical resection, survival after recurrence, and its prognostic factors. Predictors for local recurrence and distant metastasis are analyzed and discussed separately. Recent reports in the literature aiming at recurrence patterns and survival in stage I NSCLC (TNM 7) were also reviewed and included.

2. Prognostic factors for stage I NSCLC

The prognostic factors of stage I NSCLC (TNM 6) have been widely reported in the literature.[4-6,18,19] Martini et al[4] reported that T2 status and sublobar resection were the prognostic factors for poor overall survival in resected stage I NSCLC. Harpole et al[5] reported that presence of symptoms, vascular invasion, visceral pleural invasion and tumor size greater than 3 cm were the factors affecting overall survival in resected stage I NSCLC. Sawyer et al[18] reported that factors predicting poor overall survival included fewer than 15 lymph nodes dissected and tumor size greater than 3 cm. Varlotto et al[19] also reported that lymphadenectomy was associated with improved overall survival and disease-free survival in resected stage I NSCLC. Many other reports also demonstrated the prognostic value of tumor size in stage I NSCLC.[6,20] The number of mediastinal lymph nodes dissected/sampled alternatively represents the quality of lymphadenectomy and affects the survival rate for patients with resected stage I NSCLC.[19,21] Our previous studies[21,22] also showed that number of mediastinal lymph nodes dissected/sampled was a predictor of survival in stage I NSCLC. Cigarette smoking has been shown to be another prognostic factor in patients with NSCLC in the literature.[23-26] Hanagiri et al[23] reported that smoking was a significant postoperative prognostic factor in patients with NSCLC. Bryant et al[24] reported that 5-year survival rate was significantly better for never smokers compared to smokers in stage I NSCLC (TNM 6).

Only few studies reported the prognostic factors of stage I NSCLC (TNM 7).[25-28] In the report by Maeda et al, [27] 5-year overall survival rates for stage IA and IB (TNM 7) were 89.9% and 72.3%, respectively. They also demonstrated that older age, intratumoral vascular invasion, and visceral pleural invasion were poor prognostic factors in stage IB NSCLC.[27] In the report by Maeda et al,[27] 5-year disease-specific survival rates for stage IA and IB NSCLC (TNM 7) were 93.1% and 72.3%, respectively. They also demonstrated that intratumoral vascular invasion and visceral pleural invasion were poor prognostic factors for cancer-specific survival in stage IB NSCLC.[27] Maeda et al[25] reported that overall survival and recurrence-free survival in never smokers were significant better than those of ever smokers in patients with stage I NSCLC (TNM 7). Maeda et al[26] also discovered that a greater smoking extent was associated with the presence of solid components in stage I lung adenocarcinoma, which may have more aggressive biological features resulting in poorer outcomes.

3. Recurrence patterns

For stage I NSCLC (TNM 6), Martini et al[4] reported that the 2- and 5-year recurrence-free rates were 84% and 76%, respectively. Sixty percent of patients developed recurrence within the first 2 years after operation. Sawyer et al[18] reported that 5-year of local recurrence-free and distant metastasis-free rates were 85% and 83%, respectively, in patients with resected stage I NSCLC. In the study by Varlotto et al [29] regarding tumor recurrence in patients with resected NSCLC (including 82% of patients with stage I NSCLC), the 2- and 5-year local recurrence-free rates were 84% and 68%, respectively. The 2- and 5-year distant metastasis-free rates were 87% and 79%, respectively.

Martini et al[4] reported the overall incidence of recurrence in patients with resected stage I NSCLC was 27% (local or regional 7%, systemic 20%). In the study by Harpole et al,[5] the initial location of recurrence of stage I NSCLC after surgical resection was at a distant site in 19%, within the ipsilateral hemithorax in 11% or at both locations in 6% of patients. Distant recurrence rates between 14% to 23% in stage I NSCLC after surgical resection have also been reported in the literature.[6-8] Our studies[11,12] demonstrated that overall incidence of recurrence was 31.0% (distant only in 17.8%, local only in 7.9%, local and distant in 5.3%) in stage I NSCLC after surgical resection. The patterns of local recurrence included local only in 60.2%, local with distant in 15.4%, local before distant in 19.5% and distant before local in 4.9% of patients. Approximately 78% of patients with local recurrence occurred within the first 2 years after operation. We also showed that approximately 84% of patients with distant metastases occurred within the first 2 years after operation. A major proportion of patients (62%) died within one year after distant metastasis.

Most distant metastases appear as multiple foci in multiple organs after treatment of original cancer.[30] Martini et al[4] reported that the most common site of distant metastasis in patients with resected stage I NSCLC was the brain. Yoshino et al[31] demonstrated that pulmonary metastasis was most common in NSCLC patients with recurrence at distant organs, followed by bone metastasis. Our study[12] revealed that bone (32.1%) was the most common site of single organ metastasis in patients with resected stage I NSCLC, followed by the brain (29.2%). We further demonstrated that the patterns of distant metastasis included single and multiple organ metastases in approximately 64% and 36% of patients, respectively.

The recurrence-free rate of stage I NSCLC (TNM 7) has also been reported in the literature.[28,32,33] Maeda et al[32,33] reported that the 5-year recurrence-free rate in patients with stage IA NSCLC (TNM 7) ranges between 84 to 87%. In another article by Maeda et al,[28] they reported that 5-year recurrence-free rate in patients with stage I NSCLC (TNM 7) was 84.2%.

4. Predictors of recurrence

The predictors for recurrence in resected stage I NSCLC (TNM 6) has been well demonstrated in the literature.[4,5,18,29] In the report by Martini et al,[4] the factors having adverse effects on recurrence in resected stage I NSCLC included lesser resection than lobectomy, no lymph node dissection, T2 tumor, and greater tumor size. In the study by Harpole et al,[5] the factors affecting early recurrence in resected stage I NSCLC included presence of symptoms, vascular invasion, visceral pleural invasion, and tumor size greater than 3 cm. Although both Martini et al[4] and Harpole et al[5] performed elegant analysis demonstrating the factors influencing tumor recurrence in resected stage I NSCLC, they did not analyze local recurrence and distant metastasis as separate end-points. Only few studies evaluated the risk factors for local recurrence and distant metastasis separately. Varlotto et al[29] reported that local recurrence in resected NSCLC was associated with lymphatic or vascular invasion, the use of chemotherapy, and diabetes. Distant metastasis in resected NSCLC was significantly higher in patients with non-squamous cell histology, those undergoing pneumonectomy and those with more advanced TNM stage.[29] In the report by Sawyer et al,18 the factors independently predicting local recurrence in resected stage I NSCLC included fewer than 15 lymph nodes dissected and T2 tumor. Tumor size greater than 5 cm and non-squamous histology independently predicted a poor distant metastasis-free rate in resected stage I NSCLC.[18]

The predictors for recurrence in resected stage I NSCLC (TNM 7) has not been widely investigated in the literature. In the reports by Maeda et al,[28,33] they demonstrated that histologic differentiation, intratumoral vascular invasion, and visceral of pleural invasion were significant predictors for recurrence in stage I NSCLC (TNM 7).

5. Postrecurrence survival

In our previous study,[11] the 1- and 2-year post-recurrence survival rates for resected stage I NSCLC patients with local only recurrence were 48.7% and 17.6%, respectively. Tumor size and treatment for initial recurrence were significant predictors for post-recurrence survival in patients with local only recurrence in univariate analyses. The hazard of death was greater in patients with larger tumor size. Treatment for initial recurrence was still significant prognostic indicator in multivariate analysis. Patients underwent re-operation after local recurrence survived longer than those with chemotherapy or/and radiotherapy and those without treatment.

For patients with single organ metastasis, the 1- and 2-year post-recurrence survival rates were 30.2% and 15.1%, respectively.[12] The most common site of single organ metastasis was the bone, followed by the brain. Disease-free interval > 16 months and treatment for distant metastasis (including re-operation, chemotherapy and/or radiotherapy) were significant predictors of better post-recurrence survival in resected stage I NSCLC with single organ metastasis. Post-recurrence survival was not significantly different between single and multiple organ metastases groups of patients. Multiplicity of metastatic organ sites is not a significant prognostic factor in these patients. Yoshino and coworkers[31] reported that the 2-year survival rate of NSCLC patients with postoperative recurrence at distant organs was 15.7 %. Their result is similar to that in our study.

Surgical resection offers a good chance of cure for patients with stage I NSCLC.[3,5,20] However, the outcome of surgical treatment in resected stage I NSCLC after local recurrence have rarely been reported. Walsh et al[34] reported that complete surgical resection or high-dose radiotherapy with curative intent significantly prolonged post-recurrence survival in NSCLC. Sugimura et al[10] demonstrated that whether surgery or combination chemotherapy with radiation significantly improved post-recurrence survival over both no treatment and radiation alone in resected NSCLC after local recurrence. Voltolini et al[35] reported that 5-year survival after re-operation for locally recurrent bronchogenic carcinoma was 15.5%. The 5-year post-recurrence survival in our patients undergoing re-operation after local recurrence was 15%.

Treatment for recurrent NSCLC significantly prolongs overall survival and post-recurrence survival.[10,34] Yoshino et al[31] reported that patients who underwent metastatectomy for recurrence in distant organs had significantly longer survival while those with chemotherapy had marginally prolonged survival. Nakagawa et al[7] reported that treatment for the initial recurrence prolonged survival in stage I NSCLC after recurrence. In our study,[12] treatment for distant metastasis (including surgery and chemotherapy and/or radiotherapy) had a favorable survival in resected stage I NSCLC after distant metastasis than without treatment. There was no significant difference in post-recurrence survival between patients undergoing re-operation and those treated with chemotherapy and/or radiotherapy. However, there were two postoperative deaths due to respiratory failure after pulmonary resection. If the two patients were excluded, patients undergoing re-operation had significantly better post-recurrence survival than those receiving chemotherapy and/or radiotherapy (P = 0.021). The differences of therapeutic effects of surgery and chemotherapy and/or radiotherapy need larger series for further investigation.

Disease-free interval has also been shown to be a significant prognostic factor of post-recurrence survival in NSCLC. Longer disease-free interval was associated as with better post-recurrence survival in NSCLC after complete pulmonary resection.[10,34,36] Walsh et al[34] reported that disease-free interval greater than 12 months was a favorable predictor of post-recurrence survival in NSCLC after complete resection. Our study[12] showed that disease-free interval > 16 months was a significant predictor for better post-recurrence survival in patients with stage I NSCLC after distant metastasis.

Although some reports in the literature had tried to figure out the impact of specific distant metastatic organ sites on post-recurrence survival in resected NSCLC, small cohorts or mixtures with local and distant metastasis made it difficult to acquire definite results. Sugimura et al[10] reported that initial recurrence confined to the lung was associated with better post-recurrence survival in resected NSCLC. Yoshino et al[31] demonstrated that intra-pulmonary metastasis was a favorable factor for postrecurrence survival of resected NSCLC, while bone metastasis was a marginally unfavorable factor. Liver metastasis has also been reported as a worse prognostic factor in NSCLC after recurrence.[7,36] In our study, patients with distant metastases confined within the contralateral lung have significantly better post-recurrence survival than those with distant metastases outside the contralateral lung. We further showed that for patients with distant metastases outside the contralateral lung, those with bone metastasis had significantly worse post-recurrence survival.

6. Conclusion

Treatment for initial recurrence is a prognostic predictor for post-recurrence survival in resected stage I NSCLC with local recurrence. Longer disease-free interval and treatment for distant metastasis are indicators for better post-recurrence survival in resected stage I NSCLC with single organ metastasis. Complete surgical resection should be considered in selected candidates with resectable local recurrent disease. Aggressive treatment for distant metastasis in selected patients with longer disease-free interval may prolong the post-recurrence survival.

7. References

[1] Spira A, Ettinger DS. Multidisciplinary management of lung cancer. N Engl J Med. 2004;350:379-392.

[2] Scott WJ, Howington J, Feigenberg S, et al. Treatment of Non-small Cell Lung Cancer Stage I and Stage II: ACCP Evidence-Based Clinical Practice Guidelines (2nd Edition). Chest. 2007;132:234S-242S.

[3] Mountain CF. Revisions in the international system for staging lung cancer. Chest. 1997;111:1710-1717.

[4] Martini N, Bains MS, Burt ME, et al. Incidence of local recurrence and second primary tumors in resected stage I lung cancer. J Thorac Cardiovasc Surg. 1995;109:120-129.

[5] Harpole DH Jr, Herndon JE II, Young WG Jr, et al. Stage I non-small cell lung cancer. Cancer. 1995;76:787-796.

[6] Jones DR, Daniel TM, Denlinger CE, et al. Stage IB nonsmall cell lung cancers: are they all the same? Ann Thorac Surg. 2006;81:1958-1962.

[7] Nakagawa T, Okumura N, Ohata K, et al. Postrecurrence survival in patients with stage I non-small cell lung cancer. Eur J Cardiothorac Surg 2008;34:499-504.

[8] Al-Kattan K, Sepsas E, Fountain SW, et al. Disease recurrence after resection for stage I lung cancer. Eur J Cardiothorac Surg 1997;12:380-384.

[9] Martin J, Ginsberg RJ, Venkatraman ES, et al. Long-term results of combined-modality therapy in resectable non-small-cell lung cancer. J Clin Oncol 2002;20:1989-1995.

[10] Sugimura H, Nichols FC, Yang P, et al. Survival after recurrent nonsmall-cell lung cancer after complete pulmonary resection. Ann Thorac Surg 2007;83:409-418.

[11] Hung JJ, Hsu WH, Hsieh CC, et al. Post-recurrence survival in completely resected stage I non-small cell lung cancer with local recurrence. Thorax. 2009;64:192-196.

[12] Hung JJ, Jeng WJ, Hsu WH, et al. Prognostic factors of post-recurrence survival in completely resected stage I non-small cell lung cancer with distant metastasis. Thorax. 2009;65:241-245.

[13] Sobin L, Wittekind Ch, eds. TNM Classification of Malignant Tumors, Sixth Edition. New York: Wiley-Liss, 2002: 99-103.

[14] American Joint Committee on Cancer. AJCC Cancer Staging Manual. 7th ed. New York: Springer; 2010.

[15] International Union Against Cancer. TNM Classification of Malignant Tumours. 7th ed. Oxford, UK: Wiley-Blackwell; 2009.

[16] Rami-Porta R, Ball D, Crowley J, et al. The IASLC Lung Cancer Staging Project: proposals for the revision of the T descriptors in the forthcoming (seventh) edition of the TNM classification for lung cancer. J Thorac Oncol 2007;2:593-602.

[17] Goldstraw P, Crowley J, Chansky K, et al. The IASLC Lung Cancer Staging Project: proposals for the revision of the TNM stage groupings in the forthcoming (seventh) edition of the TNM Classification of malignant tumours. J Thorac Oncol 2007;2:706-714.

[18] Sawyer TE, Bonner JA, Gould PM, et al. Patients with stage I non-small cell lung carcinoma at postoperative risk for local recurrence, distant metastasis, and death: implications related to the design of clinical trials. Int J Radiat Oncol Biol Phys. 1999;45:315-321.

[19] Varlotto JM, Recht A, Nikolov M, et al. Extent of lymphadenectomy and outcome for patients with stage I nonsmall cell lung cancer. Cancer. 2009;115:851-858.

[20] Nesbitt JC, Putnam JB Jr, Walsh GL, et al. Survival in early-stage non-small cell lung cancer. Ann Thorac Surg 1995;60:466-472.

[21] Hung JJ, Wang CY, Huang MH, et al. Prognostic factors in resected stage I non-small cell lung cancer with a diameter of 3 cm or less: visceral pleural invasion did not

influence overall and disease-free survival. J Thorac Cardiovasc Surg. 2007;134:638-643.

[22] Hung JJ, Jeng WJ, Hsu WH, et al. Prognostic factors in pathological stage IB non-small cell lung cancer greater than 3 cm. Eur Respir J 2010;36:1355-1361.

[23] Hanagiri T, Sugio K, Mizukami M, et al. Significance of smoking as a postoperative prognostic factor in patients with non-small cell lung cancer. J Thorac Oncol 2008;3:1127-1132.

[24] Bryant A, Cerfolio RJ. Differences in epidemiology, histology, and survival between cigarette smokers and never-smokers who develop non-small cell lung cancer. Chest 2007;132:185-192.

[25] Maeda R, Yoshida J, Ishii G, et al. The Prognostic Impact of Cigarette Smoking on Patients with Non-small Cell Lung Cancer. J Thorac Oncol 2011;6:735-742.

[26] Maeda R, Ishii G, Yoshida J, et al. Influence of cigarette smoking on histological subtypes of stage I lung adenocarcinoma. J Thorac Oncol 2011;6:743-750.

[27] Maeda R, Yoshida J, Ishii G, et al. Poor prognostic factors in patients with stage IB non-small cell lung cancer according to the seventh edition TNM classification. Chest 2011;139:855-861.

[28] Maeda R, Yoshida J, Ishii G, et al. Risk factors for tumor recurrence in patients with early-stage (stage I and II) non-small cell lung cancer: Patient selection criteria for adjuvant chemotherapy according to the 7th edition TNM classification. Chest 2011 May 26. [Epub ahead of print]

[29] Varlotto JM, Recht A, Flickinger JC, et al. Factors associated with local and distant recurrence and survival in patients with resected nonsmall cell lung cancer. Cancer 2009;115:1059-1069.

[30] Cady B. Fundamentals of contemporary surgical oncology: biologic principles and the threshold concept govern treatment and outcomes. J Am Coll Surg 2001;192:777-792.

[31] Yoshino I, Yohena T, Kitajima M, et al. Survival of non-small cell lung cancer patients with postoperative recurrence at distant organs. Ann Thorac Cardiovasc Surg 2001;7:204-209.

[32] Maeda R, Yoshida J, Ishii G, et al. Long-term outcome and late recurrence in patients with completely resected stage IA non-small cell lung cancer. J Thorac Oncol 2010;5:1246-1250.

[33] Maeda R, Yoshida J, Ishii G, et al. Long-term survival and risk factors for recurrence in stage I non-small cell lung cancer patients with tumors up to 3 cm in maximum dimension. Chest 2010;138:357-362.

[34] Walsh GL, O'Connor M, Willis KM, et al. Is follow-up of lung cancer patients after resection medically indicated and cost-effective? Ann Thorac Surg 1995;60:1563-1570.

[35] Voltolini L, Paladini P, Luzzi L, et al. Iterative surgical resections for local recurrent and second primary bronchogenic carcinoma. Eur J Cardiothorac Surg 2000;18:529-534.

[36] Williams BA, Sugimura H, Endo C, et al. Predicting postrecurrence survival among completely resected nonsmall-cell lung cancer patients. Ann Thorac Surg 2006;81:1021-1027.

4

Lung Volume Reduction Surgery

James D. Maloney, Nicole K. Strieter and Joshua L. Hermsen
University of Wisconsin School of Medicine and Public Health,
William S. Middleton Memorial VA,
USA

1. Introduction

Lung volume reduction surgery (LVRS) was first reported by Drs Brantigan and Mueller from the University of Maryland in 1957. (1) Since that time it has enjoyed both fame and infamy but has never experienced widespread acceptance. Although subjective and often quantitative improvements in breathing were documented, early results were plagued by high mortality. Since those early reports the selection process for patients undergoing LVRS has been refined and has resulted in a safe and effective procedure. Regardless of selection criteria, however, numbers of LVR cases remain small. This is in contrast to the burgeoning population of patients with emphysema.

Chronic Obstructive Pulmonary Disease (COPD) is a major cause of morbidity and mortality in the United States. COPD includes both chronic bronchitis and emphysema as these conditions often coexist. It is estimated that 12.1 million adults aged 18 and over have a diagnosis of COPD. As many as 24 million U.S. adults have some evidence of impaired lung function This suggests that the disease in under diagnosed. (2,3) COPD is currently the fourth leading cause of death in the United States, and is projected to be the third most common by 2020. The disease no longer predominates in men. The number of women dying from the disease has surpassed the number seen in men. (2) As we move outside the United States to areas still seeing a rise in tobacco consumption millions more are affected. Chronic bronchitis and emphysema dramatically increase healthcare costs. COPD leads to high resource utilization, including frequent clinician office visits, hospitalizations due to acute exacerbations, and chronic therapy. (3) According to the National Heart Lung and Blood Institute, the national projected annual cost for COPD in 2010 was $49.9 billion. This includes $29.5 billion in direct health care expenditures, $8.0 billion in indirect morbidity costs and $12.4 billion in indirect mortality costs. (2,3)

The primary cause of COPD is smoking. COPD is under-diagnosed, with only 15 to 20 percent of smokers confirmed as having the disease although the majority develop some degree of airflow obstruction (4,6). Inhalation of tobacco smoke causes destruction of lung tissue that occurs in several ways. Tobacco exposure directly disrupts clearance of mucous secretions by injuring and destroying the cilia in turn increases mucus production from mucosal irritation leads to infection and injury. Chronic inflammation from direct irritation and subclinical infection results in elevated levels of inflammatory mediators. With continued exposure, there is loss of proteins and destruction of normal parenchymal architecture with decreased elasticity and alveolar destruction.(7)

2. Emphysema

DEFINITION — The Global Initiative for Chronic Obstructive Lung Disease (GOLD) — a report produced by the National Heart, Lung, and Blood Institute (NHLBI) and the World Health Organization (WHO) — defines COPD as follows (8):
"COPD is characterized by airflow limitation that is not fully reversible. The airflow limitation is usually progressive and associated with an abnormal inflammatory response of the lungs to noxious particles or gases."
There are commonly three distinct forms of COPD: chronic bronchitis, asthma and emphysema (9). Chronic bronchitis is characterized by chronic productive cough for three months in each of two successive years. This requires exclusion of other causes of chronic cough (9, 10). Asthma is "a chronic inflammatory disorder of the airways in which many cells and cellular elements play a role. The chronic inflammation is associated with airway responsiveness that leads to recurrent episodes of wheezing, breathlessness, chest tightness, and coughing. Asthma manifests airflow obstruction that is reversible, spontaneously or with treatment". (11) Asthma is not dependent on the noxious stimuli of smoking and does not have the same effect on survival that is seen in other forms of COPD. Emphysema is abnormal, permanent enlargement of the airspaces that are distal to the terminal bronchioles. (12)Emphysema is normally accompanied by moderate or severe airflow obstruction and destruction of alveolar walls without evidence of fibrosis. Emphysema causes dyspnea through airflow limitation, hyperinflation, and loss of gas exchanging surfaces in the lungs (13). In contrast to asthma, chronic bronchitis and emphysema typically manifest in the sixth decade of life and have a higher mortality to prevalence ratio. Emphysema is separated into radiographic definitions of centrilobular, panacinar and distal acinar(14) . In centrilobular emphysema the areas of disease are located near the center of the secondary pulmonary lobule. Arterial deficiency in the upper lobes accompanies this, but the distal acinus is unaffected. *Panacinar* emphysema affects the entire respiratory acinus, from respiratory bronchiole to alveoli. It occurs more commonly in the lower lobes, especially basal segments, and anterior margins of the lungs. Similar to centrilobular disease, affected areas demonstrate arterial defficiency. Most candidates for LVRS will have centrilobular emphysema.
COPD can be categorized as mild, moderate, severe and very severe, based primarily on forced expiratory volume in 1 second (FEV1).(8) In cases of very severe COPD, classification is impacted by pulmonary hypertension and pCO2. (table 1) Most candidates for LVRS will be classified as very severe based on GOLD criteria.

• Stage 1: Mild
FEV1 ≥ 80% predicted
• Stage 2: Moderate
80> FEV1 ≥ 50%
• Stage 3: Severe
50 > FEV1 ≥30% predicted
• Stage 4: Very Severe
FEV1 < 30% or
FEV1 < 50% + chronic respiratory failure
(PaO2 < 60mmHg, PaCO2 > 50mmHg, cor pulmonale)

Table 1. Gold executive summary for staging of emphysema.
Klaus FR, et al. Global Strategy for the Diagnosis, Management, and Prevention of Chronic Obstructive Pulmonary Disease: GOLD Executive Summary. Am L Respir Crit Care Med. Vol 176. Pp 532-55, 2007.

3. Lung Volume Reduction Surgery (LVRS)

Lung volume reduction attempts to correct loss of elastic recoil by reducing the volume of the most damaged lung segments and allowing the remaining less damaged tissues to expand within the chest. By eliminating parts of emphysematous lung with the longest expiratory time and removing dead space, dynamic air trapping is reduced and exercise capacity can be increased. The operating length of respiratory muscles is also normalized improving both inspiratory and expiratory effort. (14) Surgical removal of diseased lung restores the normal dimensions of both the chest wall and the diaphragm and augments the force exerted by the diaphragm. In addition it addresses dead space and ventilation/perfusion mismatch. The underlying mechanisms of improvement have not been fully elucidated. Increased elastic recoil, reduction in dynamic hyperinflation, and augmented force exerted by the diaphragm (15,16) have been suggested to explain the improvement in (FEV_1). There are quantitative increases in FVC, FEV_1, RV, and RV/TLC after LVRS in appropriately chosen candidates. These results support the hypothesis that the improvement in airflow rates resulted from a decrease in static hyperinflation and an increase in elastic recoil, resulting in greater radial traction on peripheral airways.(16) In short, respiratory mechanics are improved with LVRS.

Cremona and colleagues studied pulmonary gas exchange in COPD patients and recorded a very wide range of physiologic abnormality pre-operatively. (17) Post-LVRS Pa_{O2} increases were related to improvement in ventilation/perfusion mismatch, mainly due to a reduction in hyperinflation and dead space. There was no direct contribution from changes in lung mechanical properties. In contrast, the changes in Pa_{CO2} were accounted for by improvement in lung mechanical properties and not V/Q mismatch. (17) This corroborate data provided by Criner et al that also showed a downward shift in PaCo2 post LVRS in upper lobe predominant patients.(18)

Dr Joel Cooper reinvigorated the concept of lung volume reduction surgery as a successful therapy for emphysema. (19) It was in 1996 after publication of his results in the JCTVS that the volume of LVRS cases performed in the United States ballooned. Unfortunately the thoracic surgical community was not able to duplicate his results. Morbidity and mortality were excessive, and the cost to medicare and other third party payers extravagant. The outcomes were not consistent with Dr Cooper's published data. CMS took notice and quickly ceased reimbursement for the procedure. This discrepancy ultimately led to the NETT a study that was in part initiated to determine medicare reimbursement.

4. NETT (national emphysema treatment trial) review

The NETT was and continues to be the most influential trial of surgical lung volume reduction despite the fact that it was closed for accrual almost 10 years ago. To this day, it continues to be exhaustively reviewed and analyzed. This study determined not only the patient population should undergo LVRS for maximum benefit and the population who were high risk of mortality, but also criteria to circumscribe the number of centers able to offer the therapy. The NETT was a randomized, controlled, multicenter, long-term trial that examined the effects of LVRS. The primary endpoints were survival and maximum exercise performance and secondary endpoints were post surgical lung function, patient symptoms and quality of life all compared to medical therapy alone.(20) The initial data was published in 2003 and reported the effects of LVRS on survival and maximum exercise capacity.

Median follow-up was 2.4 years in its primary iteration.(21) In 2006, NETT investigators reported updated analyses with a median follow-up of 4.3 years.(22) Over 1200 patients were randomized in the trial giving it sufficient statistical power. 608 patients were randomized to the surgery arm, 70% were by median sternotomy, the remainder by VATS. Quantitative improvement was seen in the LVRS group as compared to the medically managed patients. Exercise capacity, a primary endpoint, improved following LVRS after 6, 12 and 24 months compared to medically treated patients. In comparison to medically treated patients, LVRS patients performed better in 6 minute walk distance (6MWD), percent predicted forced expiratory volume in one-second (FEV1), the severity of dyspnea, and quality of life assessments. (21) Though overall mortality was not statistically different, 90 day mortality for the surgery arm was approaching 8%, far higher than the medical arm (1.3 %). Upon further review, it was determined that there was a subgroup who posed prohibitive surgical risk. This subgroup, defined by FEV1 < 20 % predicted and either a diffusing capacity for carbon monoxide (DLCO) < 20% predicted or homogeneous emphysema represented prohibitive risks with a 30-day mortality of 16% (23). Identification of this subgroup helped to delineate the pulmonary function testing criteria appropriate for LVRS and led to categorizing non-high risk patients into four distinct groups for analysis.

The basis for grouping non high risk patients was the craniocaudal distribution of emphysema on chest CT (upper lobe predominance) and post rehabilitation exercise test maximum wattage (low or high exercise).

4.1 NETT Subgroup analysis

1.   Upper lobe predominant low exercise capacity

This group demonstrated the most benefit from LVRS. Patients with upper lobe predominant emphysema and low exercise capacity had a lower risk of death with LVRS than medical therapy. This LVRS group was more likely to achieve > 10 W improvement in maximum exercise wattage at 24 months, and > an 8 point improvement in St. George's Respiratory Questionnaire (SGRQ) score at 24 months.

2.   Upper lobe predominant high exercise capacity

Patients with upper lobe predominant emphysema and high exercise tolerance, LVRS had no effect on survival even in extended follow up. Following LVRS, however, patients were more likely to have > 10 W improvement in maximum exercise wattage at 24 months and significant improvement in SGRQ as compared to medical therapy.

3.   Non-upper lobe predominant low exercise capacity

Patients with non-upper lobe predominant disease and low exercise capacity, LVRS had no effect on the risk of death or maximum exercise capacity at 24 months. However, LVRS patients were more likely to have significant improvement in SGRQ at 24 months.

4.   Non-upper lobe predominant high exercise capacity

Patients with non-upper lobe predominant emphysema and high exercise at baseline, LVRS increased the risk for death and had no beneficial impact on maximum exercise capacity at 24 months or SGRQ.

4.2 Patient outcomes

The above groupings were instrumental in determining appropriate patients for LVRS. In the non-high risk population the 30-day mortality was 2.2% with LVRS and 0.2% with medical treatment (p< 0.001). 90-day mortality rate was 5.2% with LVRS and 1.5% with medical treatment (21). LVRS did not demonstrate short term survival benefit over medical treatment. LVRS showed significant and sustained increases in exercise capacity and 6 minute walk distance, reduction in dyspnea, and improvements in disease-specific and general quality of life measurements.(24) In patients with upper lobe predominant emphysema and low exercise capacity, total mortality rate was 0.11 deaths per person-year with LVRS and 0.13 with medical treatment, respectively. In upper lobe predominant, low exercise tolerance patients, LVRS increased survival, and improved exercise capacity and quality of life compared to medical therapy. (22)

Postoperative morbidity was not a primary endpoint in the NETT but is important in assessing the success of a procedure. 58.7% of the patients had at least one complication within 30 days of surgery. Major pulmonary and cardiovascular morbidity occurred in approximately 30% and 20% respectively during the NETT. Cardiac arryhtmia occurred in almost 25%. 18% developed pneumonia, 21% were re-intubated and 8% underwent tracheostomy.(24,25) Despite significant morbidity, quality of life measures were improved with LVRS over medical therapy. Outcomes related to mortality and morbidity continue to improve. Ginsburg et al recently published their series of 49 patients undergoing LVRS selected using the criteria defined by the NETT. Both BODE index and FEV1 showed statistically significant improvement, and operative mortality (90 day) was zero, with acceptable morbidity. (26) Boley and colleagues published a recent series with morbidity and mortality lower than that documented in the NETT. (27) Despite improved mortality, predicting response in LVRS patients continues to be difficult. Imfeld and colleagues demonstrated that post-operative BODE index accurately predicts survival, however preoperative values do not.(28) (see table 2) Similarly there is no perfect instrument to determine an expected increase in FEV1 or 6 minute walk that will positively influence BODE index and subsequently survival.

Variable	Points on BODE Index			
	0	1	2	3
FEV$_1$ (% of predicted)†	≥65	50–64	36–49	≤35
Distance walked in 6 min (m)	≥350	250–349	150–249	≤149
MMRC dyspnea scale‡	0–1	2	3	4
Body-mass index§	>21	≤21		

Table 2. Variables for BODE index a predictor of survival in COPD patients

5. Indications for LVRS

Criteria for LVRS in our institution is based on the NETT inclusion and exclusion criteria with some limited changes. We have not set firm age limitations in our patient exclusion criteria for LVRS but review them on a case by case basis in patients over 65 years of age. With few exceptions, in patients with FEV1 > 35% predicted, we have chosen to manage medically barring substantial symptoms in a patient with severe bullous disease and significant segmental or lobar compression.

History and physical exam consistent with emphysema
Imaging with evidence of heterogeneous emphysema
Pre-rehabilitation postbronchodilator TLC ≥ 100% predicted
Pre-rehabilitation postbronchodilator RV ≥ 150% predicted
FEV1 % predicted 20-35 %
Pre-rehabilitation room air, resting $PaCO_2$ ≤ 60 mm Hg (≤ 55 mm Hg in Denver)
Pre-rehabilitation room air, resting PaO_2 ≥ 45 mm Hg (≥ 30 mm Hg in Denver)
Body-mass index ≤ 32 (males) or ≤ 35 (females)
Nonsmoker for 6 months prior to initial review with negative urine cotinines
Completion pulmonary rehabilitation program (prior to surgery)

Table 3. Inclusion Criteria for LVRS at UWHC.

CT scan evidence of diffuse emphysema judged unsuitable for LVRS
Previous LVRS
Previous sternotomy (relative) or lobectomy
Significant untreated coronary disease
CHF and ejection fraction < 45%
Pulmonary hypertension: mean≥ 40 mm Hg or peak systolic >50 mm
History of recurrent infections with daily sputum production judged clinically significant
Daily use of > 20 mg of prednisone or its equivalent
Evidence of systemic disease or neoplasia that may compromise survival
Inability to complete screening, baseline data or pulmonary rehabilitation

Table 4. Exclusion Criteria for UWHC.

Questions remain regarding two patient groups, Alpha 1 antitrypsin and homogeneous emphysema. There is data to suggest benefit from LVRS in both patient populations. (29,30) The overall benefit has been less pronounced than patients with heterogeneous upper lobe predominant emphysema patients. Patients have been shown to have a slightly reduced survival without transplant when compared with upper lobe predominant group. (29) Our institution has not as yet recommended LVRS in homogeneous disease. Similarly, we recommend transplantation primarily for Alpha-1-antitrypsin, though LVRS is considered as a bridge to transplant in specific individuals.

6. Pre-operative evaluation

PreOperative assessment for LVRS should parallel evaluation for lung transplantation. The goals are similar: the patient should be physiologically capable of tolerating the procedure, there are no non-pulmonary conditions which exist that would limit the expected benefit of the procedure, and the pulmonary status is such that the patient's quality of life or overall health is positively impacted by the surgery. Referral is often through the auspices of lung transplantation at our institution. The advent of the lung allocation score has changed the lung transplant recipient profile substantially. Therefore, all patients referred with COPD/emphysema are additionally reviewed for LVRS.

Pulmonary evaluation begins with pulmonary function testing and 6 minute walk as an assessment of exercise tolerance. Clear indications for transplantation evaluation include FEV1 or DLCO ≤ 20% predicted. In patients with FEV1 ≥ 35% symptoms appear reasonably controlled with medical management alone and observation is typically recommended in our institution. Patients at higher risk of acute exacerbations post –operatively such as those with significant chronic bronchitic, asthmatic, or bronchiectatic components, may not be optimal surgical candidates. If COPD exacerbation occurs we generally delay surgery 1 month and confirm that steroid dosage is down to a level less than or equal to 10 mg /day. Computed Tomography scanning is performed with a graded degree of emphysema (1-4) in the upper, middle and lower lung fields. A change in score of 2 or more is considered significant and suggests heterogeneous disease.(14,31) We have found the lung perfusion scan to be immensely helpful in determining appropriate candidates and anecdotally in predicting response from surgery. The geometric mean of the perfusion score is quantitative and not dependent on the interpreting radiologist. CT scan quality may affect interpretation though this is less influential with improved technology and dissemination into the community.

The importance of perfusion scanning in determining appropriate patient selection has become evident. Recent analysis of the existing NETT data emphasized the importance of perfusion scintigraphy in the evaluation of potential LVRS patients. Low upper lobe perfusion was defined as less than 20% of blood flow to the upper third of the lungs. (24) We believe that this should be lateralized to 10% of perfusion per lung. In patients with upper lobe predominance and low exercise capacity who were confirmed as having low upper zone perfusion by scintigaraphy there was lower mortality with LVRS vs. medical therapy (p=0.008) Similarly, in upper lobe predominant emphysema and high exercise, patients with confirmed low upper lobe zone perfusion had lower mortality with LVRS (p=0.02). (24) Though perfusion scintigraphy this appears to be a predictor of mortality we cannot definitively state that it is a predictor of change in FEV1.

It is important to underscore the multidisciplinary nature of LVRS evaluation. In addition to meeting screening criteria and confirming an absence of comorbidity that would increase the risk of complication or mortality, patients should be medically optimized. This is crucial during pulmonary rehabilitation for the individuals to get the best response possible from this surgery. Minor modifications in COPD medications may be important such as discontinuing inhaled corticosteroid as this may be a risk factor for prolonged airleak.(32) Some have advocated preoperative initiation of B blockade or even amiodarone due to the high (approaching 25% incidence) of arrhythmia. We routinely administer prophylactic beta blockade B blockers in the immediate postoperative period in patients who are at high risk, but have not yet moved to more aggressive amiodarone regimen.

6.1 Technical considerations

Our institutional bias is to perform LVRS with bilateral thoracoscopy. We use lateral positioning, starting on the side that has greater perfusion, then repositioning for the contralateral side. The more severely affected lung is more likely to have significant air leak post resection. This may create ventilatory difficulty intraoperatively during single lung ventilation. A double lumen tube is preferred for lung isolation, though Arndt bronchial blockers have been used successfully. A three Port exposure is normally adequate. We recommend placing ports at the seventh intercostal space anterior axillary line, the fourth intercostal space anteriorly, and just inferior to the scapula. (figure 2) The amount of lung resected is based on surgeon discretion, estimating the residual pleural volume appropriate for the patient and the severity of the disease. Typically this means resection of approximately 40-50% of the left upper lobe volume and 50-60% of the right upper lobe volume. Resection is performed with a linear cutter stapling device and buttressing material. Surgeon preference dictates choice of both stapler and buttress material and there is no data suggesting significantly improved outcome with a specific model. (25,26) We do not routinely use sealant in our procedures, but perform an extended pleural tent extending from the 4th intercostal port site anteriorly around the apex and down to the hilum medially and posteriorly. Straight chest tubes are placed anteriorly and posteriorly extending to the height of the tent, not the apex of the bony thorax.

Surgical approach does not appear to significantly alter outcomes. In the NETT 90 day mortality and all cause mortality did not show significant differences. Mean operative time was less with median sternotomy (MS). Transfusion requirements were equivalent. There was a higher incidence of intraoperative complication in the VATS group related to a higher occurrence of hypoxemia. (24,27) A recent study by Boley and colleagues showed equivalent early outcomes with VATS and MS. Pain scores, narcotic requirement and incentive spirometry scores were similar (27). The NETT did show some differences. At 30 days post LVRS a higher percentage of VATS patients were living independently than MS patients, 80% vs 70% respectively. (22) Surprisingly, though functional outcomes were equivalent at 1 and 2 years, LVRS related cost and total medical costs were higher for MS patients than VATS patients. (24) My personal and institutional preference for VATS stems from the following. A more effective pleural tent can be created with VATS than median sternotomy. Second is my concern that sternal precautions limits early return to preoperative lifestyle. A VATS LVRS patient can be back to driving 2 weeks after discharge which I would not allow in MS patients.

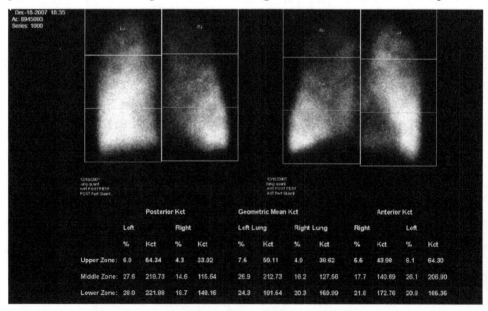

| | Posterior Kct | | | | Geometric Mean Kct | | | | Anterior Kct | | | |
| | Left | | Right | | Left Lung | | Right Lung | | Right | | Left | |
	%	Kct	%	Kct	%	Kct	%	Kct	%	Kct	%	Kct
Upper Zone:	6.9	64.34	4.3	33.92	7.6	59.11	4.9	38.62	6.6	43.98	8.1	64.30
Middle Zone:	27.6	218.73	14.6	115.64	26.9	212.73	16.2	127.56	17.7	140.69	26.1	206.90
Lower Zone:	28.0	221.98	18.7	149.16	24.3	191.64	20.3	169.99	21.8	172.76	20.9	166.36

Fig. 1. Perfusion scan demonstrating favorable upper lobe distribution of emphysema.

Unilateral LVRS in patients with anatomic or other contraindications to bilateral therapy has been reported. Meyers et al showed that FEV1 was increased 32% at 12months and 28% at 3 years.(33) Exercise capacity and QOL measures were also improved. The increase in FEV1 however, was not maintained at 5 years. (33) This reflects our experience in unilateral LVRS and patients undergoing incidental LVR effects during upper lobectomy for lung malignancy.

6.2 Peri-operative care
Perioperative care for LVRS patients in our institution is provided in an adaptable acuity care unit for cardiothoracic surgical patients. All beds within the Unit are ICU capable and require only an electronic order to change patient status. Not all patients require ICU care, however it is easily and immediately available when required. In our recent series 25% of patients required ICU care. One patient remained intubated overnight after a combined robotic off pump coronary artery bypass and LVRS. Three patients required reintubation. In all three patients, we moved quickly to tracheostomy and all were off ventilator support at the time of discharge. Average days in the ICU is 2, reflecting the few patients who have been reintubated and required tracheostomy. Overall median LOS was 7 days in our series. We have had no 30 or 90 day mortality. Mean preoperative FEV1 was 26% predicted and mean FEV1 increase was 44% over baseline. The extent of quantifiable respiratory functional improvement is variable, as demonstrated in Table 2
Pain control postoperatively is quite different from our thoracic oncology patients due to the frequent need for prolonged chest drainage and the bilateral nature of the procedure. We use a combination of epidural and oral narcotic analgesics. We try to avoid ketoralac and other NSAIDs in the early postoperative period. An aggressive respiratory therapy protocol is used for pulmonary toilet. With this approach we have reduced our need for bronchoscopy for secretion clearance. In patients where unilateral or staged LVRS is performed we employ a protocol similar to that for lobectomy. Paravertebral blocks for preemptive pain control and patient controlled or oral narcotic analgesia are utilized. Chest tubes are maintained to water seal unless subcutaneous emphysema or increasing pneumothorax develops. Air leaks are currently the most common reason for longer LOS. Examining the NETT data, following LVRS 90% of patients had air leak at some point within 30 days of surgery. (22) Median air leak duration was 7 days, but 12% had air leaks > 30 days. As expected air leak was longer in patients with lower FEV1. Post operative complications were greater in patients with a prolonged air leak and the post-operative stay was longer. With new ways of managing air leaks as an outpatient there is less effect on LOS. Easily maintained, miniature, waterless pleural drainage systems have allowed safe discharge with weekly outpatient clinic visits. These drainage systems allow extra time healing and give patients more mobility post discharge.

6.3 LVRS as alternative to lung transplant
Comparisons of LVRS to lung transplant have been reported. However, it is currently not a fair comparison as patients who undergo LVRS would not generate a LAS high enough to be considered for lung transplantation. A retrospective series compared functional outcomes (pulmonary function tests, arterial blood gas analysis, six-minute walk distance) in 33 patients who underwent LVRS versus 39 patients who had single lung transplantation and 27 patients who had bilateral sequential lung transplantation (34). The patients were evaluated before the operation and at 3, 6, and 12 months after surgery. In the LVRS group mean FEV1 improved by 79% and 82% at 6 and 9 months, respectively. Improvement in PFTS was far more dramatic

in the transplant population. Mean FEV1 increases were over 200% in the single lung transplant group and approaching 500% in the bilateral lung transplant group. 6 MW showed similar differences in response(34). While lung transplant demonstrated far superior function at 12 months than LVRS, improvements in survival for COPD patients from lung transplant have been difficult to identify though it appears from recently published reports that adjusted mortality is improved with lung transplant in COPD patients with a high LAS.(35) Overall survival after lung transplantation at one and 3 years is currently 84% and 70% respectively.(36) This is juxtaposed to the results of LVRS. Longterm follow-up of NETT data published in 2006 demonstrated improved survival in the upper lobe predominant, low exercise capacity cohort.(22) In another recent series three year survival was 95%. (26)

Organ availability is currently the major limitation in lung transplantation. Organ allocation has therefore been a matter of much controversy. The lung transplant population has had a remarkable shift in the last 5 years due to the Lung Allocation Score. Components of the score are listed in table 6 (37). Of Note FEV1 is not present within the scoring system though it appears to have an effect on mortality and is represented in the Bode Index. In 2000, 43% of lung transplants done within the US were for COPD and 14.6%for IPF. In 2008 that ratio had shifted to 28.6% and 33.5% for COPD and IPF, respectively (36). Shortly after initiation of the LAS, we reviewed patients undergoing evaluation for lung transplantation at the William S. Middleton Memorial VA Hospital to determine the need for a dedicated LVRS program. 162 patients were referred from 2002 to 2007. 69 patients were listed and 93 deferred. 60% of the deferred group (56 patients) had COPD. 29% met screening criteria for LVRS. (Maloney, unpublished abstract). We compared the functional status and overall severity of disease as measured by an estimated Lung Allocation Score (LAS) between the 29 patients who met criteria for LVRS and patients undergoing lung transplant during that time period. In addition to demographic differences there was a significant difference in LAS. (table 7) The mean age was older in the LVRS group but the value was not statistically significant.

LVRS has been used as a bridge to transplant. As with any re-operative technique there is increased complexity related to postoperative scarring and adhesion. Dissection of the hilum with phrenic nerve injury or praxia is the foremost concern. In one prospective study, LVRS prior to lung transplantation improved symptoms and lung function enough to delay lung transplantation for a median of 33 months. A second series stated LVRS could potentially delay lung transplant for up to five years.(39) Patients undergoing LVRS prior to transplant had a similar response to surgical intervention as patients not being considered for transplantation, with the exception of lower lung field predominance which had a shorter duration of improvement. (39,40)

Patient 1				
	PreOP	%	Post OP	%
FVC	1.76	59	2.53	84
FEV1	0.51	23	0.77	35
Patient 2				
	PreOP	%	Post OP	%
FVC	1.53	51	2.61	81
FEV1	0.47	21	1.09	40

Table 5. Representative Patient data demonstrating the variability of response to LVRS.

Lung Diagnosis
Date of birth
Functional Status
Assisted Ventilation
Height and Weight
Diabetes
Supplemental Oxygen
Percent predicted FVC
Six minute walk distance
Serum creatinine
PA pressures (especially systolic & mean)
Pulmonary capillary wedge mean
PCO2

Table 6. Data elements used in determining the LAS.

LVRS	Transplant	
Age 61	Age 54	NS
LAS (estimated) 31.9	LAS 43.9	P=0.0154
	FEV1 16.4 ± 3.7	

Table 7. Comparison of potential LVRS patients to transplant recipients after adopting LAS as means for recipient selection.

1.	Anatomic lobar resection of the most hyperinflated lobe is performed through an axillary muscle sparing thoracotomy.
2.	The medial anterior mediastinal parietal pleura is incised in a craniocaudal fashion, ideally from the apex to the diaphragm.
3.	Using primarily blunt, manually assisted dissection, generous pleural flaps are developed.
4.	Ideally these flaps are dissected back to the edge of remaining lung (anterior flap) and to the medial hilum (posterior flap)
5.	The pleural flaps are trimmed (if needed), overlapped (in whichever orientation seems most appropriate), and tacked in place with 3-0 braided, absorbable suture.

Table 8. Mediastinal Pexy Technique for native lung hypertrophy after Single lung transplant

7. LVRS post lung transplant

Although the optimal approach to end-stage COPD is argued, the International Society for Heart and Lung Transplantation Registry demonstrates that single lung transplant for COPD has been the most common lung transplantation procedure performed.(40) When single lung transplant is performed, there is risk of developing native lung hyperinflation. A percentage of these patients have decreased function resulting from graft compression by the native lung, which can compromise oxygenation, pulmonary function tests and exercise capacity. While the physiology of the transplanted lung becomes restrictive, the overall pulmonary function picture is one of obstruction dominated by the native lung. Chest CT scans can facilitate diagnosis in these patients, with demonstration of increasing native lung expansion at the cost of allograft volume. It is critical to identify chronic rejection or bronciolitis obliterans syndrome prior to native LVRS as mortality in this setting is prohibitive. Bronchoscpy with biopsy, lung scintigraphy, PFTs and CT imaging are helpful but clinical suspicion of confounding causes of functional decline can be difficult to rule out. Native side LVRS (nLVRS) was first described in such patients in the 1990's although it remains an uncommon procedure. (41) Both anatomic and non-anatomic resection has been described for this purpose. The largest series, comprised of 8 pts, was reported by Reece et al in 2008. (42) This experience and others show that while nLVRS can reliably relieve graft compression and improve lung function/patient symptomatology, it is high risk with considerable morbidity and mortality. It is important to note that the patterns of disease amenable to LVRS as determined by the National Emphysema Treatment Trial do not necessarily apply to the post-transplant patient given that the main problem is compression of the functional transplant lung graft. Much of the morbidity following nLVRS is owed to prolonged air leak and infectious complication in the native lung. We have developed a technique of mediastinal pexy that fixes the mediastinum towards, and minimizes pleural space on the volume reduced side.

2004	2010
27 transplants total	37 transplants total
12/27 COPD = 44.4%	8/37 COPD = 21.6 %
7/27 IPF = 25.9%	15/37 IPF = 40.5%

Table 9. UW distribution of Lung transplants by disease

7.1 Technique
1.   Anatomic lobar resection of the most hyperinflated lobe is performed through an axillary muscle sparing thoracotomy.
2.   The medial anterior mediastinal parietal pleura is incised in a craniocaudal fashion, ideally from the apex to the diaphragm.
3.   Using primarily blunt, manually assisted dissection, generous pleural flaps are developed.
4.   Ideally these flaps are dissected back to the edge of remaining lung (anterior flap) and to the medial hilum (posterior flap)
5.   The pleural flaps are trimmed (if needed), overlapped (in whichever orientation seems most appropriate), and tacked in place with 3-0 braided, absorbable suture.
The 20% mortality rate in the largest series of this technique underscores the high-risk nature of this procedure. Both patient mortalities in Reece's series ultimately died of infectious respiratory complications, one in the setting of bronchial stump leak and the other was ultimately diagnosed with bronchiolitis obliterans at autopsy. The average ICU LOS was 13d and average hospital LOS was 21 days. Their functional results were excellent with 87.5% of patients having significant and sustained pulmonary function and symptom improvement. Other authors have reported smaller experiences with 1-yr survival rates of 50% or less. (41,42) We propose that the mediastinal pexy technique allows for both minimization and fixation of pleural space on the volume reduced side greater than can be

achieved with standard pleural tenting and/or physiologic shifting following volume reduction. Our experience is small but encouraging. ICU length of stay is less than previously reported and there seems to be at least a trend towards decreased chest tube duration. Other authors have reported use of endobronchial valves acutely for native lung hyperinflation (43).

8. Endobronchial treatments for LVRS

Bronchoscopic techniques for volume reduction of emphysematous lung are inherently attractive because of decreased periprocedural mortality and morbidity. Currently available data on efficacy of bronchoscopic lung volume reduction are not conclusive. Patients appear to derive a subjective benefit in relief of dyspnea, however improvements in spirometry or exercise tolerance have not been demonstrated. Endobronchial technique for LVR include; one-way endobronchial valves implanted into the airway, self-activating coils, targeted destruction and remodeling of emphysematous tissue and bypass tract airway stenting. Of the multiple forms of bronchoscopic therapy we will concentrate on endobrochial valves which have the most data, and touch briefly on other options.

8.1 Endobronchial valves

Endobronchial valves are designed to exclude the most emphysematous regions from ventilation and reduce air trapping. Valves allow expiration, but prevent any distal flow during inspiration (44). There are two distinct endobronchial valve designs; duckbill (zephyr) and umbrella-shaped (spiration) valves. The VENT trial was a prospective multicenter randomized trial comparing endobronchial valve therapy to medical management.(44,45) Post procedure (6 month) FEV1 increased 4.3% over baseline and an increase in 6MW of 2.5%. Though both were statistically significant it is hard to determine the clinical value of these increases. In patients with complete fissures, the increase in FEV1 was 17%. Patients showed subjective improvements based on St. George Respiratory Questionnaire (SGRQ). Major complications occurred in 6% demonstrating safety. Acute COPD exacerbations however were increased substantially over the medically managed group. The Spiration IBV valve did not demonstrate increased FEV1 or quantitative functional assessment. Subjective improvements were seen in some patients. Morbidity and mortality also were low demonstrating feasibility and safety of the device. (44) Lobar atelectasis appears to be evidence of clinically favorable response to valve placement. Less than 25% of reported cases achieved this effect. (45,46) Of note neither device is approved in the US for volume reduction in emphysema. The spiration IBV valve is approved for persistent air leaks and there is good documentation of its efficacy in that arena.(47)

The greatest limitation in effective endobronchial LVR is crossventilation. Incomplete fissures between lobes of the lung and collateral ventilation accounts for this finding. However, the greatest benefits appear to be found in patients who actually do develop such target lobe atelectasis because of favorable changes in chest wall dimensions. (22,48) If valves are to be used in the future, bronchoscopic LVR trials may need to incorporate assessment techniques to preferentially select patients with high collateral ventilation resistance as they are more likely to obtain greater benefit. Other means of bronchoscopic LVR are not as affected by cross ventilation and may have greater long term value.

8.2 Biological lung volume reduction

Biological agents aim to reduce lung volume by sealing off the most emphysematous areas. The rapidly polymerizing sealant is designed to work at the alveolar level rather than in the airways. The mechanism of action involves resorption atelectasis from airway occlusion, subsequent airspace inflammation, and then remodeling resulting in contraction of lung parenchyma. This therapy should not be affected by collateral ventilation as it works on an alveolar level.

The sealant, a mixture of fibrinogen suspension and thrombin solution, is instilled into targeted areas determined by preoperative imaging. Serious adverse events were limited and no fatalities documented. Improvement was identified in FEV_1 (38% to 44%); 6-minute walk (27%), and in SGRQ (32% to 46%). Concern has been expressed regarding the longevity of the treatment as smaller dose therapy did not appear to maintain results even with short term follow up. (49)

8.3 LVRC

Lung volume reduction coils (LVRS) are wire implants placed into the parenchyma bronchoscopically. The coil once deployed, acts to contract the tissue leading to a volume reduction effect. This concept is not affected by the influence of cross ventilation, so may have an advantage over endobronchial valves. A small series has been reported that demonstrated safety and additional trials are necessary to confirm efficacy. (50)

9. Cost-effectiveness of LVRS

As discussed previously the costs of caring for patients with COPD are staggering and increase as the severity of emphysema worsens regardless of therapy used to palliate the disease. However, it is a small portion of patients with emphysema and even smaller percentage that are candidates for LVRS. A review of the NETT data showed that costs for LVRS was higher than best medical care and this was confirmed in a different healthcare system in a Canadian trial. (51,52) The mean total costs per person ($98,952 vs. $62,560, p<0.001) and per-person medical costs ($80,818 vs. $43,689, p<0.001) at three years.(49,51) Cost effectiveness for LVRS improves over time as care for a medically managed patient increases in expense. There is a significant difference in costs for the four groups defined by the NETT. The cost-effectiveness of LVRS vs. medical therapy was $140,000 per quality-adjusted life-year (QALY) gained at 5 years, and was projected to be $54,000 per QALY gained at 10 years. In the subgroup with upper lobe–predominant emphysema and low baseline exercise capacity, which showed the greatest overall benefits after LVRS, the cost per quality-adjusted life year gained was $98,000 at 3 years and $21,000 at 10 years.(53) Bronchoscopic LVR is less costly initially, but without a significant change in BODE score that decrease in amount per QALY seen in surgical LVRS over time may not occur. The financial impact of endobronchial therapy is not trivial as workup, implants, and surveillance are costly, and potentially without the quantifiable improvement of surgical therapy. As healthcare dollars become less available we must make sure that emerging therapies are measured against the gold standard of surgical LVRS instead of being driven by market forces. At the same time we must continue to improve morbidity and mortality in LVRS which will limit costs related to adverse events.

10. Summary

LVRS along with supplemental oxygen and smoking cessation is only one of few therapies that can improve survival in selected patients with severe emphysema. Despite the impressive conclusions demonstrated by the NETT data and more recent trials that show substantial benefit, relatively few patients undergo LVRS relative to the prevalence of emphysema.(24) In 2009 118 medicare patients underwent the procedure based on STS data. This number is down from approximately 250 patients in 2004, shortly after the initial NETT data was published. At that time in 2004 there were 42 approved centers. This number has decreased as participation in the NETT no longer results in automatic center approval. Only CMS certified centers and transplant centers now may be reimbursed through medicare for the procedure. In addition, some of the LVRS literature has stigmatized the surgery, suggesting that the risk is prohibitive. Many pulmonologists remain unaware of the benefits of LVRS and the consistently improving procedure related morbidity, mortality and LOS. Also as non-surgical options consistently achieve below expected results and remain investigational, the pulmonary community loses interest. One appropriate ongoing concern is the cost of therapy to the healthcare system as funds become increasingly limited. This will minimize cost and improve the QALY in comparison to best medical treatment. Education of the community pulmonologist and availability of information to patients will limit referrals to patients who are likely to benefit from surgery. This too will minimize costs in patient evaluation. Another is that LVRS functional and quantitative PFTS results show substantial variation between patients. Ongoing assessment of more recent LVRS series will be crucial in determining predictive capabilties of preoperative testing and minimizing morbidity and streamlining care and hospital stay.

11. References

[1]   Brantigan OC, Mueller E, Kress MB. A surgical approach to pulmonary emphysema. Am Rev Respir Dis 1959; 80:194.

[2]   National Heart Lung and Blood Institute. Morbidity and Mortality: 2009 Chart Book on Cardiovascular, Lung and Blood Diseases.

[3]   Centers for Disease Control and Prevention. National Center for Health Statistics. National Health & Nutrition Examination Survey, 1988-1994.

[4]   Rennard SI, Vestbo J. COPD: the dangerous underestimate of 15%. Lancet 2006; 367:1216.

[5]   Buist AS, McBurnie MA, Vollmer WM, et al. International variation in the prevalence of COPD (the BOLD Study): a population-based prevalence study. Lancet 2007; 370:741.

[6]   Petty, RL, Nett, LM. COPD: Prevention in the primary care setting, The National Lung Health Education Program, 2001. p.341.

[7]   Bridges RB, Wyatt RJ, Rehm SR. Effects of smoking on inflammatory mediators and their relationship to pulmonary dysfunction Eur J Respir Dis Suppl. 1986;146:145-52.

[8]   Global strategy for the diagnosis, management, and prevention of chronic obstructive pulmonary disease: Executive summary 2006. Global Initiative for Chronic Obstructive Lung Disease (GOLD). http://www.goldcopd.org (Accessed on December 14, 2009).

[9]   Standards for the diagnosis and care of patients with chronic obstructive pulmonary disease. American Thoracic Society. Am J Respir Crit Care Med 1995; 152:S77.

[10] BTS guidelines for the management of chronic obstructive pulmonary disease. The COPD Guidelines Group of the Standards of Care Committee of the BTS. Thorax 1997; 52 Suppl 5:S1.

[11] GINA report, global strategy for asthma management and prevention 2006. Global Initiative for Asthma (GINA) http://www.ginasthma.com (Accessed on August 31, 2007).

[12] Hogg JC. Pathophysiology of airflow limitation in chronic obstructive pulmonary disease. Lancet 2004; 364:709.

[13] Obstructive lung disease. Med Clin North Am 1990; 74:547.

[14] Radiology paper

[15] Travaline j, Sudarshan S, Obrien G, Kuzma AM, Furukawa S. Effect of lung volume reduction surgery on diaphragm strength. Am J Respir Crit Care Med 157: 1578–1585, 1998.

[16] Martinez FJ, deOca MM, Whyte RI, Stetz J, Gay SE, Celli BR. Lung-volume reduction improves dyspnea, dynamic hyperinflation, and respiratory muscle function. Am J Respir Crit Care Med 155: 1984–1990, 1997.

[17] Cremona G, Barbara J, Melgosa T, Appendini L, Roca J, Casaio C. Mechanisms of gas exchange response to lung volume reduction surgery in severe emphysema. J Appl Physiol. 2011 Apr;110(4):1036-45. Epub 2011 Jan 13

[18]

[19] J.D. Cooper, A.G. Patterson, S.R. Sundaresan, E.P. Trulock, R.D. Yusen, M.S. Pohl and S.S. Lefrak, Results of 150 consecutive bilateral lung volume reduction procedures in patients with severe emphysema, J Thorac Cardiovasc Surg 112 (1996), pp. 1319–1330.

[20] NETT Research Group. Rationale and design of the national emphysema treatment trial,A prospective randomized trial of lung volume reduction surgery. Chest. 1999;116:1750

[21] A. Fishman, F. Martinez, K. Naunheim et al., "A randomized trial comparing lung-volume-reduction surgery with medical therapy for severe emphysema," The New England Journal of Medicine, vol. 348, no. 21, pp. 2059–2073, 2003.

[22] Naunheim KS, Wood DE, Mohsenifar Z, et al. Long-term follow-up of patients receiving lung-volume-reduction surgery versus medical therapy for severe emphysema by the National Emphysema Treatment Trial Research Group. Ann Thorac Surg 2006; 82:431.

[23] National Emphysema Treatment Trial Research Group. Patients at high risk of death after lung-volume-reduction surgery. N Engl J Med 2001; 345:1075.

[24] Criner GJ, Cordova F, Sternberg AL, Martinez FJ. The NETT: Part II- Lessons learned about lung volume reduction surgery. Am J Respir Crit Care Med. 2011 Jun 30. [Epub ahead of print]

[25] M. M. DeCamp, R. J. McKenna, C. C. Deschamps, and M. J. Krasna, "Lung volume reduction surgery: technique, operative mortality, and morbidity," Proceedings of the American Thoracic Society, vol. 5, no. 4, pp. 442–446, 2008

[26] Ginsburg ME, Thomashow BM, Yip CK, DiMango AM, Maxfield RA, Bartels MN, Jellen P, Bulman WA, Lederer D, Brogan FL, Gorenstein LA, Sonett JR. Lung volume reduction surgery using the NETT selection criteria. Ann Thorac Surg. 2011 May;91(5):1556-60; discussion 1561. Epub 2011 Apr 2

[27] Boley TM, Reid A, Manning BT, Markwell SJ, Vassileva CM, Hazelrigg SR.Sternotomy or bilateral thoracospy: pain and post-operative complicationsafter lung-volume reduction surgery. Eur J Cardiothorac Surg. 2011 May 19. [Epub ahead of print]

[28] Imfeld S, Bloch KE, Weder W, Russi EW. The BODE index after lung volume reduction surgery correlates with survival. Chest 2006; 129:873.

[29] Weder W, Tutic M, Bloch KE. Lung volume reduction surgery in nonheterogeneous emphysema. Thorac Surg Clin. 2009 May;19(2):193-9.

[30] Donahue JM, Cassivi SD. Lung volume reduction surgery for patients with alpha-1 antitrypsin deficiency emphysema. Thorac Surg Clin. 2009 May;19(2):201-8.

[31] Washko GR, Hoffman E, Reilly JJ. Radiographic evaluation of the potential lung volume reduction surgery candidate. Proc Am Thorac Soc 2008; 5:421.

[32] DeCamp MM Jr, Lipson D, Krasna M, Minai OA, McKenna RJ Jr, Thomashow BM The evaluation and preparation of the patient for lung volume reduction surgery. Proc Am Thorac Soc. 2008 May 1;5(4):427-31

[33] Meyers BF, Sultan PK, Guthrie TJ, et al. Outcomes after unilateral lung volume reduction. Ann Thorac Surg 2008; 86:204.

[34] Gaissert HA, Trulock EP, Cooper JD, et al. Comparison of early functional results after volume reduction or lung transplantation for chronic obstructive pulmonary disease. J Thorac Cardiovasc Surg 1996; 111:296.

[35] OPTN/SRTR database annual report 2009

[36] Chest. 2007 Nov;132(5):1646-51

[37] Tutic M, Lardinois D, Imfeld S, et al. Lung-volume reduction surgery as an alternative or bridging procedure to lung transplantation. Ann Thorac Surg 2006; 82:208.

[38] Meyers BF, Yusen RD, Guthrie TJ, et al. Outcome of bilateral lung volume reduction in patients with emphysema potentially eligible for lung transplantation. J Thorac Cardiovasc Surg 2001; 122:10.

[39] Nathan SD, Edwards LB, Barnett SD, et al. Outcomes of COPD lung transplant recipients after lung volume reduction surgery. Chest 2004; 126:1569.

[40] E.P. Trulock, L.B. Edwards, D.O. Taylor, M.M. Boucek, B.M. Keck and M.I. Hertz et al., Registry of the International Society for Heart and Lung Transplantation: twenty-third official adult lung and heart-lung transplantation report—2006, J Heart Lung Transplant 25 (2006), pp. 880–892.

[41] Fitton, B.T. Bethea, M.C. Borja, D.D. Yuh, S.C. Yang and J.B. Orens et al., Pulmonary resection following lung transplantation, Ann Thorac Surg 76 (2003), pp. 1680–1685.

[42] Reece TB, Mitchell JD, Zamora MR, Fullerton DA, Cleveland JC, Pomerantz M, Lyu DM, Grover FL, Weyant MJ. Native lung volume reduction surgery relieves functional graft compression after single-lung transplantation for chronic obstructive pulmonary disease. J Thorac Cardiovasc Surg. 2008 Apr;135(4):931-7.

[43] Crespo MM, Johnson BA, McCurry KR, Landreneau RJ, Sciurba FC. Use of endobronchial valves for native lung hyperinflation associated with respiratory

failure in a single-lung transplant recipient for emphysema. Chest. 2007 Jan;131(1):214-6.

[44] I. Y. P. Wan, T. P. Toma, D. M. Geddes et al., "Bronchoscopic lung volume reduction for end-stage emphysema: report on the first 98 patients," Chest, vol. 129, no. 3, pp. 518-526, 2006.

[45] F. C. Sciurba, A. Ernst, F. J.F. Herth et al., "A randomized study of endobronchial valves for advanced emphysema," The New England Journal of Medicine, vol. 363, no. 13, pp. 1233-1244, 2010.

[46] S. C. Springmeyer, C. T. Bolliger, T. K. Waddell, X. Gonzalez, and D. E. Wood, "Treatment of heterogeneous emphysema using the spiration IBV valves," Thoracic Surgery Clinics, vol. 19, no. 2, pp. 247-253, 2009.

[47] J. M. Travaline, R. J. McKenna, T. De Giacomo et al., "Treatment of persistent pulmonary air leaks using endobronchial valves," Chest, vol. 136, no. 2, pp. 355-360, 2009.

[48] E. J. Cetti, A. J. Moore, and D. M. Geddes, "Collateral ventilation," Thorax, vol. 61, no. 5, pp. 371-373, 2006.

[49] Berger RL, Decamp MM, Criner GJ, Celli BR Lung volume reduction therapies for advanced emphysema: an update. Chest. 2010 Aug;138(2):407-17.

[50] F. J. Herth, R. Eberhard, D. Gompelmann, D. -J. Slebos, and A. Ernst, "Bronchoscopic lung volume reduction with a dedicated coil: a clinical pilot study," Therapeutic Advances in Respiratory Disease, vol. 4, no. 4, pp. 225-231, 2010.

[51] Ramsey SD, Berry K, Etzioni R, et al. Cost effectiveness of lung-volume-reduction surgery for patients with severe emphysema. N Engl J Med 2003; 348:2092.

[52] Miller JD, Malthaner RA, Goldsmith CH, et al. A randomized clinical trial of lung volume reduction surgery versus best medical care for patients with advanced emphysema: a two-year study from Canada. Ann Thorac Surg 2006; 81:314.

[53] Ramsey SD, Shroyer AL, Sullivan SD, Wood DE. Updated evaluation of the cost-effectiveness of lung volume reduction surgery. Chest 2007; 131:823.

5

Role of Thoracomyoplasty Procedures in Modern Surgery for Intrathoracic Suppurations

Petre Vlah-Horea Botianu and Alexandru Mihail Botianu
Surgical Clinic 4, University of Medicine and Pharmacy from Targu-Mures,
Romania

1. Introduction

Both thoracoplasty and muscle transposition are rarely performed procedures in modern thoracic surgery (Deslauriers et al., 2002). Their importance comes from the fact that these procedures are usually indicated in desperate cases, with failed medical treatments and who cannot be cured through standard procedures such as resection or decortication. For these patients, thoracomyoplasty operations are often the last chance for cure and sometimes even life-saving procedures (Botianu et al., 2010a).

2. Modern indications of thoracomyoplasty procedures

In our days, most of the intrathoracic suppurations can be managed without surgery, through antibiotics and minor procedures such as thoracocenthesis or tube-thoracostomy (Davies et al., 2011). Overall, about 10-15% of patients with intrathoracic suppurations still require some form of major surgical treatment. Out of them, most can be managed through less invasive and mutilating procedures (Pardos-Gea et al., 2011, Zahid et al., 2011), which make thoracomyoplasty a quite rarely indicated procedure:

- for pleural empyema: in cases not amenable to decortication – usually chronic cases with no cleavage plane and subjacent lesions in the parenchyma limiting the re-expansion of the lung;
- for pulmonary lesions (abscesses, tuberculosis, aspergilloma etc.): in cases not amenable to lung resection – usually a combination of poor biological and cardio-pulmonary status (including pulmonary hypertension), contralateral disease, fixed and adherent lesions with major technical difficulties.

Tuberculosis (TB) requires a special attention. Although TB infection by itself is not an indication for such procedures, many cases with chronic disease present with features making them candidates for thoracomyoplasty procedures. In our experience, almost half of the patients requiring thoracomyoplasty operations had different forms of TB lesions (Botianu P. et al., 2010a).

Bronchial fistula is frequently solved with the use of muscle flaps, alone or in combination with thoracoplasty. Simple closure by suturing through an inflamed tissue has very few chances of success, making reinforcement with a viable flap almost mandatory in most cases. In many cases, the muscle flaps are used as a plug to close the bronchial defect, without direct suture of the edges of the fistula (Hollaus et al., 1999, Zaheer et al., 2009).

Postoperative empyema is also an indication for thoracomyoplasty procedures in selected cases (Garcia-Yuste et al., 1998, Regnard et al., 2000). A particular technical aspect is that the previous thoracotomy reduces the availability of the neighbourhood flaps. The need to have some flaps available in case of postoperative complications is the main argument for the use of muscle-sparing thoracotomies (Nosotti et al., 2010).

Intrathoracic muscle transposition (without thoracoplasty) has also some other indications such as reinforcement of high-risk sutures (Abolhoda et al., 2009, Thingnam et al., 2011), repair of esophageal and tracheal defects (Kotzampassakis et al., 2009, Meyer et al., 2004), pericardial and diaphragmatic reconstruction (Kobayashi et al., 2009), dynamic cardiomyoplasty for end-stage heart failure (Chachques et al., 2008), salvage of infected vascular prosthesis (Mitra et al., 2005) etc.

3. Thoracoplasty

3.1 Historical background

The term "thoracoplasty" was introduced by Estlander (1879) who performed resection of multiple fragments of ribs ("resectio costorum multiplex") to achieve obliteration of an underlying empyema (Estlander, 1879). The operation became popular mainly as a method of lung collapse to achieve healing of tuberculosis before the introduction of modern TB chemotherapy. In fact, thoracoplasty procedures dominated chest surgery before the 1950's and played an essential role in the development of thoracic surgery as a distinct specialty. After 1950-60's, the interest for this procedure decreased due to the introduction of medical treatment (antibiotics and specific TB drugs) and development of other less mutilating and more effective surgical procedures (Deslauriers et al., 2002, Horrigan & Snow, 1990).

3.2 Terminology

Thoracoplasty is a procedure that targets the resolution of a cavity (pleural or pulmonary) by collapsing the chest wall through rib resection and/or plombage; according to the way this collapse is achieved, there are different terms which are used to describe the procedure:

- **in one or more stages** – according to the number of operative steps used. In the past many authors preferred to perform the thoracoplasty in more steps, with resection of 2-3 ribs in each step, in order to lower the magnitude of the operative aggression and to reduce mortality (Alexander 1936). This was a reasonable attitude in the early years of thoracic surgery, when a lot of things that are today standard were not available (general anesthesia, oro-tracheal intubation, blood transfusion, antibiotics, electrocautery etc). Besides the need for more procedures, a specific disadvantage is the cavity movement phenomenon, in which the cavity just moves in one direction without any resolution; at the end, the patient will have some ribs resected and the same cavity in another position (Archibald 1926). In our days, most of these procedures are done in a single step.

- **extra-pleural or intra-pleural** – according to the intact preservation or opening of the parietal pleural. In the past, opening of the pleural space during thoracoplasty was considered as a major accident (fear for wound contamination, pneumothorax etc.) (Archibald 1926). In our days, in most cases the pleura is opened deliberately to achieve a direct access to the pleural and/or pulmonary lesion.

- **sub-periostal or extra-periostal** – according to the plane used for rib resection, with or without preservation of the periosteum. In our days, in most cases the ribs are resected using a subperiostal plane. Leaving the periosteum intact allows some form of bone regeneration which helps the long-time stabilization of the chest wall (Alexander 1936).

Many authors use the term "classic" thoracoplasty, with different meanings depending on time and geographical location. For example, in Europe, in the 1910-20's, "classic" thoracoplasty referred to the procedures described by Estlander and Schede, which were then replaced by the procedures described by Andre Maurer and Sauerbruch; the later became also "classic" for the American surgeons who trained in Europe. In the USA, after 1930, the technique described by Alexander became the standard thoracoplasty performed for lung collapse in order to heal lung TB. In the 1950's, the osteoplastic techniques and plombage with different materials became popular, being then almost abandoned.

In our days, most thoracoplasties are done in a single operative step, intrapleural and using a subperiosteal plane for rib resection (Hopkins et al., 1985).

3.3 Main types of thoracoplasty

Over the time, more than 100 thoracoplasty procedures were described, many of them being in fact minor modifications or combinations of previously described techniques; such a big number of techniques is by itself an indication for the dificulties encountered in this kind of surgery. We present a brief description of the most important techniques, all of them being very popular at a certain moment of the development of thoracic surgery.

The Schede thoracoplasty is a very "radical" procedure developed for empyema and involving the resection of ribs, intercostal spaces and parietal pleura overlying the empyema cavity. The wound was left opened and the visceral pleura from the empyema cavity was placed in direct contact with healthy tissues represented by extracostal chest wall muscles and subcutaneous tissue (Schede 1890). For small empyema cavities it may be a reasonable procedure but for big cavities the procedure is a very mutilant one. With different modifications, it is still used today for highly selected cases of empyema (Stobernack et al., 1997, Botianu 2005, 2008).

The Sauerbruch thoracoplasty (paravertebral) was indicated for empyema cavities that extended more in the vertical axis than in the horizontal one and involved a 4-6 cm length resection of the posterior part of the ribs. The main disadvantages were the risk of respiratory failure due to the paradoxical movements of the chest wall and the secondary scoliosis.

The Andre Maurer thoracoplasty (descendant) involves complete excision of the first 2 ribs and partial removal of the ribs 3-5, leaving intact only the anterior part of them; it was performed extrapleurally, in one or more steps according to the patient's biological status.

The Alexander thoracoplasty was designed for treatment of lung TB and involved a subperiosteal and extrapleural removal of the first 8-9 ribs; for a better collapse the removal of the first rib and the transverse vertebral apophyses was considered to be mandatory. For a better tolerance of the procedure, it was performed in 3 steps at 3 weeks intervals. With this strategy and a good selection of the patients, Alexander achieved an important improvement of the results, with a 10% mortality and 90% rate of healing in survivors (Alexander 1936).

The Archibald thoracoplasty involved resection of the first 3 ribs and introduction of the pectoral muscles in the extrapleural space to maintain the collapse of the lung; a particular aspect is the ingenious separate mobilization of the two flaps: the pectoralis major was mobilized based on the branches from the internal mammary vessels and the pectoralis minor was mobilized based on the thoraco-acromial pedicle (Entin 1995).

Extrapleural plombage (plombage thoracoplasty) achieves lung collapse with the use of different materials that are introduced inside the chest using an extrafascial or extraperiosteal plane (fig. 1). The main advantages of the plombage thoracoplasties are the absence of chest wall mutilation and the fact that the procedure is easy, quick and well-tolerated, even by patients with poor biological status; the procedure was quite popular in the 1950-60's, with immediate good results (Wilson et al., 1956). The main disadvantage is the high risk of complications related to the introduction inside the chest of a foreign material, including overinfection, migration and erosion of major vessels, which may frequently require the removal of the plombage material (Massard et al., 1997).

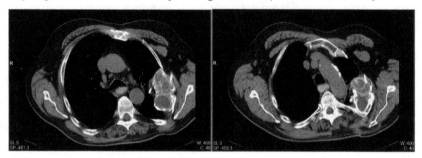

Fig. 1. CT aspect of an 81 years-old patient who underwent a plombage thoracoplasty 46 years ago for left upper lobe tuberculosis. The patient presented no TB recurrence and no chest complaints.

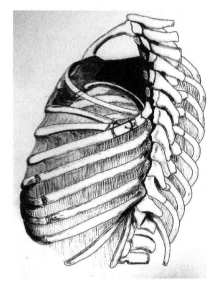

Fig. 2. Osteoplastic thoracoplasty developed by Naftali (1964) for apical TB lesions. Note the rib grafts placed in a paramediastinal position which induce also a transversal collapse.

The osteoplastic thoracoplasty was popularized by Holst and Björk in the 1950's and aimed to create a new roof for the chest cavity. The posterior parts of the upper ribs were resected in a growing length, from superior towards inferior and their new posterior ends were sutured to the first rib that was left intact. This resulted in a smaller thoracic cage with a stable wall that prevented the reexpansion of the lung above the new roof (Holst 1952, Bjork 1954, Krasnov et al., 1989). Besides lung TB, these procedures were also frequently performed for the prophylaxis or treatment of pleural space problems after upper lobectomies. In our unit, Naftali Zoltan has developed and used in the 1960's an original technique of osteoplastic thoracoplasty (fig. 2) which involved also the use of rib grafts placed in a paramediastinal position, achieving a collapse not only in the vertical plane, but also in the transversal one – from medial towards lateral (Naftali, 1964).

Apycolisis was introduced by Semb (1937) and involved the division of the adhesions between the pleural dome at the apex and the soft tissues from the base of the neck. This manoeuver, which was used by many surgeons during thoracoplasties for apical TB lesions, allowed a more complete collapse of the lung apex.

Resection of the first rib was mandatory in many of the classic thoracoplasties, being considered the key to achieve an adequate collapse in the vertical plane. However, it's resection is associated with severe adverse effects such as scoliosis, asymmetry and functional impairment of the shoulder and upper extremity. For these reasons, we believe that it's preservation is nowadays manatory; if there is a space below the first rib it can be easily filled with local flaps (Botianu P. et al., 2010a, c, Deslauriers et al., 2002).

3.4 Modern thoracoplasty – The Andrews procedure and it's modifications

In our time, thoracoplasty is almost always performed for pleural or pleuro-pulmonary cavities, with opening of the pleura and subperiostal rib resection. Most surgeons use the Andrews thoracoplasty, with or without various modifications (Cornet et al., 1965, Icard et al., 1999). The technique was first described as a solution for postpneumonectomy empyema / thoracomediastinal plication (Andrews 1961) and then used for other types of empyema (Andrews 1965).

The original technique involved:
- thoracotomy;
- subperiostal rib resection, limited to the portion of the chest wall located above the empyema cavity;
- wide opening of the suppurated pleural cavity with careful removal of the pus and detrituses;
- closure of the bronchial fistula (if present);
- removal of the parietal pleura;
- obliteration of the cavity by fixation of the remaining periosto-intercostal plane to the visceral/mediastinal pleura; this is achieved by mattressing using separate "U" stitches;
- drainage of the subscapulary space and closure of the wound.

The main original idea of this technique was to open the infected pleural cavity, clean it and obliterate it, with primary wound closure.

In our unit, we have tried to improve the results of the Andrews thoracoplasty by several modifications which resulted in a personal procedure (Botianu A.M., 1996 - licence no. 100297/1989/RO) which was used with good results in the last 25 years. The main steps of the procedure are:

- postero-lateral incision and opening of the empyema cavity (fig. 3a);
- wide debridement and toilet of the cavity; if bronchial fistulas are present, they are temporary closed using small gauzes to avoid bronchial inundation.
- subperiosteal removal of ribs overlying the empyema cavity (fig. 3b);
- the remaining chest wall (consisting of parietal pleura, periosteum and intercostal spaces) is sectioned using several cranio-caudal and transversal incisions, which are placed according to how we plan to use the resulting intercostal flaps. The transversal incisions are made through the bed of the resected ribs to avoid damage to the intercostal vessels. The parietal pleura is carefully cleaned but without attempting a complete excision. The resulting pleuro-periosto-intercostal flaps must remain well vascularised and are used for:
    - closure-reinforcement of the bronchial fistulas, using always atraumatic needles and late resorbable suture materials;
    - plombage of the cul-de-sacs and dead angles (such as below the first rib or paravertebral), diminishing the extent of the rib resection;
    - plombage of intrapulmonary cavities (fig. 3c);

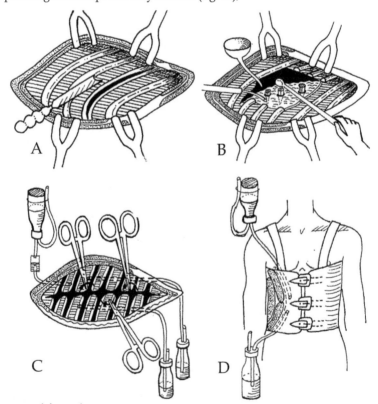

Fig. 3. Main steps of the thoracopleuroplasty procedure used in Surgical Clinic 4, University of Medicine and Pharmacy from Targu-Mures, Romania (Botianu A.M., 1996 /licence no. 100297/1989/RO).

- installation of a closed-circuit irrigation-aspiration system which consists of 1-2 usual drains which are placed in a declive position and are connected to a standard chest drainage system and a separate smaller drain placed in the upper part of the cavity and connected to a standard perfusion set (fig. 3d). This system allows postoperative elimination of pus and secretions, as well as lavages with different antibiotic and antiseptic solutions; in case of postoperative bleeding, local hemostatics may also be introduced in the cavity. Before having CT and US highly available, we also used this system to introduce contrast inside the chest to follow the resolution of the lesion.
- we have completely abandoned the matressing described by Andrews by suturing with "U" stitches the remaining chest wall to the visceral or mediastinal pleura. We consider that this manoeuver is not only time-consuming but has several disadvantages such as the danger to damage the underlying lung or mediastinal structures, ischemia of the remaining pleuro-periosto-intercostal plane and an overall fixation of the chest wall in a non-physiologic position.
- suturing of the remaining planes (skin, subcutaneous fat and chest wall muscles) in a single layer with separate stitches;

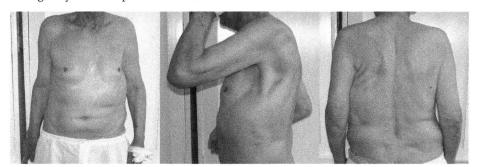

Fig. 4. Postoperative aspect at 10 years after a thoracomediastinal plication for a left post-pneumonectomy empyema, performed according to the technique described previously. The cosmetic result is acceptable, with no soliosis and no major chest difformity.

- temporary fixation of the chest wall using compressive bandage and an external contention (fig. 3d); this allows a definitive fixation of the new chest wall in a more natural position, after the cavity is obliterated and the patient starts to breathe normally (fig. 4).

4. Intrathoracic muscle transposition

4.1 Historical background

The idea to bring muscle flaps inside the chest is not a new one, as it was described at the beginning of the 20th century by surgeons like Abrashanoff (1911), Robinson (1915) or Archibald (1921). However, these techniques did not become very popular, mainly due to the fear of infection (large dissections without the possibility to use antibiotics) and absence of precise anatomical knowledge (Arnold & Pairolero, 1989).

In the 1960-70's, plastic and reconstructive surgeons developed the techniques for extensive mobilization of muscle and musculo-cutaneous flaps, based on precise anatomic knowledge.

The use of muscle flaps in thoracic surgery was popularized in the 1990's mainly through the work of the Mayo Rochester team of surgeons, with an excellent cooperation between thoracic and plastic surgeons (Arnold & Pairolero, 1989, Pairolero et al., 1990).

4.2 Basic principles

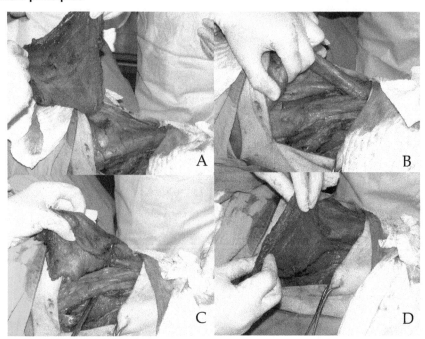

Fig. 5. Intrathoracic transposition of a latissimus dorsi flap. A: The flap raised from the chest wall with preservation of the thoraco-dorsal vessels B: Aspect of the small opening ("second thoracotomy") C: introduction of the flap inside the chest D: final aspect of the flap after intrathoracic transposition.

The basic idea is that muscle flaps bring a well vascularized tissue able to fight actively against infection and promote angiogenesis and healing. These characteristics were proven by the experience of plastic and reconstructive surgeons, who have used them with good results in a great variety of defects – including chronic infections, traumatic lesions or irradiated wounds (Mathes et al., 1977). In order to maintain the aforementioned qualities, the entire muscle flap should remain viable at the end of the procedure and in the postoperative period. A correct mobilization requires precise anatomic knowledge about vascularization and cleavage planes and an accurate dissection with preservation of the vascular pedicles - both arterial and venous (Mathes & Nahai, 1979). As a general rule, in most cases of intrathoracic transposition the flaps do not require such an extensive mobilization as it is needed in plastic surgery procedures.

The surgeon who performs intrathoracic muscle transposition must be familiar with the anatomy of the local flaps, in terms of cleavage planes, relationships with other structures and blood supply, as well as with the dimensions of the flap and its limits of mobilization.

Most muscles have several vascular sources, not all of them allowing a complete mobilization of the flap. Anatomical variations may also play an important role. The nutritive pedicle must be carefully prepared using a combination of blunt and sharp dissection, avoiding any damage since this is equivalent to the loss of the flap (McCraw & Arnold, 1987).

At the end of the mobilization, the viability of the entire flap must be carefully evaluated. In case of ischemic changes, the affected portion of the flap must be resected; from our experience, severe ischemia of extended portions of the flap is very rare if the mobilization is correctly performed. Any severe ischemia leads to flap necrosis with subsequent recurrence of the intrathoracic suppuration and failure of the surgical procedure.

Introduction of the flap inside the thorax requires usually a second window created through a limited rib resection (less than 10 cm length, no more than one rib). When introducing the flap inside the chest, care must be taken to avoid any compression, kinking or twisting of the vascular pedicle in order to avoid thrombosis and loss of the flap. The muscle must reach the defect without any tension and without torsion. Haemostasis must be carefully checked, since postoperative bleeding from the flap will lead to hemothorax. The wound is usually closed, with separate chest and subcutaneous drainage to avoid the postoperative development of seroma in the space resulted from muscle flap dissection (fig. 5).

Mobilization of any flap and it's transposition in a different position involves a certain degree of functional morbidity. For most of the flaps used for intrathoracic transposition, these functional sequelae are minor, since there are some other muscles with synergic action that compensate their absence. When put in balance, these functional sequelae are minor compared to the gravity of the situation of the patients that require thoracomyoplasty procedures. However, these aspects must be discussed with the patient before the procedure and a signed informed consent should be obtained (Pairolero & Arnold, 1989, Arnold & Pairolero, 1989).

4.3 Surgical anatomy and techniques of mobilization of the most important flaps

The techniques of muscle flap mobilization were described in detail by the plastic surgeons (Mathes & Nahai, 1979, McCraw & Arnold, 1987), and are based on very precise anatomical knowledges concerning the blood supply (Mathes & Nahai, 1981).

The latissimus dorsi flap is probably the most used flap in thoracic surgery. It may be prepared using a skin incision running parallel with the anterior border of the muscle or through a standard postero-lateral skin incision. The standard latissimus dorsi flap involves detachment of the muscle from the iliac crest and sacrum and mobilization from the chest wall keeping intact the main blood supply represented by the thoraco-dorsal vessels, which run parallel with the anterior margin on the deep side of the muscle. If necessary, the insertion tendon and the vascular branch for the serratus anterior may be sectioned in order to increase the length. The flap is quite easy to prepare since there are distinct cleavage planes and the nutrient blood vessels are large enough and with very few anatomical variants; it has a large volume and a long arch of rotation, which allows it to reach almost every part of the thorax (Abolhoda et al., 2008, Seify et al., 2007).

The reversed latissimus dorsi flap is much rarely used. It involves sectioning of the flap in the upper part and mobilization based on the secondary blood supply represented by some perforator branches from the last intercostal and first lumbar vessels; these branches are small and have an extremely variable anatomy, which make this mobilization more limited and difficult compared to the standard one. However, it may be used with good results in certain circumstances, the main indication being repair or filling of defects located in the supradiaphragmatic area (Botianu P et al., 2010b).

Due to the synergic activity of other muscles, mobilization of the latissimus dorsi is not associated with serious functional impairment, having no impact on daily activities.

The serratus anterior flap has two main sources of blood supply: the thoracic lateral artery (originating from the axillary artery) and a branch originating from the thoraco-dorsal artery. Since the two vessels have an almost parallel traject, we prefer to preserve both of them if the entire muscle is mobilized; the veins run parallel to the arteries, draining in the axillary vein. The muscle can be easily dissected from the surrounding structures and detached from the chest wall and the scapula. It reaches easily the hilum and is excellent for defects located in the upper half of the thorax. Another advantage is that almost the entire muscle remains intact after the standard postero-lateral thoracotomy, making it suitable for postoperative complications. A specific complication described in the literature is the winged scapula ("scapula allata"), which is very unpleasant for the patient and difficult to treat (Arnold et al., 1984). If several prophylactic measures are taken, this complication is very rare. In our personal experience with over 70 serratus anterior flaps, we had no case of true winged scapula, only some cases of minor asymmetry (Botianu P et al., 2010c).

If necessary, the serratus anterior and the latissimus dorsi can be mobilized together using the common thoraco-dorsal vascular pedicle.

The pectoralis flap may also be mobilized in more ways. The most used is the mobilization of the pectoralis major, with or without the pectoralis minor muscle, by detachment from the chest wall and subcutis using the thoracoacromial vessels for blood supply. For an increased mobilization, it is necessary to section the insertion tendon on the humerus. Another common way of mobilization is based on the perforator branches that arise from the internal thoracic and anterior intercostal vessels in the parasternal region. The pectoralis flap is usefull for defects located in the apical region (Kalweit et al., 1994, Nomori et al., 2001), although it's mobilization is difficult through a standard thoracotomy incision; it is also frequently used to prevent and treat infectious complications after median sternotomy (Gao et al., 2010).

The rectus abdominis flap can be mobilized based on the superior epigastric vessels, which continue the internal thoracic ones. The second pedicle, represented by the inferior epigastric vessels, can also support the entire flap but does not allow it's mobilization inside the chest and therefore cannot be used for intrathoracic transposition. Usually, a paramedian vertical incision is made in the abdominal wall and the anterior rectus sheath is opened, allowing exposure of the muscle. The rectus abdominis is raised from the posterior sheath and the inferior epigastric vessels are ligated. A special care must be taken when the flap is turned towards the chest in order to avoid damaging of the vascular pedicle. Specific complications for this flap are represented by the abdominal wall problems, with the risk of developing an incisional hernia. It is preferred by some authors for the treatment of sterno-mediastinal infections following sternotomy (Oh et al., 2004) but it is also usefull for different infections located in the inferior part of the thorax (Ojika et al., 1995).

Intercostal flaps are very easy to prepare during thoracomyoplasty procedures (Sarkar et al., 1985). These flaps usually contain the intercostal spaces (including the muscles), the parietal pleura and the periosteum remaining after the rib resection. The arterial blood supply is represented by the posterior intercostal arteries arising from the thoracic aorta and the anterior intercostal arteries arising from the internal thoracic artery; the veins have a parallel traject and drain into the azygos veins, respectively the internal thoracic veins. There is a very rich network connecting the anterior and the posterior intercostal vessels, as well as the vessels from adjacent intercostal spaces and neighbourhood muscles. According to the location of the defect, both the anterior and the posterior intercostal vessels may be used as blood supply for the flaps. When creating the intercostal flaps, the incision should be always made through the bed of the resected ribs in order to minimize the risk of damaging the main intercostal vessels. We found these intercostal flaps particularly usefull for bronchial fistula closure and filling of some dead angles and cul-de-sacs (Botianu P et al., 2010a, c).

The omentum flap – although it is not a muscle, it should be included here since it is preferred in many instances with the same purposes and principles as the muscle flaps (Petrov et al., 1999). The main vessels are represented by the left gastro-epiploic artery (originating from the splenic artery) and the right gastro-epiploic artery (originating from the gastro-duodenal artery). These two arteries create the gastro-epiploic arcade which runs along the great curvature of the stomach and gives small branches for the stomach and the so-called epiploic arteries for the omentum. The veins run parallel with the arteries, creating similar arcades. These epiploic vessels have a descendant traject and form a second arcade along the inferior edge of the omentum (Barkow's arcade). There are many ways to mobilize the omentum based on the vessels and arcades described. However, the anatomy of the omental vascularization is extremely variable and it should be carefully evaluated before planning the flap and making any incision (Kirikuta, 1980). Specific complications are related to the risk of incisional hernia and development of adhesions with intestinal obstruction. The omentum flap is preferred by some authors for sterno-mediastinal infections (Hountis et al., 2009), closure of large bronchial fistulas - especially after pneumonectomy (Chichevatov & Gorshenev, 2005) and reinforcement of high-risk sutures (D'Andrilli et al., 2009). Recent publications have shown good results with the laparoscopic mobilization, which makes the omental flap more attractive (van Wingerden et al., 2010).

Other rarely used flaps have been reported in case-reports or small series, with more or less good results: trapezius, subscapularis, infraspinatus, external oblique, teres major etc. Such flaps should be taken into consideration especially when other standard flaps are not available or have failed (Fuchs et al., 2010, Schreiner et al., 2010).

5. Thoracomyoplasty – combining thoracoplasty and muscle flaps

The idea of this kind of procedures is to combine thoracoplasty with intrathoracic muscle transposition in an attempt to achieve safe obliteration of the diseased intrathoracic space. Since for suppurated defects complete filling is mandatory for safe primary wound closure, combining thoracoplasty and muscle transposition acts as a compromise between:

- an extended thoracoplasty (rib resection) with major chest wall mutilation;
- the use of multiple muscle flaps, with added donor-site morbidity and postoperative functional deficits.

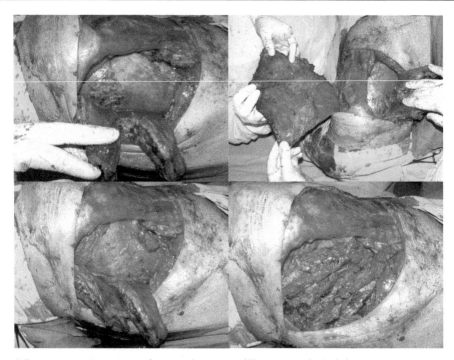

Fig. 6. Intraoperative aspects of a complex space-filling procedure / thoracomyoplasty: a limited 5-ribs thoracoplasty, transposition of the latissimus dorsi based on the thoracodorsal vessels and 2 intercostal flaps with posterior vascularization.

There is no standardized technique of thoracomyoplasty. Both rib resection and muscle transposition should be performed trying to reduce the chest wall mutilation and functional morbidity to minimum, but without compromising the definitive obliteration of the cavity (fig. 6).

The local anatomy should be carefully evaluated when planning the procedure:
- location and dimensions of the cavity, which can be easily assessed on preoperative CT scans;
- presence of bronchial fistula, whose safe closure is mandatory. The presence of a bronchial fistula may be suggested preoperatively by the clinical course; bronchoscopy and CT may detect some large and centrally located fistula but the exact position of the smaller ones can be evaluated only intraoperative.
- available flaps – in many cases, the neighbourhood muscles may be compromised by previous procedures; typical examples are postero-lateral thoracotomy which divides the latissimus dorsi, upper digestive surgery which compromises the omentum, subcostal laparotomy or myocardial revascularization with the internal mammary artery which compromise the rectus abdominis flap.

The terminology used for this kind of procedures is not very clear. The term "thoracoplasty" should be reserved for cases not associating any muscle flap mobilization. Some authors talk about myoplasty, muscle flaps or intrathoracic muscle transposition, which can quite rarely solve alone a large suppurated cavity without associating any rib resection. As well as other authors, we find the terms "thoracomyoplasty" and "complex space-filling procedures" are the most appropriate to describe this kind of procedures (Botianu P et al., 2010a, García-Yuste et al., 1998, Naumov et al., 1991, Riquet 2010).

6. Personal experience and results from the literature

During the last 8 years we have performed thoracomyoplasty procedures in 102 patients, with almost one half of them having different TB lesions. The procedure was adapted to the local anatomy of the lesion, with an average of 5 resected ribs/patient and 1.9 flaps/patient. Our recently published analysis of the first 76 patients showed an acceptable mortality (5%) and rate of recurrence requiring an open-window procedure (5%); other minor local complications included a few skin necrosis and persistent small thoracic fistulae solved under local anesthesia with no need for a major reoperation.

Postoperative hospitalization ranged between 4 and 180 days, with an average of 40 ± 5 days; all the patients with hospitalizations longer than 60 days presented recurrence of the infection requiring on open-window procedure. At the moment of discharge, all the patients had healed wounds with no need for any other surgical care. TB patients were referred to our pneumology colleagues to continue the specific chemotherapy.

Five patients presented a mild impairment of the shoulder function, but without interfering with the daily activities; 4 patients presented a minor asymmetry of the two shoulders and scapulas but we had no case of true winged scapula and no major functional disturbance secondary to the extrathoracic muscle flap mobilization. None of our patients presented severe scoliosis or a major chest deformity. At 3 months follow-up, 91% (66 patients) of the survivors returned to an almost normal life compared with their preoperative status.

A comparative evaluation showed no statistically significant difference between the pre- and post-operative values of the the functional respiratory tests (VC preoperative – mean 1050 ml/62% of predicted vs postoperative – mean 1100 ml/63% of predicted, FEV1 preoperative – mean 850 ml/61% of predicted vs postoperative - mean 890 ml/62% of predicted, Wilcoxon signed-rank test, $p>0.05$). The main explanation is that the parenchyma underlying the thoracomyoplasty is more or less diseased, therefore with a lower contribution to the respiration; also, closure of the bronchial fistula improves the respiratory function (Botianu P et al., 2010a).

Other authors have also recently published important series with quite similar results, with mortality, morbidity and hospitalization falling within an acceptable range of values. These data recommend the use of thoracomyoplasty procedures to solve difficult cases of intrathoracic suppurations (García-Yuste et al., 1998, Icard et al., 1999, Jadczuk 1998, Krassas et al., 2010, Regnard et al., 2000, Stefani et al., 2011).

7. Future challenges

During the recent years, a few new ideas emerged:
-   the use of free-transfers, which increases the number and volume of the flaps available for filling of the infected spaces (Walsh et al., 2011). However, they involve a multidisciplinary approach and complicated procedures; the microsurgical anastomoses of the vessels require experience and special technical skills, are time-consuming and involve a specific morbidity.

-   the use of less-invasive procedures for flap mobilization, using special retractors, light sources, instruments and dissection techniques borrowed from endoscopic surgery. Proponents consider that with the use of these techniques the mobilization of the muscle flaps may be performed using shorter skin incisions and less donor-site morbidity, making them more acceptable (Blidisel et al., 2008).

A major problem is the difficulty to study these procedures according to the modern principles of evidenced-based medicine. These procedures are rarely performed and address to a small number of desperate cases, not comparable to those submitted to the standard treatment consisting of lung resection and/or pleural decortication. The rarity of these procedures and the great heterogenicity of the patients (in terms of local anatomy, etiology and biological status) makes any kind of randomised trial or fair comparison impossible (Botianu P. et al., 2010a, b).

The most important challenge remains probably training, since many surgeons are not familiar with the techniques of thoracoplasty or muscle flaps mobilization; most young surgeons have neither performed, nor seen such procedures. Specific training and/or a good cooperation with a plastic and reconstructive surgery colleague is mandatory.

8. Conclusions

Both thoracoplasty and muscle transposition remain in the armamentarium of modern thoracic surgery (Riquet 2010). Due to the recrudescence of TB and other infectious diseases of the chest, it is possible that the number of patients requiring this kind of surgery will increase in the near future. We believe that sooner or later any thoracic surgeon will meet a patient requiring such a procedure. Thoracomyoplasty may solve a complicated case with good immediate and long-term outcome. In such situations, training, careful evaluation and an accurate surgical technique are essential to achieve good results (Botianu P. et al., 2010a, Krassas et al., 2010, Stefani et al., 2011).

9. References

Abolhoda A,; Bui T.D.; Milliken J.C. & Wirth G.A. (2009) *Pedicled latissimus dorsi muscle flap: routine use in high-risk thoracic surgery,* Tex Heart Inst J; 36(4):298-302

Abolhoda A.; Wirth G.A.; Bui T.D. & Milliken J.C. (2008) *Harvest technique for pedicled transposition of latissimus dorsi muscle: an old trade revisited,* Eur J Cardiothorac Surg; 33(5):928-30

Abrashanoff G. (1911) *Plastische Methode der Schliessung von Fistelgangen, welche von inneren Organen kommen,* Zentralbl Chir; 38:186-7

Alexander J. (1936) *Some advances in the technic of thoracoplasty,* Ann Surg; 104(4):545-51

Andrews NC. (1961) *Thoracomediastinal plication: a surgical technique for chronic empyema,* J Thorac Cardiovasc Surg; 41:809-16

Andrews NC. (1965) *The surgical treatment of chronic empyema,* Dis Chest; 47:533-8

Archibald E. (1926) *On extra-pleural thoracoplasty,* Can Med Assoc J;16(4)433-5

Arnold P.G. & Pairolero P.C. (1989) *Intrathoracic muscle flaps: a 10-year experience in the management of life-threatening infections,* Plast Reconstr Surg; 84(1):92-8

Arnold P.G.; Pairolero P.C. & Waldorf J.C. (1984) *The serratus anterior muscle: intrathoracic and extrathoracic utilization,* Plast Reconstr Surg; 73(2):240-8

Bjork V.O. (1954) *Thoracoplasty, a new osteo plastic technique,* J Thorac Surg; 28(2):194-211

Blidisel A.; Maciuceanu B.; Jiga L.; Papurica M. & Ionac M. (2008) *Endoscopy-assisted harvesting and free latissimus dorsi muscle flap transfer in reconstructive microsurgery*, Chirurgia (Bucur); 103(1):67-72

Botianu A.M. (1996) *Procedeu de toracopleuroplastie pentru tratamentul chirurgical al empiemului toracic cu sau fara fistula bronsica/Personal procedure of thoracopleuroplasty for the treatment of the thoracic empyema, with or without bronchial fistula*, Jurnalul de Chirurgie toracică/Journal of Thoracic Surgery; 1:3:251-260

Botianu P. V.-H. (2005) *Re-evaluation of the Schede thoracoplasty*, Jurnalul de Chirurgie Toracica - Journal of Thoracic Surgery; 7(1):71-78

Botianu P.V.-H.; Butiurca A.; Dobrica A.; Damian V.; Ionica S.; Lupu C. & Stoica S. (2008) *Schede procedure and muscular plombage for a multirelapsed TB empyema with pleuro-cutaneous fistula*, Revista de Medicina şi Farmacie-Orvosi es Gyogyszereszeti Szemle (Acta Medica Marisiensis); 54(S3): 69-72

Botianu P.V.-H.; Botianu A.M.; Bacarea V. & Dobrica A.C. (2010) *Thoracodorsal versus reversed mobilisation of the latissimus dorsi muscle for intrathoracic transposition*, Eur J Cardiothorac Surg; 38(4):461-5

Botianu P.V.-H.; Botianu A.M.; Dobrica A.C. & Bacarea V. (2010) *Intrathoracic transposition of the serratus anterior muscle flap--personal experience with 65 consecutive patients*, Eur J Cardiothorac Surg; 38(6):669-73

Botianu P.V.-H.; Dobrica A.C.; Butiurca A. & Botianu A.M. (2010) *Complex space-filling procedures for intrathoracic infections - personal experience with 76 consecutive cases*, Eur J Cardiothorac Surg; 37(2):478-81

Chachques J.C.; Jegaden O.J.; Bors V.; Mesana T.; Latremouille C.; Grandjean P.A.; Fabiani J.N. & Carpentier A. (2008) *Heart transplantation following cardiomyoplasty: a biological bridge*, Eur J Cardiothorac Surg; 33(4):685-90

Chichevatov D. & Gorshenev A. (2005) *Omentoplasty in treatment of early bronchopleural fistulas after pneumonectomy*, Asian Cardiovasc Thorac Ann; 13(3):211-6

Cornet E.; Dupon H.; Coiffard P. & Rembeaux A. (1965) *Thoracopleuroplasties for empyema according to Andrews' method (18 cases)*, Ann Chir Thorac Cardiovasc; 4(4):509-15

D'Andrilli A.; Ibrahim M.; Andreetti C.; Ciccone A.M.; Venuta F. & Rendina E.A. (2009) *Transdiaphragmatic harvesting of the omentum through thoracotomy for bronchial stump reinforcement*, Ann Thorac Surg; 88(1):212-5

Davies H.E.; Rosenstengel A. & Lee Y.G. (2011) *The diminishing role of surgery in pleural disease*, Curr Opin Pulm; 17(4):247-54

Deslauriers J.; Jacques L.F. & Grégoire J. (2002) *Role of Eloesser flap and thoracoplasty in the third millennium*, Chest Surg Clin N Am; 12(3):605-23

Entin MA. (1995) *Romance and tragedy of tuberculosis: Edward Archibald's contribution to the surgical treatment of pulmonary tuberculosis*, The Canadian Journal of Plastic Surgery; 3(4):213-6

Estlander J.A. (1879) *Résection des côtes dans l'empyème chronique*, Rev Med Chir (Paris); 3:157-70

Fuchs P.; Schreiner W.; Wolter T.P.; Autschbach R.; Sirbu H. & Pallua N. (2011) *A four-muscle-flap for thoracomyoplasty in patients with sacrificed thoracodorsal vessels*, J Plast Reconstr Aesthet Surg; 64(3):335-8

Gao J.; Wang Y.L.; Lu S.Q.; Cai A.B., Yang Z.F., Han Z.Y., Li J.J., Wen Y.M., Geng F.Y. & Wang W.Z. (2010) *Management of sternal osteomyelitis and mediastinal infection following median sternotomy*, Chin Med J (Engl); 123(20):2803-6

García-Yuste M.; Ramos G.; Duque J.L.; Heras F.; Castanedo M.; Cerezal L.J. & Matilla J.M. (1998) *Open-window thoracostomy and thoracomyoplasty to manage chronic pleural empyema,* Ann Thorac Surg; 65(3):818-22

Hollaus P.H.; Huber M.; Lax F.; Wurnig P.N.; Böhm G. & Pridun N.S. (1999) *Closure of bronchopleural fistula after pneumonectomy with a pedicled intercostal muscle flap,* Eur J Cardiothorac Surg; 16(2):181-6

Holst J. (1952) *Technique of so-called dome thoracoplasty; preliminary report,* Nord Med; 19:48(38):1290-3

Hopkins R.A.; Ungerleider R.M.; Staub E.W. & Young W.G. Jr. (1985) *The modern use of thoracoplasty,* Ann Thorac Surg; 40(2):181-7

Horrigan T.P. & Snow N.J. (1990) *Thoracoplasty: current application to the infected pleural space,* Ann Thorac Surg; 50(5):695-9

Hountis P.; Dedeilias P. & Bolos K. (2009) *The role of omental transposition for the management of postoperative mediastinitis: a case series,* Cases J; 23;2(1):142

Icard P.; Le Rochais J.P.; Rabut B.; Cazaban S.; Martel B. & Evrard C. (1999) *Andrews thoracoplasty as a treatment of post-pneumonectomy empyema: experience in 23 cases,* Ann Thorac Surg; 68(4):1159-63

Jadczuk E. (1998) *Posptneumonectomy empyema,* Eur J Cardiothorac Surg; 14(2):123-6

Kalweit G.; Feindt P.; Huwer H.; Volkmer I. & Gams E. (1994) *The pectoral muscle flaps in the treatment of bronchial stump fistula following pneumonectomy,* Eur J Cardiothorac Surg; 8(7):358-62

Kirikuta I. (1980) *Use of the omentum in plastic surgery,* Ed. Medicala/Medical Publishing House, Bucuresti

Kobayashi H.; Nomori H.; Mori T.; Shibata H.; Yoshimoto K. & Ohba Y. (2009) *Extrapleural pneumonectomy with reconstruction of diaphragm and pericardium using autologous materials,* Ann Thorac Surg 2009; 87(5):1630-2

Kotzampassakis N.; Christodoulou M.; Krueger T.; Demartines N.; Vuillemier H.; Cheng C.; Dorta G. & Ris H.B. (2009) *Esophageal leaks repaired by a muscle onlay approach in the presence of mediastinal sepsis,* Ann Thorac Surg; 88(3):966-72

Krasnov V.A.; Kozhevnikov N.N.; Gorbunov G.M. & Andrenko A.A. (1989) *Long-term results of the use of osteoplastic thoracoplasty in the treatment of destructive tuberculosis of the lungs in patients with antisocial behavior,* Probl Tuberk; (1):41-4

Krassas A.; Grima R.; Bagan P.; Badia A.; Arame A.; Barthes F.P. & Riquet M. (2010) *Current indications and results for thoracoplasty and intrathoracic muscle transposition,* Eur J Cardiothorac Surg; 37(5):1215-20

Massard G.; Thomas P.; Barsotti P.; Riera P.; Giudicelli R.; Reboud E.; Morand G.; Fuentes P.A. & Wihlm J.M. (1997) *Long-term complications of extraperiosteal plombage,* Ann Thorac Surg; 64(1):220-4

Mathes S.J. & Nahai F. (1981) *Classification of the vascular anatomy of muscles: experimental and clinical correlation,* Plast Reconstr Surg; 67(2):177-87

Mathes S.J. & Nahai S. (1979) *Clinical atlas of muscle and musculocutaneous flaps,* CV Mosby Co, St. Louis

Mathes S.J.; Vasconez L.O. & Jurkiewicz M.J. (1977) *Extensions and further applications of muscle flap transposition,* Plast Reconstr Surg; 60:6-13

McCraw J.B. & Arnold P.G. (1987) *McCraw and Arnold's Atlas of Muscle and Musculocutaneous Flaps,* Hampton Press, Norfolk, VA

Meyer A.J.; Krueger T.; Lepori D.; Dusmet M.; Aubert J.D.; Pasche P. & Ris H.B. (2004) *Closure of large intrathoracic airway defects using extrathoracic muscle flaps,* Ann Thorac Surg; 77(2):397-404

Mitra A.; Spears J.; Perrotta V.; McClurkin J. & Mitra A. (2005) *Salvage of infected prosthetic grafts of the great vessels via muscle flap reconstruction,* Chest; 128(2):1040-3

Naftali Z. (1964) *Toracoplastia osteoplastica cu transplant paramediastinal de coastă in tratamentul tuberculozei cavernoase (Osteoplastic thoracoplasty with paramediastinal transplantation of rib grafts in the treatment of cavernous tuberculosis),* PhD Thesis

Naumov V.N.; Shaikhaev A.I. & Testov V.V. (1991) *Thoracomyoplastic operations in the surgery of tuberculosis of the lungs,* Grud Serdechnososudistaia Khir; (7):46-8

Nomori H.; Horio H.; Hasegawa T. & Suemasu K. (2001) *Intrathoracic transposition of a pectoralis major and pectoralis minor muscle flap for empyema in patients previously subjected to posterolateral thoracotomy,* Surg Today; 31(4):295-9

Nosotti M.; Baisi A.; Mendogni P.; Palleschi A.; Tosi D. & Rosso L. (2010) *Muscle sparing versus posterolateral thoracotomy for pulmonary lobectomy: randomised controlled trial,* Interact Cardiovasc Thorac Surg; 11(4):415-9

Oh A.K.; Lechtman A.N.; Whetzel T.P. & Stevenson T.R. (2004) *The infected median sternotomy wound: management with the rectus abdominis musculocutaneous flap,* Ann Plast Surg; 52(4):367-70

Ojika T.; Mukoyama N.; Suzuki M.; Senda Y. & Namiki Y. (1995) *Two cases of empyema treated with rectus abdominis myocutaneous flap and muscle flap,* Kyobu Geka; 48(5):394-6

Pairolero P.C. & Arnold P.G. (1989) *Intrathoracic transfer of flaps for fistulas, exposed prosthetic devices, and reinforcement of suture lines,* Surg Clin North Am; 69(5):1047-59

Pairolero P.C.; Arnold P.G.; Trastek V.F.; Meland N.B. & Kay P.P. (1990) *Postpneumonectomy empyema. The role of intrathoracic muscle transposition.* J Thorac Cardiovasc Surg; 99(6):958-66

Pardos-Gea J.; Maza Ú.; Pérez-López J. & San José Laporte A. (2011) *Home intravenous antibiotic therapy of empyema and lung abscess: safety and efficacy,* Enferm Infecc Microbiol Clin; 29(3):237-9

Petrov D.; Dzhambazov V.; Minchev T.; Plochev M.; Goranov E.; Krupev M. & Petkov R. (1999) *Omentoplasty in surgical management of postpulmonectomy pleural empyema,* Khirurgiia (Sofiia); 55(6):13-5

Regnard J.F.; Alifano M.; Puyo P.; Fares E.; Magdeleinat P. & Levasseur P. (2000) *Open window thoracostomy followed by intrathoracic flap transposition in the treatment of empyema complicating pulmonary resection,* J Thorac Cardiovasc Surg; 120(2):270-5

Riquet M. (2010) *Thoracomyoplasty (Editorial comment),* Eur J Cardiothorac Surg; 37(2):482

Sarkar S.K.; Sharma T.N.; Singh H.; Singh A.; Purohit S.D. & Sharma V.K. (1985) *Thoracoplasty with intercostal myoplasty for closure of an empyema cavity and bronchopleural fistula,* Int Surg; 70(3):219-21

Schede M. (1890) *Die behandlung der empyeme,* Verh Long Innere Med Wiesbaden; 9:41-141

Schreiner W.; Fuchs P.; Autschbach R.; Pallua N. & Sirbu H. (2010) *Modified technique for thoracomyoplasty after posterolateral thoracotomy,* Thorac Cardiovasc Surg; 58(2):98-101

Seify H.; Mansour K.; Miller J.; Douglas T.; Burke R.; Losken A.; Culbertson J.; Jones G.; Nahai F. & Hester T.R. (2007) *Single-stage muscle flap reconstruction of the postpneumonectomy empyema space: the Emory experience,* Plast Reconstr Surg; 120(7):1886-91

Semb C. (1937) *Thoracoplasty with extrafascial apicolysis*, Br Med J; 2(4004):650-6

Stefani A.; Jouni R.; Alifano M.; Bobbio A.; Strano S.; Magdeleinat P. & Regnard J.F. (2011) *Thoracoplasty in the current practice of thoracic surgery: a single-institution 10-years experience*, Ann Thorac Surg; 91(1):263-8

Stobernack A.; Achatzy R. & Engelmann C. (1997) *Delayed complications after extrapleural pneumonolysis for lung tuberculosis*, Chirurg; 68(9):921-7

Thingnam S.K.; Mohite P.N.; Raju G.; Ranade S.D. & Saklani R. (2011) *Triple reinforcement of bronchial stump*, Thorac Cardiovasc Surg; 59(3):169-71

van Wingerden J.J.; Coret M.E.; van Nieuwenhoven C.A.; Totté E.R. (2010) *The laparoscopically harvested omental flap for deep sternal wound infection*, Eur J Cardiothorac Surg 2010; 37(1):87-92

Walsh M.D.; Bruno A.D.; Onaitis M.W.; Erdmann D.; Wolfe W.G.; Toloza E.M. & Levin L.S. (2011) *The role of intrathoracic free flaps for chronic empyema*, Ann Thorac Surg; 91(3):865-8

Wilson N.J.; Armada O.; Vindzberg V. & O'Brien WB (1956) *Extraperiosteal plombage thoracoplasty: operative technique and results with 161 cases with unilateral surgical problems*, J Thorac Surg; 32:797-813

Zaheer S.; Allen M.S.; Cassivi S.D.; Nichols F.C. 3rd; Johnson C.H.; Deschamps C. & Pairolero P.C. (2006) *Postpneumonectomy empyema: results after the Clagett procedure*, Ann Thorac Surg; 82(1):279-86

Zahid I.; Nagendran M.; Routledge T. & Scarci M. (2011) *Comparison of video-assisted thoracoscopic surgery and open surgery in the management of primary empyema*, Curr Opin Pulm Med; 17(4):255-9

6

Endoscopic Lung Volume Reduction for Emphysema

Paulo F. Guerreiro Cardoso
Department of Cardio-Pneumology, Division of Thoracic Surgery,
Heart Institute (InCor)-Hospital das Clínicas,
Faculdade de Medicina, Universidade de São Paulo,
Brazil

1. Introduction

In advanced stages of emphysema there is a sequence of events that start with hyperinflation, followed by a reduction in diaphragmatic mobility, an increase in resting pleural pressures that intensifies expiratory muscle recruitment and reduces elastic recoil of the lungs.

During exercise, the limitation to expiratory flow prolongs the expiratory phase causing dynamic hyperinflation and ultimately reducing exercise tolerance. Such factors altogether will predispose to respiratory infections, will cause body mass consumption, muscular deconditioning and weight loss. This ominous cycle of events in the emphysema patient impacts negatively and progressively on the quality of life. The patient experiences breathlessness during ordinary activities and even at rest. At this stage of the disease process, palliation becomes a more relevant goal than increased longevity (Berger, Decamp et al. 2010).

The medical treatment of this condition includes bronchodilators, costicosteroids, oxygen and the management of exacerbations and infections. The pulmonary rehabilitation programs, when added to the medical management has been shown to reduce dyspnea, improve quality of life, reduce the frequency of hospital admitions but it does not impact on survival (ATS 1999).

The current options for the surgical treatment are surgical ablation of bulous disease (bullectomy), lung volume reduction surgery (LVRS) and lung transplantation. Despite its unequivocal benefits in selected patients, all such procedures carry a considerable morbidity and mortality.

The LVRS was initially proposed by Brantigan in the 1950's, but mortality was a major issue in the early years (Brantigan, Mueller et al. 1959). In the 1990's, Cooper et al published the first successful, series of pacientes submitted to LVRS (Cooper, Patterson et al. 1996). This was followed by randomized studies that demonstrated functional benefits and acceptable mortality in patients with low exercise capacity and upper lobe predominant heterogeneous disease (Ciccone, Meyers et al. 2003). Despite the promising results of LVRS, mortality has remained high and duration of the benefits remained a controversial issue as shown in the National Emphysema Treatment Trial (NETT) (Fishman, Martinez et al. 2003). The application of LVRS for homogeneous emphysema has added to the controversy (Weder,

Tutic et al. 2009). A recent reassessment of the NETT results revealed that only 45% of the LVRS were actually performed in upper lobe predominant heterogeneous emphysema, and more that one half of the patients were lost to follow up at 5 years, both in the medical and the surgical arms of the trial (Sanchez 2009).

The loss of enthusiasm in LVRS was followed by the development of several endoscopic methods and devices for lung volume reduction. There have been several experimental and clinical studies on such devices based on the asumption that a bronchoscopic procedure is less invasive and a safer alternative for achieving LVR. Furthermore, a non-surgical procedure will probably extend the current indications for LVR, resulting in a broader access to a larger number of patients with emphysema (Herth, Gompelmann et al. 2010).

This chapter focuses on the description of the current methods and devices for bronchoscopic lung volume reduction for emphysema and the results of the clinical trials.

2. Principles of bronchoscopic lung volume reduction (BLVR)

Some procedures have shared the same principle of LVRS in which, by reducing the hyperinflated lung size, there is an improvement in elastic recoil of the emphysematous lungs and consequently in the breathing mechanics (Ingenito, Wood et al. 2008).

The one-way valves promote size reduction as a result of selective atelectasis mostly when the devices are applied in the upper lobes. However, this relies upon poor collateral ventilation in order to function properly and to provide sizeable volume reduction (Gompelmann, Eberhardt et al. 2010). A complete fissure is a feature that ensures that there is little or no connection with the ajacent lobe, and therefore less collateral ventilation.

Biologic lung volume reduction (BioLVR) uses polymers administered endobronchially to produce a similar effect. It causes selective occlusion of segmental areas where it is instilled, and blocks collateral ventilation because of the inflammatory reaction it causes across the area treated and permeates deeply into the alveoli. Such properties makes BioLVR amenable to be used for either homogeneous or heterogeneous emphysema.

The production of local fibrosis has also been attempted using endobronchial thermal vapor ablation. The principle here is a definitive volume reduction, only achieved at the cost of an inflammatory response and subsequent local scarring that is not reversible (Snell, Hopkins et al. 2009).

The emphysema with predominantly homogeneous destruction calls for different measures. The principle is opposed to what is found in heterogeneous emphysema. Collateral ventilation is usually abundant in homogeneous emphysema, and the procedure must take advantage of it. The production of extra-anatomic passages communicating the distal bronchi with the lung parenchyma is known as airway bypass. This was originally proposed as communications or "spiracles" between the lung and the chest wall (Macklem 1978; Moore, Cetti et al. 2010). Recently, this procedure was then modified to accomodate such passages within the bronchi, thus enabling it to be performed bronchoscopically (Choong, Macklem et al. 2008). This procedure will reduce hyperinflation and provide a diaphragmatic remodelling that will ultimately improve ventilatory mechanics.

3. Devices and results

The devices developed for endoscopic treatment of heterogeneous emphysema can be divided into 3 categories: Blocking devices (e.g. one-way valves); Reversible non-blocking or removable (e.g. *coils*); Non-reversible or non-blocking definitive (e.g. vapor thermoablation, endobronchial polymers, airway bypass).

3.1 Blocking devices
3.1.1 One-way valves
These devices have been validated for clinical use in some countries. The Zephyr® (Pulmonx, Redwood City-CA, EUA) (FIGURE 1) is a model that can be placed bronchoscopically.

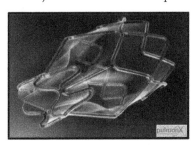

Fig. 1. The Zephyr® one-way valve (Pulmonx, Redwood City-CA, USA)

The success of the procedure is related to presence of complete fissures, high heterogeneity and the presence of atelectasis of the treated lobe. The manufaturer has recently introduced a device for measuring collateral flow which is composed of a catheter with a baloon tip and a flow transducer Chartis™, Pulmonx, Redwood City-CA, EUA) (Figure 2).

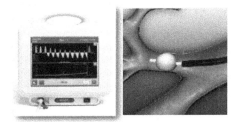

Fig. 2. The console and catheter for the measurement of collateral ventilation (Chartis® system; Pulmonx, Redwood City-CA, USA).

Once the target area is identified radiologically, the catheter is passed through the working channel of the bronchoscope, advanced into the lobar bronchus, the baloon tip is inflated in place occluding the bronchus. The collateral ventilation is then measured on site by the flow transducer connected to the tip of the catheter (Aljuri and Freitag 2009). This allows the examiner to choose the area with the least collateral ventilation for installing the valves. A study with 25 patients using this method of measuring collateral flow showed that in 90% of the cases the resistance measurements correlated with the post-implantation atelectasis visualized on a chest X-ray (Gompelmann, Eberhardt et al. 2010).

The clinical studies carried out so far have been done in a heterogeneous population of emphysema patients and this has impacted the results negatively. A safety and efficacy non-randomized study showed that 90 days post-implant of one-way valves has revealed a 4,9% decrease in residual volume (RV) and a 10% increase in FEV1. There were 8% serious adverse events and 1% mortality (Wan, Toma et al. 2006).

To date, the largest randomized study with one-way valves was the **VENT** study (**V**alve for **E**mphysema **P**alliatio**N** **T**rial). There were 321 patients included accross 31 centers in the United States and 23 centers in Europe. Major inclusion criteria were: FEV1 between 15-45%; RV ≥ 150% and total lung capacity (TLC) ≥ 100% predicted. All patients underwent a full pulmonary rehabilitation program before and after the procedure. A 2:1 randomization (treatment with valves : control with best medical care) resulted in 214 patients receiving valves and the results have been published recently (Sciurba, Ernst et al.). At 6 months there was a small but significant improvement in FEV1 of 4,3% with a mean difference between treatment versus control group of 6,8% ($p<0.005$). There was a 2,5% increase in exercise tolerance on the 6-minute walk test (6MWT) in the treatment group, versus a decrease of -3,4% in the control group (mean difference of 5,8% $p=0.04$). There were small improvements in dyspnea, a reduction in suplemmental O_2 requirements (-12L/day), and better quality of life (-3,4 points in the St. George Respiratory Questionnaire).

The high heterogeneity (> 15% between lobes by CT) subset analysis at 6 months post-procedure showed that enhanced effects on FEV1 improvements of 10,7% ($p=0,004$) and of 12,4% in the 6MWT ($p=0,002$).

The presence of complete fissure also yielded improvements in FEV1 difference between treatment and control at 6 months (16,2%; $p<0,001$) and at 12 months (17,9%; $p<0,001$). The results at 6 months are summarized in (Figure 3). Major adverse events occurring within 90 days after placement of the one-way valves were mostly COPD exacerbations requiring hospitalization (7,9% in the treated group versus 1,1% in controls; $p=0,03$). Pneumothorax occurred in 4.2% of patients in the treated group early post-procedure follow-up and it was similar between groups in the late follow-up (valves=1%; control=2,4%). All but one resolved spontaneously (Hopkinson, Toma et al. 2005) (de Oliveira, Macedo-Neto et al. 2006).

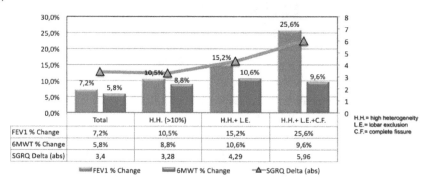

Compiled from Sciurba et al. New Engl J Med 2010;363:1233

Fig. 3. Overall % changes (left axis) in FEV1 (orange), 6 MWT (purple) and the delta in the points (right axis) of the Saint George Respiratory Questionnaire (SGRQ) triangle (gray) are shown. The subset of high heterogeneity above 10% increased in about 30% the differences from baseline. When high heterogeneity was added to lobar exclusion, the functional parameters have doubled the differences and, in the subset that congregates high heterogeneity with lobar exclusion and low collateral flow, FEV1 jumped to 25%, 6 MWT to 10% and the delta in SGRQ went up to 6 points.

Hopkinson et al (Hopkinson, Toma et al. 2005) demonstrated that in a series of 19 patients patients treated with one-way valves who developed persisting lobar atelectasis at 1 month after the procedure, showed an improved survival at 6 years of follow-up.

One-way valves have been employed for BLVR as a bridge to lung transplantation in severe COPD patients. There is one report on 4 patients undergoing Zephyr® valve placement (average on 3,5 valves/patient), that showed no procedure related morbidity or mortality. BLVR was able to reduce RV and improve the 6MWT mMRC score. Three out of the four patients were transplanted successfully between 6-7 months, and one patient died 13 months after valve placement still on the transplant waiting list. The authors concluded that in a selected group of COPD patients awaiting lung transplantation, BLVR with one-valves can improve functional status and help patients awaiting lung transplantation for severe emphysema (Venuta, Diso et al. 2011).

Another valve device with a different design has been developed and tested (IBV®, Olympus Co., Spiration, Redmond-WA, EUA) (FIGURE 4). It has the ability of obstructing the airflow selectively in the segments where it is placed and, by the same token, allows secretions to exit the segment. One study with 30 patients showed improvements in quality of life, however without significant differences in pulmonary function (Wood, McKenna et al. 2007). This study has used outcome measures similar to LVRS. An expansion of this study has been published recently and included 91 patients with severe obstruction, hyperinflation and upper lobe predominant emphysema (Sterman, Mehta et al. 2010). A total of 609 bronchial valves placed bilaterally into the upper lobes. There were no procedure-related deaths. Thirty-day morbidity and mortality were 5.5 and 1.1%, respectively and pneumothorax was the most frequent serious device-related complication. There were no significant differences at 1,3,6 and 12 months in pulmonary function, exercise tolerance and gas exchange. There was a significant health-related quality of life improvement (-8.2+/-16.2) change at 6 months and it was associated with a decreased volume in the treated lobes without visible atelectasis.

In another recent study, the IBV® valves were tested and validated for clinical use in persistent air leaks (Wood, Cerfolio et al. 2010).

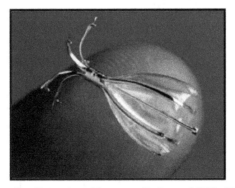

Fig. 4. The IBV® one-way valve (Spiration-Olympus, Redmond-WA, USA)

The studies using one-way valves concluded that this procedures have a good safety profile with low mortality and can be effective in selected subgroups of patients.

3.2 Removable non-blocking devices
3.2.1 Coils
This device is made out of a single nitinol wire with a memory (RePneu® Lung Volume Reduction Coil, PneumRx Inc., Mountain View, CA-EUA) (FIGURE 5). It is placed in a straight position within an introducer sheath that fits in the working channel of the flexible bronchoscope. Once the target segmental bronchus is reached, the device is deployed and its memory causes it to curve around its own axis, forcing the bronchus along with the adjacent lung parenchyma. Volume reduction is achieved when several of such devices are placed within the same lobe.

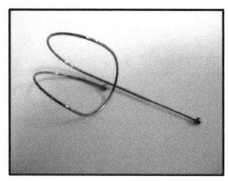

Fig. 5. Endobronchial nitinol coil utilized for BLVR (RePneu® Lung Volume Reduction Coil, PneumRx Inc, Mountain View, CA-USA)

The device a used in a preliminary safety trial on 11 patients, in whom 21 procedures were required to place the coils (average of 4.9 ± 0.6 coils per procedure), lasting 45 minutes each in average. After a follow-up of 7-11 months, efficacy was superior in patients with heterogeneous emphysema (Herth, Eberhardt et al. 2009; Herth, Eberhard et al. 2010).

3.3 Definitive (non-removeable) non-blocking devices
3.3.1 Bronchial thermal vapor ablation (BTVA)
This is a new technology that uses hot water vapor administered via a flexible bronchoscope by means of a baloon occlusion catheter (BTVA-*bronchial thermal vapor ablation*; Uptake Medical Corporation, Seattle-WA, EUA) (FIGURE 6). The system was designed to deliver a precise amount of vapor per gram of lung tissue. The early experimental studies carried out in animal models concluded that an amount of 5cal/gram of lung tissue was sufficient to cause a thermal lesion with subsequent fibrotic scarring and lung volume reduction. A preliminary clinical study on 11 patients with severe heterogeneous emphysema showed no significant improvements in FEV1 or RV at 6 months. However, gas transfer improved, the Medical Research Council Dyspnea Score (mMRC) improved 0,5 points from baseline, and the St. George Respiratory Questionnaire Score improved from 64,4 at baseline to 49,1 (Snell, Hopkins et al. 2009). The complication most frequently found with this procedure was bacterial pneumonia and COPD exacerbation. This technology is still under clinical testing, and new studies with higher amounts of vapor are under way.

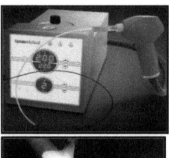

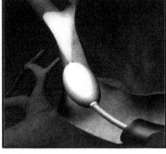

Fig. 6. Vapor generator (top) and catheter (bottom) used for bronchial thermal vapor ablation (BTVA-Uptake Medical Corporation, Seattle-WA, EUA).

3.3.2 Biological lung volume reduction (BioLVR) with polymers

This procedure consists of achieving lung volume reduction after obstruction with biodegradeable polymers instilled endobronchially under flexible bronchoscopy. This substance is a polymer mixed with fibrin and thrombin (*Aeriseal®*, Aeris Therapeutics Woburn-MA, EUA). Once it is delivered via a catheter into the segmental bronchi, its components polymerize resulting in a gel that blocks the bronchi. This substance progresses into the alveoli causing a local inflammatory reaction that causes scarring formation which will ultimately perpetuate the lung volume reduction (Ingenito and Tsai 2007).

The BioLVR has been applied to upper lobe predominant emphysema, both homogeneous and heterogeneous. Experimental data has shown that, by reaching deep into the alveoli, the polymer promotes blockage of the collateral ventilation. A clinical study on patients with homogeneous emphysema has been concluded recently (Reilly, Washko et al. 2007; Refaely, Dransfield et al. 2010). Among the 25 patients that underwent BioLVR, 17 received a dose of 10ml per treated site and 8 received 20ml. The higher dose group had the best results at 6 months. FEV1 reduced 8%, the mMRC dyspnea score reduced by 0,4 points and the St.George's Respiratory Questionnaire reduced by 4.9%. The authors concluded that in homogeneous emphysema the higher dose and the number of segmental bronchi treated were related to a better functional result (Murgu and Colt 2010).

The largest series published on BioLVR included 50 patients with upper lobe predominant emphysema. The FEV1 increased 15.6% at 6 months relative to pre-treatment values ($p=0.002$). On the other hand, subjects receiving higher doses of the polymer experienced more serious adverse events (8%), including pneumonia, pulmonary thromboembolism ad aspiration (Criner, Pinto-Plata et al. 2009).

3.3.3 Airway bypass

As mentioned earlier in this chapter, this procedure was designed to take advantage of the collateral ventilation that occurs naturally and is greatly enhanced in homogeneous emphysema.

This procedure evolved from the earlier concept of extra-anatomical communications between the lung parenchyma and the skin created by Macklem (Macklem 1978), to the production of fenestrations between the segmental bronchi and the adjacent lung proposed by Macklem and Cooper (Macklem, Cardoso et al. 2006).

The procedure consists of the production of orifices in the wall of the distal segmental and subsegmental bronchi (fenestrations), which are kept open with small self-expandable metal stents covered with a thin layer of medical silicone (Choong, Haddad et al. 2005).

The airway bypass procedure uses a proprietary system (Exhale Emphysema Treatment System™, Broncus Technologies Inc., Mountain View, CA-EUA) that includes: a doppler probe, catheter and a processor used for the location of extraluminal vessels through the bronchial wall; a needle-baloon dilator and a baloon catheter that expands the stents and the drug eluting stents loaded with paclitaxel. All devices described above were designed to pass through the 2mm or larger working channel of a flexible bronchoscope (FIGURE 7).

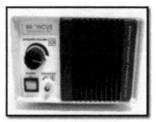
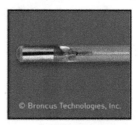

Doppler processor   Doppler probe

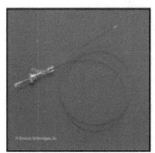
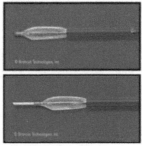
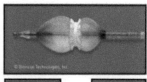

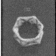

Needle-baloon dilator   Baloon + needle   Catheter & Stents

Fig. 7. The Exhale Emphysema Treatment System™, Broncus technologies Inc., Mountain View, CA-USA) used for the airway bypass procedure: doppler processor and probe (top row); needle-baloon dilator and a baloon catheter that expands the stents and the drug eluting stents loaded with paclitaxel (bottom row).

The proof of concept was achieved in a preliminary study on 12 explanted emphysematous lungs extracted from recipients of lung transplants. The lungs were placed in an airtight negative pressure ventilation chamber and connected to a pneumotachometer. Passages were created in the distal bronchi using a radiofrequency probe and stents were placed to hold the passage open. The creation of the passages resulted in an increase in the cumulative expiratory volumes in a direct proportion to the number of passages created (Lausberg, Chino et al. 2003). Further studies in the same model concluded that airway bypass was able to improve mechanics of breathing in severely emphysematous lungs, therefore supporting that it can improve ventilatory function in patients by reducing gas trapping and flow resistance (Choong, Macklem et al. 2008).

This was followed by a feasibility and safety study in humans prior to lobectomy and lung transplantation using radiofrequency generators to create the passages communicating the distal bronchi with the emphysematous lung parenchyma (Rendina, De Giacomo et al. 2003). The next step was to prolong the patency of the stents. This was achieved experimentally with the use of mitomycin-C in the stents (Choong, Haddad et al. 2005) and later by the development of drug eluting stents loaded with paclitaxel (Choong, Phan et al. 2006).

Prior to the procedure itself, the preferred sites for stent placement were identified on the chest CT scans based on the areas of most emphysematous destruction within the lung parenchyma (FIGURE 8). Efforts were made to place a minimum of three stents in each lung bilaterally. The middle lobe was not treated.

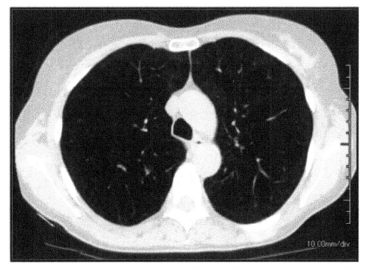

Fig. 8. CT scan showing homogeneous destruction by emphysema in a potentially suitable candidate for the airway bypass procedure.

The creation of each stented passage requires the following steps: 1) identification of a blood vessel-free location with a Doppler probe at the level of segmental bronchi; 2) fenestration of the bronchial wall by means of the needle-baloon dilator; 3) re-scanning the fenestration and its adjacent area with the the doppler probe to ascertain that no vessels were in the vicinity of the puncture site; 4) passage of the stent loaded catheter and deployment of the paclitaxel-eluting stent into the hole by expanding the hidrostatic baloon with a comercially available inflation syringe (FIGURES 9, 10).

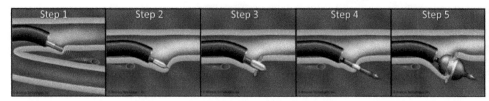

Fig. 9. Steps of the airway bypass procedure: 1- flexible bronchoscope is advanced into the distal airway, the area is scanned by the doppler probe; 2- the needle is passed, the airway pierced; 3- the passage is dilated with the baloon, and scanned again with the doppler probe to ascertain the absence of blood vessels in the vicinity of the passage; 4- the stent is then positioned into the passage; 5- the stent is deployed using a special baloon coupled to the catheter.

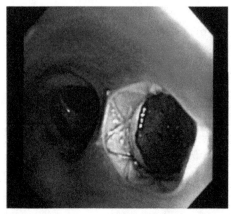

Fig. 10. Paclitaxel eluting stent (right) placed adjacent to a segmental bronchus (left).

The initial feasibility studies were followed by the first clinical studies to evaluate efficacy and safety (Macklem, Cardoso et al. 2006; Cardoso, Snell et al. 2007). A multicentric study included 35 patients with a RV ≥ 220%, FEV1 ≤ 40% and mMRC ≥ 2. Two hundred and sixty four stents were implanted, with an average of 8 stents per patient. There was 1 death secondary to bleeding in this series (mortality of 2,6%). This event triggered an extensive safety revision that resulted in several recommendations made, including re-scanning puncture sites, and the placement of a stand-by bronchial blocker into the airway during the procedure. At 1 month after the procedure there were significant differences in all functional parameters, however such changes got smaller and were restricted to rv ($p=0,04$) and mmrc ($p=0.02$) at 6 months. The subset of patients with RV/TLC ≥ 0.67 sustained the best benefits with significant changes in RV (-14,1% ; $p=0,02$) and mMRC (-0,5% ; $p=0,03$). The most frequent serious adverse events were COPD exacerbation (32%) and respiratory infection (27%), most of them have occurred in the first monthy after procedure. One additional death occurred due to bowel obstruction in the late follow up, which was considered as unrelated to the procedure.

These results led to the design of the *Exhale Airway Stents for Emphysema* (*EASE* Trial) (Shah, Slebos et al. 2011). This was a multicenter phase III trial of airway bypass with paclitaxel-eluting stents. The EASE trial was the first double-blind, randomised, sham-controlled study on bronchoscopic lung volume reduction in severe homogeneous emphysema.

The EASE Trial used a 2:1 (treatment:sham) randomization. Double-blinding was maintained by dividing the investigators into two teams (blinded Team A with access to pre and post-procedure assessments ; and blinded Team B that performed only the bronchoscopic procedures without further patient contact). All patients underwent a full 6-10 week program of pulmonary rehabilitation prior to the procedure and 8 weeks after the procedure. Follow-up visits were scheduled for 1, 3, 6 and 12 months emphysema (Shah, Slebos et al. 2011).

The 6-month efficacy endpoints required both an improvement greater than 12% in FVC, and a more than 1 point decrease in mMRC over baseline. This trial enrolled 315 patients at 38 centers with homogeneous emphysema and severe hyperinflation (RV ≥ 180% predicted; RV/TLC ≥ 0.65). There were 208 patients randomised for airway bypass and 107 for sham bronchoscopy.

The results of the EASE trial were submitted for publication recently (Shah, Slebos et al. 2011). The airway bypass group received a mean of 4.7±1.4 stents per patient. The 6-month co-primary endpoint was 14.4%for AB vs 11.2% for SC. On day 1, RV decreased significantly in the airway bypass group (change of 379mL from baseline ; $p=0,006$), and this was associated with increases in FEV_1 and FVC. At months 1, 3, 6 and 12 the changes were no longer significant between the groups on FVC, FEV1, mMRC. The functional assessment by Saint George Respiratory Questionnaire was better in the airway bypass group at 1 month, but this coincided with the post-procedural rehabilitation program. The 6MWT showed no significant differences after the first month of follow-up between the groups.

Composite safety endpoints at 6 months were 14,4% in the airway bypass group and 11,2% in the sham controls ($p=1,0$). There was one death after the airway bypass procedure due to a ruptured abdominal aortic aneurysm. Overall mortality at 12 months was similar between airway bypass and sham controls (6,7% and 6,5% respectively).

Further CT analysis showed that there were lobar volume decreases after stent placement at day 1. However, at month 6 the RV increased coincidently with stent loss by expectoration or stent occlusion. Such findings have suggested that the loss of stents or its occlusion were the limiting factors for achieving long term benefit. Further studies must be redesigned with special attention to the functional endpoints and focus on new imaging methods.

Targeting trapped air regions with more accurate mapping in COPD patients is another issue that has to be addressed. Better monitoring for loss of effect and sequential interventions to prolong effect durability with the current technology are therefore required.

In summary, despite the early promising results in the first clinical trial with the airway bypass procedure, the paclitaxel eluting stents used in the EASE trial showed only short term good results. The trial exposed both the need for technical improvements in the stents and for preventing its early occlusion. This will then prolong effect durability if this technology is to be pursued in the future.

The common denominator in all procedures and the few trials on BLVR is the lack of common endpoints and the need for new assessment methods that are both non-invasive and accurate.

4. New methods for the assessment in BLVR

The assessment methods used in BLVR today are essentially the same used a decade ago for LVRS and during the NETT trial.

As BLVR has evolved, this has led the centers to enroll patients with worse pulmonary function and poor performance requiring a more thorough evaluation. On the other hand, all major trials on BLVR did not share the same endpoints, making interpretation of results not only difficult, but sometimes confusing.

All procedures proposed for BLVR so far are based on lung deflation. Surprisingly, none of the methods currently employed have the ability to provide dynamic information as the procedure is being carried out along with the pattern of lung deflation.

Based on the facts abovementioned, new methods for patient selection and post-treatment evaluation must be studied to correct this idiosyncrasy. Such new methods shall be ideally less invasive, able to provide meaningful information and add on to the current evaluation strategy (PFTs, performance testing, Chest CT scan, etc).

4.1 Chest CT scan imaging analysis

Advanced helical scanners have enabled much better imaging management. This has been particularly useful for the detection of target areas in emphysema and airway navigation for bronchoscopy planning. The ability to quantify emphysema based on the CT scan is also a powerful tool for post-treatment assessment.

There are commercially available softwares able to provide an accurate volumetry of each lobe. This is accomplished by mapping the emphysematous areas using the -910 and -950 Hounsfield unit cut-offs and applying the information to complex algorithms. The software will calculate many parameters such as air and tissue volumes. It will generate histograms with the less dense (and more emphysematous) areas, comparing them between the lobes and giving numerical information about heterogeneity. This has become a key for the success of certain procedures such as BLVR with one-way valves (Coxson, Nasute Fauerbach et al. 2008). The software can generate multiplannar images of the airway and its relation to the emphysematous areas, in addition to schematic depictions of the target emphysematous areas with accurate volume calculations (Figure 11). This is particularly useful for obtaining post-procedure static volumetry and to determine heterogeneity between lobes.

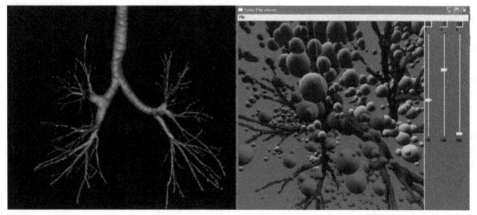

Fig. 11. Images of the airway (left) and a schematic depiction of the emphysematous lobes and its distribution (right) to facilitate navigation and device placement (Apollo®-Vida Diagnostics, Iowa-USA).

The problem limiting repeat CT scans for post-treatment assessment is the cumulative radiation dose. Standard-dose CT for follow-up of BLVR is limited by the risk of administration of a radiation dose of 8-12 mSv for each CT examination. Low-dose CT, in which the radiation dose is six to ten fold less than in conventional CT, has been used for the evaluation of emphysema patients (Gierada, Pilgram et al. 2007). This technique was recently used for the evaluation of the feasibility of thin-section low-dose CT in the radiologic monitoring of patients after placement of bronchial stents for airway bypass (Grgic, Wilkens et al. 2008).

4.2 Electrical impedance tomography (EIT)

EIT uses the injection of high frequency and low amplitude electrical currents through 16 or 32 electrodes placed around the chest to obtain images of a cross section of the lungs. These currents travel through the thorax following pathways that vary according to chest wall shape and thoracic distribution of impeditivities. The resulting electric potentials on the surface of the chest wall are measured and used to obtain the electric impedance distribution within the thorax using a reconstruction algorithm (Figure 12). The output image of such algorithms is usually a 32 by 32 or a 64 by 64 array from which each element corresponds to a pixel on the image and contains the change in impedance in relation to a reference frame, expressed as a percentage (Costa, Lima et al. 2009). This method has been extensively investigated in the intensive care setting for patients undergoing mechanical ventilation.

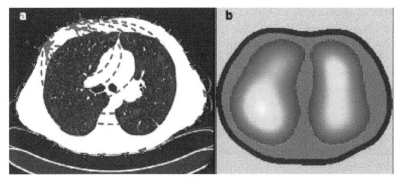

Fig. 12. Electrical impedance tomography (EIT): a) the 32 electrode belt around the chest and the electrical current between 2 electrodes; b) image generated by the software representing the average variation of impedance.

EIT combines two interesting features: it is not invasive and can be performed at the bedside. It has been proven useful for PEEP titration, to optimize ventilation strategies by detecting the imbalances in regional lung ventilation, as well as to detect pneumothorax and small pleural effusions (Victorino, Borges et al. 2004; Costa, Lima et al. 2009). More recently there have been studies showing that EIT can assess lung perfusion through intravenous injection of hypertonic saline, which is a contrast agent for EIT images because of its extremely low impeditivity (Tanaka, Ortega et al. 2008).

The characteristics of EIT makes it a potentially useful tool for the assessment of BLVR. It combines the ability of quantifying lung deflation, to show the redistribution of ventilation during and after the procedure and, by the same token, to detect pneumothorax..

Furthermore, this is the only procedure that can be done at the bedside. We have recently embarked on an experimental study of the patterns on lung deflation after BLVR to detect its feasibility prior to its clinical application.

4.3 Diaphragmatic mobility by ultrasound (US)

One of the hallmarks of advanced COPD is diaphragmatic flattening and dysfunction, both caused by chronic hyperinflation. This causes muscular deconditioning of the diaphragm, that contributes to dyspnea and low exercise tolerance. It is therefore expected that the improvements in diaphragmatic mobility should follow the improvements in breathing mechanics after BLVR in severe COPD patients. Surprisingly, insofar this has not been studied in BLVR protocols.

The US measurement of craniocaudal displacement of the left intrahepatic branches of the portal vein was described as an indirect assessment of right hemidiaphragmatic mobility (Toledo, Kodaira et al. 2003). Paulin et al (Paulin, Yamaguti et al. 2007) created a classification of diaphragmatic dysfunction based on the degree of its mobility. They showed that COPD patients with less than 33.9mm of diaphragm mobility as measured by US had greater dyspnea upon exertion and covered shorter 6MWT distances if compared to patients with more than 34mm of diaphragmatic mobility. Based on this assumption, Yamaguti et al (Yamaguti, Paulin et al. 2009) published an interesting study on the risk of death on COPD individuals with and without diaphragmatic dysfunction based on US evaluation of mobility. They concluded that COPD patients with lower diaphragm mobility had a higher risk of death than COPD patients without diaphragmatic dysfunction and that quality of life was unrelated to the decline in diaphragmatic function in their studies COPD subjects. This has yielded to another major study currently under way at the University of Sao Paulo, Brazil to specifically assess the "Evaluation of ins and expiratory muscles in respiratory diseases".

The US for the measurement of diaphragmatic mobility is also non-invasive and its reproducibility and reliability in COPD patients has been demonstrated. Its use for the assessment of BLVR shall be contemplated in future studies.

4.4 Opto-electronic plethismography (OEP) method

OEP is a new noninvasive technique that is highly accurate method for measuring the total chest wall volume variations, allowing partitioning of the complex shape of the chest wall into basically three different functional compartments (upper chest, thoraco-abdominal and abdominal). It measures breathing patterns and, if combined with pressure measurements, can be used to study statics, dynamics and energetics of the respiratory system (Aliverti, Dellaca et al. 2001). It uses non-invasive video imaging capturing the movement of skin markers while the patient breathes spontaneously. Studies on severe COPD patients using OPE have shown that dynamic hyperinflation is not the only mechanism limiting exercise performance. The measurement of chest wall volumes by OPE can identify the different patterns of respiratory muscle activation during exercise (Aliverti, Stevenson et al. 2004). Another important feature of OPE is its ability to evaluate coordination. One of the semiologic features of COPD is the paradoxical ventilation. This is also known as the Hoover's sign, in which the flattened diaphragm contracts inwards instead of downwards, thereby pulling the inferior ribs inwards with its movement. In normal subjects the expansion of both rib cage and abdomen happen synchronously and in phase. In COPD a less effective diaphragm alters this mechanism. Lower ribcage paradox at rest is associated with early-onset hyperinflation of the chest wall and predominant dyspnea at exercise. When paradox is absent, the sense of leg effort has been shown to be a more important symptom limiting exercise. On the other hand, COPD patients with an asynchronous abdominal rib cage breathing pattern showed more dynamic hyperinflation and dyspnea as the exercise limiting factor (Aliverti, Quaranta et al. 2009).

Given this is a non-invasive method of measuring both breathing, coordination and chest wall volumes, it makes OPE an excellent tool for screening and evaluating patients for BLVR. We are currently using OPE to measure coordination and lung volume integration in the assessment of COPD patients in our bronchoscopic lung volume reduction program.

5. Conclusion

Bronchoscopic lung volume reduction is an emerging non-surgical alternative for palliation in severe emphysema patients. Despite all the efforts and resources spent into trials and device development, BLVR remains mostly investigational. With the exception of the one-way valves that have been approved for use in Europe and Latin America, all other devices are still under scrutiny. A number of new devices have been proposed and only a few have shown modest benefits if compared to surgical lung volume reduction. Nevertheless, most of the devices have shown a good safety profile and their effectiveness depends greatly on the technology used and on subject selection. The need for development of new methods for evaluation and follow-up following BLVR is another issue that must be addressed in conjunction to the creation of a more uniform data aquisition and interpretation accross the clinical trials.

6. References

Aliverti, A., R. Dellaca, et al. (2001). "Optoelectronic plethysmography: a new tool in respiratory medicine." Recenti Prog Med 92(11): 644-647.

Aliverti, A., M. Quaranta, et al. (2009). "Paradoxical movement of the lower ribcage at rest and during exercise in COPD patients." Eur Respir J 33(1): 49-60.

Aliverti, A., N. Stevenson, et al. (2004). "Regional chest wall volumes during exercise in chronic obstructive pulmonary disease." Thorax 59(3): 210-216.

Aljuri, N. and L. Freitag (2009). "Validation and pilot clinical study of a new bronchoscopic method to measure collateral ventilation before endobronchial lung volume reduction." J Appl Physiol 106(3): 774-783.

ATS (1999). "Pulmonary rehabilitation-1999. American Thoracic Society." Am J Respir Crit Care Med 159(5 Pt 1): 1666-1682.

Berger, R. L., M. M. Decamp, et al. (2010). "Lung volume reduction therapies for advanced emphysema: an update." Chest 138(2): 407-417.

Brantigan, O. C., E. Mueller, et al. (1959). "A surgical approach to pulmonary emphysema." Am Rev Respir Dis 80(1, Part 2): 194-206.

Cardoso, P. F., G. I. Snell, et al. (2007). "Clinical application of airway bypass with paclitaxel-eluting stents: early results." J Thorac Cardiovasc Surg 134(4): 974-981.

Choong, C. K., F. J. Haddad, et al. (2005). "Feasibility and safety of airway bypass stent placement and influence of topical mitomycin C on stent patency." J Thorac Cardiovasc Surg 129(3): 632-638.

Choong, C. K., P. T. Macklem, et al. (2008). "Airway bypass improves the mechanical properties of explanted emphysematous lungs." Am J Respir Crit Care Med 178(9): 902-905.

Choong, C. K., L. Phan, et al. (2006). "Prolongation of patency of airway bypass stents with use of drug-eluting stents." J Thorac Cardiovasc Surg 131(1): 60-64.

Ciccone, A. M., B. F. Meyers, et al. (2003). "Long-term outcome of bilateral lung volume reduction in 250 consecutive patients with emphysema." J Thorac Cardiovasc Surg 125(3): 513-525.

Cooper, J. D., G. A. Patterson, et al. (1996). "Results of 150 consecutive bilateral lung volume reduction procedures in patients with severe emphysema." J Thorac Cardiovasc Surg 112(5): 1319-1329; discussion 1329-1330.

Costa, E. L., R. G. Lima, et al. (2009). "Electrical impedance tomography." Curr Opin Crit Care 15(1): 18-24.

Coxson, H. O., P. V. Nasute Fauerbach, et al. (2008). "Computed tomography assessment of lung volume changes after bronchial valve treatment." Eur Respir J 32(6): 1443-1450.

Criner, G. J., V. Pinto-Plata, et al. (2009). "Biologic lung volume reduction in advanced upper lobe emphysema: phase 2 results." Am J Respir Crit Care Med 179(9): 791-798.

de Oliveira, H. G., A. V. Macedo-Neto, et al. (2006). "Transbronchoscopic pulmonary emphysema treatment: 1-month to 24-month endoscopic follow-up." Chest 130(1): 190-199.

Fishman, A., F. Martinez, et al. (2003). "A randomized trial comparing lung-volume-reduction surgery with medical therapy for severe emphysema." N Engl J Med 348(21): 2059-2073.

Gierada, D. S., T. K. Pilgram, et al. (2007). "Comparison of standard- and low-radiation-dose CT for quantification of emphysema." AJR. American journal of roentgenology 188(1): 42-47.

Gompelmann, D., R. Eberhardt, et al. (2010). "Predicting atelectasis by assessment of collateral ventilation prior to endobronchial lung volume reduction: a feasibility study." Respiration 80(5): 419-425.

Grgic, A., H. Wilkens, et al. (2008). "Low-dose MDCT for surveillance of patients with severe homogeneous emphysema after bronchoscopic airway bypass." AJR. American journal of roentgenology 191(3): W112-119.

Herth, F., R. Eberhardt, et al. (2009). "Pilot Study of an Improved Lung Volume Reduction Coil for the Treatment of Emphysema." Am J Respir Crit Care Med 179: A6160.

Herth, F. J., R. Eberhard, et al. (2010). "Bronchoscopic lung volume reduction with a dedicated coil: a clinical pilot study." Ther Adv Respir Dis 4(4): 225-231.

Herth, F. J., D. Gompelmann, et al. (2010). "Endoscopic lung volume reduction." Respiration 79(1): 5-13.

Hopkinson, N. S., T. P. Toma, et al. (2005). "Effect of bronchoscopic lung volume reduction on dynamic hyperinflation and exercise in emphysema." Am J Respir Crit Care Med 171(5): 453-460.

Ingenito, E. P. and L. W. Tsai (2007). "Evolving endoscopic approaches for treatment of emphysema." Semin Thorac Cardiovasc Surg 19(2): 181-189.

Ingenito, E. P., D. E. Wood, et al. (2008). "Bronchoscopic lung volume reduction in severe emphysema." Proc Am Thorac Soc 5(4): 454-460.

Lausberg, H. F., K. Chino, et al. (2003). "Bronchial fenestration improves expiratory flow in emphysematous human lungs." Ann Thorac Surg 75(2): 393-397; discussion 398.

Macklem, P., Cardoso P., et al. (2006). Airway Bypass: A New Treatment for Emphysema. Annual Meeting of the American Thoracic Society, San Diego-CA.

Macklem, P. T. (1978). "Collateral ventilation." N Engl J Med 298(1): 49-50.

Moore, A. J., E. Cetti, et al. (2010). "Unilateral extrapulmonary airway bypass in advanced emphysema." Ann Thorac Surg 89(3): 899-906.

Murgu, S. D. and H. G. Colt (2010). "Interventional bronchoscopy from bench to bedside: new techniques for central and peripheral airway obstruction." Clin Chest Med 31(1): 101-115, Table of Contents.

Paulin, E., W. P. Yamaguti, et al. (2007). "Influence of diaphragmatic mobility on exercise tolerance and dyspnea in patients with COPD." Respir Med 101(10): 2113-2118.

Refaely, Y., M. Dransfield, et al. (2010). "Biologic lung volume reduction therapy for advanced homogeneous emphysema." Eur Respir J 36(1): 20-27.

Reilly, J., G. Washko, et al. (2007). "Biological lung volume reduction: a new bronchoscopic therapy for advanced emphysema." Chest 131(4): 1108-1113.

Rendina, E. A., T. De Giacomo, et al. (2003). "Feasibility and safety of the airway bypass procedure for patients with emphysema." J Thorac Cardiovasc Surg 125(6): 1294-1299.

Sanchez, P. (2009). "NETT trial: a reassessment." AATS meeting-Abstracts.

Sciurba, F. C., A. Ernst, et al. (2010). "A randomized study of endobronchial valves for advanced emphysema." N Engl J Med 363(13): 1233-1244.

Shah, P., D. Slebos, et al. (2011). "Bronchoscopic lung volume reduction with Exhale Airway Stents for Emphysema (EASE): A Randomised, Sham Controlled Multicenter Trial." Lancet 378: 997-1005.

Shah, P. L., D. J. Slebos, et al. (2011). "Design of the exhale airway Stents for emphysema (EASE) trial: an endoscopic procedure for reducing hyperinflation." BMC Pulm Med 11(1): 1.

Snell, G. I., P. Hopkins, et al. (2009). "A feasibility and safety study of bronchoscopic thermal vapor ablation: a novel emphysema therapy." Ann Thorac Surg 88(6): 1993-1998.

Sterman, D. H., A. C. Mehta, et al. (2010). "A multicenter pilot study of a bronchial valve for the treatment of severe emphysema." Respiration 79(3): 222-233.

Tanaka, H., N. R. Ortega, et al. (2008). "Fuzzy modeling of electrical impedance tomography images of the lungs." Clinics 63(3): 363-370.

Toledo, N. S., S. K. Kodaira, et al. (2003). "Right hemidiaphragmatic mobility: assessment with US measurement of craniocaudal displacement of left branches of portal vein." Radiology 228(2): 389-394.

Venuta, F., D. Diso, et al. (2011). "Bronchoscopic lung volume reduction as a bridge to lung transplantation in patients with chronic obstructive pulmonary disease." Eur J Cardio-Thorac Surg 39(3): 364-367.

Victorino, J. A., J. B. Borges, et al. (2004). "Imbalances in regional lung ventilation: a validation study on electrical impedance tomography." Am J Respir Crit Care Med 169(7): 791-800.

Wan, I. Y., T. P. Toma, et al. (2006). "Bronchoscopic lung volume reduction for end-stage emphysema: report on the first 98 patients." Chest 129(3): 518-526.

Weder, W., M. Tutic, et al. (2009). "Persistent benefit from lung volume reduction surgery in patients with homogeneous emphysema." Ann Thorac Surg 87(1): 229-236; discussion 236-227.

Wood, D. E., R. J. Cerfolio, et al. (2010). "Bronchoscopic management of prolonged air leak." Clin Chest Med 31(1): 127-133, Table of Contents.

Wood, D. E., R. J. McKenna, Jr., et al. (2007). "A multicenter trial of an intrabronchial valve for treatment of severe emphysema." J Thorac Cardiovasc Surg 133(1): 65-73.

Yamaguti, W. P., E. Paulin, et al. (2009). "Diaphragmatic dysfunction and mortality in patients with COPD." J Bras Pneumol 35(12): 1174-1181.

7

Mediastinal Parathyroidectomy: Preoperative Management of Hyperparathyroidism

Dariusz Sagan[1*], Jerzy S. Tarach[2], Andrzej Nowakowski[2], Maria Klatka[3],
Elżbieta Czekajska-Chehab[4], Andrzej Drop[4],
Beata Chrapko[5] and Janusz Klatka[6]

[1]*Department of Thoracic Surgery,*
[2]*Department of Endocrinology,*
[3]*Department of Paediatric Endocrinology and Neurology,*
[4]*1st Department of Radiology,*
[5]*Department of Nuclear Medicine,*
[6]*Department of Otolaryngology and Laryngeal Oncology,*
Medical University of Lublin,
Poland

1. Introduction

1.1 Anatomy and embryology of parathyroid glands

The normal parathyroid gland is oval or spherical in shape, has a distinct yellowish color, and averages 2x3x7 mm. The total mean weight of four normal parathyroids is about 150 mg. Majority of the population have four parathyroid glands typically located at the posterior capsule of the thyroid gland (Fig. 1; Fig.2), however in nearly 15% of individuals more than four glands are present. Phylogenetically, the parathyroid glands appear in amphibia, and arise from pharyngeal pouches III and IV. They may be arrested in the development as high as

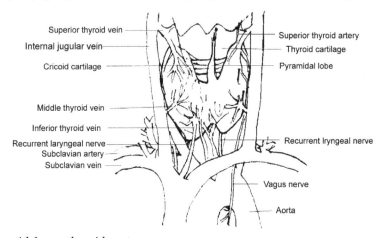

Fig. 1. Thyroid & parathyroid anatomy

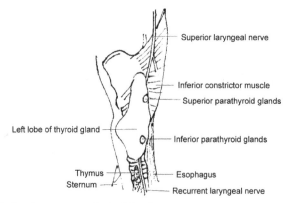

Fig. 2. Parathyroid glands anatomy. Left side view

at the level of the hyoid bone on the way of their descent to their typical location. Occasionally, parathyroids may be incorporated into the thyroid gland or thymus (intrathyroidal or mediastinal location). Lower (inferior) parathyroid glands (parathyroid III) may be found in the anterior mediastinum, while the upper (superior) parathyroids (parathyroid IV) usually remain in close association with the upper portion of the lateral thyroid lobes but may descend caudally along the esophagus into the posterior mediastinum (Fig. 3).

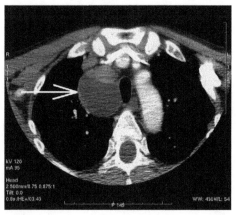

Fig. 3. Computed tomography scan showing a large mediastinal parathyroid adenoma (indicated with an arrow)

The parathyroid glands may lie in front of or behind the internal jugular vein and common carotid artery. Parathyroids are usually supplied by a branch of the inferior thyroid artery but may be supplied by the superior thyroid or, rarely, the thyroid ima arteries. The vessels can be seen entering a hilum-like structure, a feature that may be practically utilized to differentiate parathyroid glands from fat.

2. Physiology

Parathyroid glands secrete parathyroid hormone (PTH), which together with vitamin D, and calcitonin plays a vital role in precise regulation of calcium and phosphorus metabolism in bone, kidney, and gut. PTH and calcitonin work in concert to regulate plasma levels of ionized calcium. Fall in the ionized calcium level stimulates the parathyroids to secrete more PTH, and inhibits the parafollicular cells within the thyroid to produce less calcitonin. The rise in PTH and fall in calcitonin stimulate increased resorption of calcium in the renal tubules and from bones, thus more calcium enters the blood, and ionized calcium levels normalize. PTH in the blood stream is heterogeneous and consists of the intact hormone, the amino terminal (N-terminal) fragment and the carboxyl terminal (C-terminal) fragment. C-terminal fragment is biologically inert, whereas N-terminal fragment maintains hormonal activity, however substantially lower than the intact hormone. Currently available diagnostic tests are capable of intact hormone level determination, which is important for reliability of the measurement in particular for intraoperative use.

3. Primary hyperparathyroidism

Primary hyperparathyroidism is a disease characterized by autonomous overproduction of PTH resulting in hypercalcemia. In majority of cases it is caused by a single parathyroid adenoma (80-85%), and less frequently by hyperplasia (10%), multiple adenomas (6%), or carcinoma (1%). Currently, primary hyperparathyroidism occurs in 0.1-0.3% of the general population and in unselected patients is considered the most common cause of hypercalcemia. It is almost three times more common in women than in men, with peak incidence between the third and fifth decades.

Excess production of PTH results in mobilization of calcium from bone and inhibition of the renal reabsorption of phosphate, leading to hypercalcemia and hypophosphatemia. Besides, it causes a wasting of calcium and phosphorus, which eventually may result in osseous mineral loss and osteoporosis. Other conditions which may be associated with hyperparathyroidism include nephrocalcinosis, nephrolithiasis, osteitis fibrosa cystica, pancreatitis, peptic ulcer, hypertension, and gout. Diagnosis of any of these diseases should evoke suspicion for hyperparathyroidism and the patient should be referred for more precise tests.

Hyperparathyroidism is occasionally associated with multiple endocrine neoplasia (MEN) type 1, or type 2. MEN type 1 is characterized by tumors of the parathyroid, pituitary, and pancreas (hyperparathyroidism, pituitary tumors, and islet cell pancreatic tumors) that may lead to gastrinoma (Zollinger-Ellison syndrome), glucagonoma, insulinoma (hypoglycemia), somatostatinoma, lipoma and pancreatic polypeptide tumors (PPomas). Adrenocortical tumors, carcinoid tumors, and multiple lipomas have also been reported in these patients. MEN type 2 is divided into 2 subtypes: MEN 2a and MEN 2b. MEN 2a is characterized by hyperparathyroidism associated with pheochromocytoma and thyroid medullary carcinoma. Hyperparathyroidism is rare in MEN 2b patients who often have multiple neuromas and a marfanoid habitus.

Parathyroid adenomas may range in weight from 65 mg to over 35 g, but occasionally the weight of these tumors may exceed 35g. Usually the size of the tumor parallels the degree of hypercalcemia (the larger the tumor, the more severe hypercalcemia). Microscopic examination of parathyroid adenomas shows chief cell, water cell, or, rarely, oxyphil cell type.

Primary parathyroid hyperplasia may be another cause of hyperparathyroidism. This condition involves all of the parathyroid glands, which vary considerably in size but are usually larger than normal. Microscopic examination may reveal two types: chief cell hyperplasia and water-clear cell hyperplasia. Parathyroid carcinoma is rare but usually leads to severe hypercalcemia, and should be suspected at operation when the parathyroid gland is hard, has a whitish or irregular capsule, or shows signs of invasiveness. Rupture of the parathyroid tumor or breaching of the tumor capsule during rough dissection may result in seeding hyperactive tissue. This, and less frequently multiple embryologic rests may lead to a rare condition called parathyromatosis characterized by persistent hypercalcemia.

4. Signs and symptoms

Clinical signs and symptoms of hyperparathyroidism range from barely recognizable by patients, like muscle fatigablility, weakness, psychiatric disturbances, constipations, polydipsja and polyuria to severely impairing normal activities, like bone and muscle pains, nephrolithiasis, nephrocalcinosis, hypertension, peptic ulcer, pancreatitis or gout. Osteitis fibrosa cystica with bone pains and deformities, which was a prevailing symptom in patients with hyperparathyroidism a few decades ago, now became less frequent because majority of cases are detected early in the course of the disease. Also the incidence of renal complications decreased markedly and many patients are diagnosed by routine screening while still asymptomatic.

5. Laboratory tests

Serum calcium, parathyroid hormone and phosphates level are the principal laboratory tests used for the diagnosis of hyperparathyroidism. Elevated serum calcium and low phosphates are highly suggestive of hyperparathyroidism, however in about 50% of patients serum phosphates level is normal. Measurement of serum intact parathyroid hormone (PTH) concentration is the key test in diagnostic workout for patients with hypercalcemia, because the PTH level is low or nil in all cases except for those caused by primary hyperparathyroidism and familial hypocalciuric hypercalcemia, where PTH is markedly elevated.

Complementary laboratory tests include chlorides, protein electrophoretic pattern, alkaline phosphatase, creatinine, uric acid and urea nitrogen, urinary calcium, blood hematocrite and pH, serum magnesium and ESR. Sometimes, when previous tests are equivocal, measurement of nephrogenous cAMP, 1,25-hydroxy vitamin D levels and tubular resorption of phosphates may be helpful. Serum chloride concentration is elevated in nearly half of patients with hyperparathyroidism and may be a useful diagnostic clue. It's due to direct influence of PTH on the proximal renal tubule decreasing the resorption of bicarbonate, which leads to increased resorption of chloride. Other causes of hypercalcemia do not give rise in chloride concentration.

6. Secondary hyperparathyroidism

Secondary hyperparathyroidism (sHPT) is a condition characterized by excess secretion of parathyroid hormone stimulated by external factors, mainly hypocalcemia. Chronic renal failure is the most common cause of secondary hyperparathyroidism, as it results in hypocalcemia due to impaired conversion of vitamin D into active form, and excessive loss of calcium with urine. Sporadically sHPT may be caused by malabsorption, like chronic pancreatitis, small bowel disease or malabsorbtion-dependent bariatric surgery. Prolonged stimulation of parathyroid tissue by hypocalcemia results in enlargement of parathyroids in the form of their hyperplasia and less frequently parathyroid adenoma.

7. Tertiary hyperparathyroidism

Tertiary hyperparathyroidism (tHPT) is a condition of autonomic excessive secretion of parathyroid hormone developing from secondary parathyroidism, that maintains despite restoration of renal function. It is caused by development of autonomous (unregulated) parathyroid function following a prolonged period of persistent parathyroid stimulation. It is no longer responsive to treatment by medication and requires surgical removal of three and a half parathyroid glands.

8. Indications for surgical treatment

Parathyroidectomy is currently recognized as the treatment of choice for patients with primary hyperparathyroidism. For virtually all these patients surgical resection of hyperactive parathyroid tissue is curative. It provides both metabolic improvement and symptoms relief. Medical observation is contraindicated. Furthermore, parathyroidectomy is recommended as early as possible in the course of the disease because once systemic complications such as renal dysfunction or hypertension develop, they tend to progress despite elimination of the underlying hyperparathyroidism.

9. Preoperative imaging techniques

Various techniques are currently available for parathyroid glands imaging. Noninvasive studies include ultrasonography, scintigraphy, computed tomography (CT) scanning, and magnetic resonance imaging (MRI). Scintigraphy with use of the radiopharmaceuticals technetium ^{99m}Tc sestamibi or technetium ^{99m}Tc tetrofosmin is widely recommended as the preferred imaging technique for parathyroids. Parathyroid selective arteriography or selective parathyroid venous sampling have been used occasionally as invasive techniques in select cases.

9.1 Ultrasonography

Parathyroid ultrasonography is currently the most easily accessible and a relatively inexpensive non-invasive test that is routinely used for the assessment of the thyroid and parathyroid glands. It is utilized for preoperative investigation in patients with hyperparathyroidism not only to localize and visualize enlarged parathyroids, but also to rule out thyroid nodules that may need to be evaluated prior to parathyroid surgery. For best results a high-frequency (7.5- or 10-MHz) linear ultrasound transducer should be available. The patient should be supine with the neck moderately hyperextended. It is recommended to start the evaluation from the carotid bifurcation superiorly and proceed down to the sternal notch inferiorly and to the carotid artery laterally.

Normal parathyroids are barely visualized with ultrasonography. Parathyroid adenomas appear on gray-scale images as hypoechoic or anechoic, discrete, oval masses. They are located posterior to the lobe of the thyroid gland and anterior to the longus colli muscles. Usually, the common carotid artery confines the parathyroid-bearing region laterally. An echogenic line separating the thyroid tissue from the enlarged parathyroid gland can be often visualized. Cystic changes, lobulations, increased echogenicity due to fatty deposition, and occasional calcifications are more frequent in larger adenomas.

Parathyroid adenomas, in particular lesions larger than 1 cm in diameter, tend to be hypervascular, and therefore color Doppler ultrasonography is useful in localizing these enlarged glands. Besides, Doppler ultrasound can easily disclose the extrathyroidal vessel supplying parathyroid and this finding may constitute a road map to the otherwise inconspicuous gland.

Ultrasonography is efficient in diagnosing cervical parathyroid lesions with reported sensitivity up to 80% and specificity up to 90%, but fails to detect majority of parathyroid adenomas located in the mediastinum. Additionally, intrathyroidal lesions cannot be differentiated as a parathyroid adenoma or thyroid nodule based on imaging only, and a biopsy is required.

9.2 ^{99m}Tc sestamibi imaging

Nuclear imaging with use of ^{99m}Technetium (^{99m}Tc) sestamibi is currently approved as a standard technique for preoperative imaging of parathyroid glands. ^{99m}Tc sestamibi is a complex of the radioisotope technetium-^{99m}Tc with the ligand methoxyisobutylisonitrile (MIBI). ^{99m}Tc sestamibi, first applied as a myocardial perfusion agent, for parathyroids assessment is combined with either sodium iodide I^{123} or ^{99m}Tc pertechnetate in a procedure called subtraction scintigraphy. It is based on a fenomenon that ^{99m}Tc sestamibi is accumulated by both thyroid and abnormal parathyroids, whereas sodium iodide I^{123} and ^{99m}Tc pertechnetate are taken up by only thyroid tissue. To visualize parathyroids and differentiate them from thyroid tissue the sodium iodide I^{123} or ^{99m}Tc -pertechnetate image is subtracted from the ^{99m}Tc-sestamibi image.

Another, more recent imaging modality is the dual-phase technique with ^{99m}Tc sestamibi as the sole imaging agent. Both thyroid tissue and abnormal parathyroid tissue incorporate ^{99m}Tc sestamibi from circulating blood rapidly after intravenous administration. The test is based on the differential washout of ^{99m}Tc sestamibi from thyroid compared with abnormal parathyroids. The rate of washout from hyperactive parathyroid tissue, such as parathyroid adenoma, is much slower than that of normal thyroid tissue. Routine protocol includes intravenous administration of 20mCi of ^{99m}Tc Sestamibi and sequential acquisition of early and delayed images of the neck and upper mediastinum. The early image, obtained 10-15 minutes after the injection, is called the thyroid phase as ^{99m}Tc sestamibi is rapidly taken up in the thyroid gland at this time. 1.5-3 hours after the injection the delayed image called the parathyroid phase is recorded. At this phase, ^{99m}Tc sestamibi has been washed out from thyroid but remains accumulated in the hyperactive parathyroid tissue, and this allows for localization of abnormal parathyroid glands. Planar images may be complemented with lateral or oblique acquisitions, or even SPECT images when appropriate equipment is applied. Sensitivity of the ^{99m}Tc sestamibi dual phase protocol has been reported to achieve 70-100%. Small or pedunculated, mobile adenomas may, however, be missed at this test.

^{99m}Tc sestamibi may also be used in minimally invasive parathyroid surgery, as an intraoperative adjunct facilitating localization of hyperactive parathyroid adenoma and confirming curative resection. The radionuclide is injected 1.5 to 3 hours prior to surgery, and a hand-held gamma probe is used to guide the incision, localize the abnormal gland and confirm identity of the resected parathyroid tissue ex-vivo. This technique called intraoperative nuclear mapping proved to be successful, and is a standard procedure in a number of centers.

99mTc tetrofosmin is another radiopharmaceutical agent recently introduced into parathyroid imaging. It has a slightly different mechanism of accumulation in tissues, but imaging characteristics similar to those of 99mTc sestamibi. Also imaging protocols are similar with intravenous injections of 20-25 mCi of radionuclide prior to early (10-30 minutes) and delayed (1.5-3 hours) acquisition images.

9.3 Computed tomography (CT) scanning

Assessment of parathyroid glands with use of a typical CT protocol involves the acquisition of contiguous axial 2- to 3-mm images ranging from the hyoid bone down to the carina. Nonenhanced images of parathyroid adenomas have an attenuation similar to that of muscle. Substantial degree of enhancement is usually shown in parathyroid adenomas after administration of contrast material, as these lesions tend to be hypervascular structures. Typically, parathyroid adenomas present at CT as enlarged, enhancing, soft-tissue masses in the expected location of the parathyroids. The sensitivity of CT in detecting parathyroid adenomas attains 90%. However, the use of ionizing radiation and required intravenous administration of contrast material accompanied by associated risks are considered remarkable disadvantages of this imaging technique. Besides, thyroid nodule, tortuous vessel, or laterally displaced esophagus may be misidentified as a false-positive finding, whereas small or ectopic lesion, poor visualization of neck structures or distorted neck anatomy due to prior surgery may lead to false-negative result.

9.4 Magnetic resonance imaging

MRI is occasionally used for parathyroid imaging. A typical MRI protocol for the assessment of parathyroids involves axial images of the neck and mediastinum. Images are acquired using T1-weighted spin-echo sequences (short recovery time [TR], short echo time [TE]) followed by T2-weighted spin-echo sequences (long TR, long TE). Parathyroid adenomas are seen on MRI images as soft-tissue masses, whereas normal parathyroids are usually not detected. Parathyroid adenomas commonly have low-to-medium signal intensity on T1-weighted images and high signal intensity on T2-weighted images. After gadolinium contrast administration, abnormal parathyroid glands show strong enhancement on T1-weighted images, comparable to conventional T2-weighted imaging.

9.5 Parathyroid arteriography and venous sampling

Parathyroid arteriography and parathyroid venous sampling are invasive tests burdened by a remarkable risk of embolic stroke and spinal cord injury, and therefore should be considered only when the findings of noninvasive imaging modalities are nondiagnostic. Parathyroid adenomas, like many endocrine tumors, tend to be hypervascular and have a characteristic appearance on angiograms. They appear as round or oval lesions with smooth margins and dense vascular blush. Localization of parathyroid adenoma may be visualized with use of digital subtraction angiography (DSA) and/or conventional arteriography. Thyrocervical trunks and common carotid arteries should be subject to selective arteriography in typical cases. Ectopic mediastinal or thymic glands may be better identified by examination of internal thoracic arteries.

Selective venous sampling with parathyroid hormone measurement may be performed to determine the general location of hypersecreting parathyroid tissue. Right and left thymic veins, inferior thyroid veins, and vertebral veins have been reported to be sampled in this regimen. A 2-fold gradient in PTH concentration in the sampled vein as referenced to that of the peripheral vein confirms the location of hyperactive parathyroid tissue. Similar technique may also be used intraoperatively to confirm curative resection of parathyroid adenoma.

10. Preoperative anesthetic management

Since renal function is likely to be impaired in hyperparathyroidism, prior to surgical treatment hypercalcemic patients require thorough rehydration. In some of these patients urinary catheterization and central venous pressure monitoring may be indicated. After rehydration, loop diuretics may be administered to decrease renal calcium reabsorption and promote urinary excretion, which in result will alleviate hypercalcaemia. Excessive diuresis may in turn lead to increased maintenance fluid requirements. Corticosteroids, bisphosphonates, calcium chelators such as trisodium edentate, calcitonin, or even dialysis are occasionally indicated in severe cases. Hypertension, if present, should be controlled with fast-acting antihypertensive medication. In patients with end-stage renal failure, perioperative invasive central venous pressure monitoring may be helpful for thorough monitoring of circulatory system. Occasionally, tumors of other organs may secrete PTH, for example, bronchial or tracheal carcinomas. This condition is called pseudohyperparathyroidism and should be brought to attention preoperatively to avoid intreaoperative ventilatory problems in theses rare cases when the lesion occludes bronchial or tracheal lumen.

11. References

[1] Fernández-Fernández FJ, Sesma P. Primary hyperparathyroidism. N Engl J Med. 2012 Mar 1;366(9):860; author reply 860-1.

[2] Afzal A, Gauhar TM, Butt WT, Khawaja AA, Azim KM. Management of hyperparathyroidism: a five year surgical experience. J Pak Med Assoc. 2011 Dec;61(12):1194-8.

[3] Wang CC, Hsu YJ, Wu CC, Yang SS, Chen GS, Lin SH, Chu P. Serum fetuin-A levels increased following parathyroidectomy in uremic hyperparathyroidism. Clin Nephrol. 2012 Feb;77(2):89-96. doi: 10.10.5414/CN106757.

[4] Emilion E, Emilion R. Estimation of the 25(OH) vitamin D threshold below which secondary hyperparathyroidism may occur among African migrant women in Paris. Int J Vitam Nutr Res. 2011 Jul;81(4):218-24.

[5] Francucci CM, Ceccoli L, Caudarella R, Rilli S, Vescini F, Boscaro M. Asymptomatic primary hyperparathyroidism: surgical and medical management. J Endocrinol Invest. 2011 Jul;34(7 Suppl):50-4.

[6] Nuti R, Merlotti D, Gennari L. Vitamin D deficiency and primary hyperparathyroidism. J Endocrinol Invest. 2011 Jul;34(7 Suppl):45-9. Review.

[7] Pepe J, Cipriani C, Pilotto R, De Lucia F, Castro C, Lenge L, Russo S, Guarnieri V, Scillitani A, Carnevale V, D'Erasmo E, Romagnoli E, Minisola S. Sporadic and

hereditary primary hyperparathyroidism. J Endocrinol Invest. 2011 Jul;34(7 Suppl):40-4. Review.

[8] Cetani F, Pardi E, Borsari S, Marcocci C. Molecular pathogenesis of primary hyperparathyroidism. J Endocrinol Invest. 2011 Jul;34(7 Suppl):35-9. Review.

[9] Francucci CM, Ghigo E, Boscaro M. Primary hyperparathyroidism and skeleton. Foreword. J Endocrinol Invest. 2011 Jul;34(7 Suppl):1-2.

[10] Ardito G, Revelli L, Giustozzi E, Giordano A. Radioguided parathyroidectomy in forearm graft for recurrent hyperparathyroidism. Br J Radiol. 2012 Jan;85(1009):e1-3.

[11] Peiris AN, Youssef D, Grant WB. Secondary hyperparathyroidism: benign bystander or culpable contributor to adverse health outcomes? South Med J. 2012 Jan;105(1):36-42. Review.

[12] Marcocci C, Cetani F. Clinical practice. Primary hyperparathyroidism. N Engl J Med. 2011 Dec 22;365(25):2389-97.

[13] Piedra M, García-Unzueta MT, Berja A, Paule B, Lavín BA, Valero C, Riancho JA, Amado JA. "Single nucleotide polymorphisms of the OPG/RANKL system genes in primary hyperparathyroidism and their relationship with bone mineral density". BMC Med Genet. 2011 Dec 20;12:168.

[14] Duh QY. The Bayes theorem wins: comment on "Impact of localization studies and clinical scenario in patients with hyperparathyroidism being evaluated for reoperative neck surgery". Arch Surg. 2011 Dec;146(12):1403.

[15] Shin JJ, Milas M, Mitchell J, Berber E, Ross L, Siperstein A. Impact of localization studies and clinical scenario in patients with hyperparathyroidism being evaluated for reoperative neck surgery. Arch Surg. 2011 Dec;146(12):1397-403.

[16] Sorensen MD, Duh QY, Grogan RH, Tran TC, Stoller ML. Urinary parameters as predictors of primary hyperparathyroidism in patients with nephrolithiasis. J Urol. 2012 Feb;187(2):516-21. Epub 2011 Dec 15.

[17] Shlapack MA, Rizvi AA. Normocalcemic primary hyperparathyroidism-characteristics and clinical significance of an emerging entity. Am J Med Sci. 2012 Feb;343(2):163-6. Review.

[18] Bhadada SK, Bhansali A, Shah VN, Rao DS. Changes in serum leptin and adiponectin concentrations and insulin resistance after curative parathyroidectomy in moderate to severe primary hyperparathyroidism. Singapore Med J. 2011 Dec;52(12):890-3.

[19] Wang TS, Cheung K, Farrokhyar F, Roman SA, Sosa JA. Would scan, but which scan? A cost-utility analysis to optimize preoperative imaging for primary hyperparathyroidism. Surgery. 2011 Dec;150(6):1286-94.

[20] Perrier ND, Evans DB. Population-level predictors of persistent hyperparathyroidism. Surgery. 2011 Dec;150(6):1120-1.

[21] Yeh MW, Wiseman JE, Chu SD, Ituarte PH, Liu IL, Young KL, Kang SJ, Harari A, Haigh PI. Population-level predictors of persistent hyperparathyroidism. Surgery. 2011 Dec;150(6):1113-9.

[22] Wallace LB, Parikh RT, Ross LV, Mazzaglia PJ, Foley C, Shin JJ, Mitchell JC, Berber E, Siperstein AE, Milas M. The phenotype of primary hyperparathyroidism with normal parathyroid hormone levels: how low can parathyroid hormone go? Surgery. 2011 Dec;150(6):1102-12.

[23] Press D, Politz D, Lopez J, Norman J. The effect of vitamin D levels on postoperative calcium requirements, symptomatic hypocalcemia, and parathormone levels following parathyroidectomy for primary hyperparathyroidism. Surgery. 2011 Dec;150(6):1061-8.

[24] Mshelia DS, Hatutale AN, Mokgoro NP, Nchabaleng ME, Buscombe JR, Sathekge MM. Correlation between serum calcium levels and dual-phase (99m)Tc-sestamibi parathyroid scintigraphy in primary hyperparathyroidism. Clin Physiol Funct Imaging. 2012 Jan;32(1):19-24. doi: 10.1111/j.1475-097X.2011.01048.x. Epub 2011 Aug 24.

[25] Lumachi F, Camozzi V, Luisetto G, Zanella S, Basso SM. Arterial blood pressure, serum calcium and PTH in elderly men with parathyroid tumors and primary hyperparathyroidism. Anticancer Res. 2011 Nov;31(11):3969-72.

[26] El-Shafey EM, Alsahow AE, Alsaran K, Sabry AA, Atia M. Cinacalcet hydrochloride therapy for secondary hyperparathyroidism in hemodialysis patients. Ther Apher Dial. 2011 Dec;15(6):547-55. doi: 10.1111/j.1744-9987.2011.00994.x.

[27] Cheungpasitporn W, Suksaranjit P, Chanprasert S. Acute kidney injury from bilateral ureteral calcium stones in the setting of primary hyperparathyroidism. Am J Emerg Med. 2012 Feb;30(2):383-4. Epub 2011 Nov 17.

[28] Schmidt MC, Kahraman D, Neumaier B, Ortmann M, Stippel D. Tc-99m-MIBI-negative parathyroid adenoma in primary hyperparathyroidism detected by C-11-methionine PET/CT after previous thyroid surgery. Clin Nucl Med. 2011 Dec;36(12):1153-5.

[29] Sanadgol H, Bayani M, Mohammadi M, Bayani B, Mashhadi MA. Effect of vitamin C on parathyroid hormone in hemodialysis patients with mild to moderate secondary hyperparathyroidism. Iran J Kidney Dis. 2011 Nov;5(6):410-5.

[30] Carneiro-Pla D, Solorzano C. A summary of the new phenomenon of normocalcemic hyperparathyroidism and appropriate management. Curr Opin Oncol. 2012 Jan;24(1):42-5.

[31] Suwan N. Secondary hyperparathyroidism and risk factors in patients undergoing peritoneal dialysis in a tertiary hospital. J Med Assoc Thai. 2011 Sep;94 Suppl 4:S101-5.

[32] Iwata S, Walker MD, Di Tullio MR, Hyodo E, Jin Z, Liu R, Sacco RL, Homma S, Silverberg SJ. Aortic valve calcification in mild primary hyperparathyroidism. J Clin Endocrinol Metab. 2012 Jan;97(1):132-7. Epub 2011 Oct 26.

[33] Amin AL, Wang TS, Wade TJ, Quiroz FA, Hellman RS, Evans DB, Yen TW. Nonlocalizing imaging studies for hyperparathyroidism: where to explore first? J Am Coll Surg. 2011 Dec;213(6):793-9. Epub 2011 Oct 19.

[34] Pilz S, Kienreich K, Drechsler C, Ritz E, Fahrleitner-Pammer A, Gaksch M, Meinitzer A, März W, Pieber TR, Tomaschitz A. Hyperparathyroidism in patients with primary aldosteronism: cross-sectional and interventional data from the GECOH study. J Clin Endocrinol Metab. 2012 Jan;97(1):E75-9. Epub 2011 Oct 19.

[35] Jabiev AA, Lew JI, Garb JL, Sanchez YM, Solorzano CC. Primary hyperparathyroidism in the underinsured: a study of 493 patients. Surgery. 2012 Mar;151(3):471-6. Epub 2011 Oct 13.

[36] Wilson SD, Doffek KM, Wang TS, Krzywda EA, Evans DB, Yen TW. Primary hyperparathyroidism with a history of head and neck irradiation: the consequences of associated thyroid tumors. Surgery. 2011 Oct;150(4):869-77.

[37] Lu KC, Wu CC, Ma WY, Chen CC, Wu HC, Chu P. Decreased blood lead levels after calcitriol treatment in hemodialysis patients with secondary hyperparathyroidism. Bone. 2011 Dec;49(6):1306-10. Epub 2011 Oct 1.

[38] Witteveen JE, van Lierop AH, Papapoulos SE, Hamdy NA. Increased circulating levels of FGF23: an adaptive response in primary hyperparathyroidism? Eur J Endocrinol. 2012 Jan;166(1):55-60. Epub 2011 Oct 7.

[39] Udelsman R. Approach to the patient with persistent or recurrent primary hyperparathyroidism. J Clin Endocrinol Metab. 2011 Oct;96(10):2950-8.

[40] Bollerslev J, Marcocci C, Sosa M, Nordenström J, Bouillon R, Mosekilde L. Current evidence for recommendation of surgery, medical treatment and vitamin D repletion in mild primary hyperparathyroidism. Eur J Endocrinol. 2011 Dec;165(6):851-64. Epub 2011 Sep 29.

[41] Adachi M, Miyoshi T, Shiraishi N, Shimada H, Sakaguchi S, Tomita K, Kitamura K. A study of maintenance therapy after intravenous maxacalcitol for secondary hyperparathyroidism. Clin Nephrol. 2011 Oct;76(4):266-72.

[42] Ishimura E, Okuno S, Tsuboniwa N, Ichii M, Yamakawa K, Yamakawa T, Shoji S, Nishizawa Y, Inaba M. Effect of cinacalcet on bone mineral density of the radius in hemodialysis patients with secondary hyperparathyroidism. Clin Nephrol. 2011 Oct;76(4):259-65.

[43] Shapey IM, Jaunoo SS, Hanson C, Jaunoo SR, Thrush S, Munro A. Primary hyperparathyroidism: how many cases are being missed? Ann R Coll Surg Engl. 2011 May;93(4):294-6.

[44] Pyram R, Mahajan G, Gliwa A. Primary hyperparathyroidism: Skeletal and non-skeletal effects, diagnosis and management. Maturitas. 2011 Nov;70(3):246-55. Epub 2011 Sep 23.

[45] Jithpratuck W, Garrett LH, Peiris AN. Treating vitamin D insufficiency in primary hyperparathyroidism: a cautionary tale. Tenn Med. 2011 Aug;104(7):47-9.

[46] Espiritu RP, Kearns AE, Vickers KS, Grant C, Ryu E, Wermers RA. Depression in primary hyperparathyroidism: prevalence and benefit of surgery. J Clin Endocrinol Metab. 2011 Nov;96(11):E1737-45. Epub 2011 Sep 14.

[47] Boucher BJ. Re Yu et al. The natural history of treated and untreated primary hyperparathyroidism: the Parathyroid Epidemiology and Audit Research Study. Q J Med 2011; 104:513-521. QJM. 2011 Dec;104(12):1107-8. Epub 2011 Sep 10.

[48] Sorensen MD, Duh QY, Grogan RH, Tran TC, Stoller ML. Differences in metabolic urinary abnormalities in stone forming and nonstone forming patients with primary hyperparathyroidism. Surgery. 2012 Mar;151(3):477-83. Epub 2011 Sep 3.

[49] Frazão JM, Messa P, Mellotte GJ, Geiger H, Hagen EC, Quarles LD, Kerr PG, Baños A, Dehmel B, Urena P. Cinacalcet reduces plasma intact parathyroid hormone, serum phosphate and calcium levels in patients with secondary hyperparathyroidism irrespective of its severity. Clin Nephrol. 2011 Sep;76(3):233-43.

[50] Stephani J, Akinli AS, von Figura G, Barth TF, Weber T, Hartmann B, Adler G, von Boyen GB. Acute Pancreatitis in a patient with hypercalcemia due to tertiary hyperparathyroidism. Z Gastroenterol. 2011 Sep;49(9):1263-6. Epub 2011 Sep 1.

[51] Kovesdy CP, Lu JL, Malakauskas SM, Andress DL, Kalantar-Zadeh K, Ahmadzadeh S. Paricalcitol versus ergocalciferol for secondary hyperparathyroidism in CKD stages 3 and 4: a randomized controlled trial. Am J Kidney Dis. 2012 Jan;59(1):58-66. Epub 2011 Aug 31.

[52] Hoi WH, Leow MK, Sule A, Lee HY, Mmed TA, Tay JC. Hyperparathyroidism due to eutopic PTH secretion from an ectopic intrathymic parathyroid cyst. Ann Thorac Cardiovasc Surg. 2011 Oct 25;17(5):511-3. Epub 2011 Jul 13.

[53] Zitt E, Woess E, Mayer G, Lhotta K. Effect of cinacalcet on renal electrolyte handling and systemic arterial blood pressure in kidney transplant patients with persistent hyperparathyroidism. Transplantation. 2011 Oct 27;92(8):883-9.

[54] Macfarlane DP, Yu N, Donnan PT, Leese GP. Should 'mild primary hyperparathyroidism' be reclassified as 'insidious': is it time to reconsider? Clin Endocrinol (Oxf). 2011 Dec;75(6):730-7. doi: 10.1111/j.1365-2265.2011.04201.x.

[55] Lucchi L, Carboni C, Stipo L, Malaguti V, Ferrari F, Graziani R, Arletti S, Graziosi C. Early initiation of cinacalcet for the treatment of secondary hyperparathyroidism in hemodialysis patients: a three-year clinical experience. Artif Organs. 2011 Dec;35(12):1186-93. doi: 10.1111/j.1525-1594.2011.01270.x. Epub 2011 Aug 17.

[56] Plosker GL. Cinacalcet: a pharmacoeconomic review of its use in secondary hyperparathyroidism in end-stage renal disease. Pharmacoeconomics. 2011 Sep;29(9):807-21. doi: 10.2165/11207220-000000000-00000.

[57] Akizawa T, Kido R, Fukagawa M, Onishi Y, Yamaguchi T, Hasegawa T, Fukuhara S, Kurokawa K. Decreases in PTH in Japanese hemodialysis patients with secondary hyperparathyroidism: associations with changing practice patterns. Clin J Am Soc Nephrol. 2011 Sep;6(9):2280-8. Epub 2011 Aug 11.

[58] Hansen D, Rasmussen K, Danielsen H, Meyer-Hofmann H, Bacevicius E, Lauridsen TG, Madsen JK, Tougaard BG, Marckmann P, Thye-Roenn P, Nielsen JE, Kreiner S, Brandi L. No difference between alfacalcidol and paricalcitol in the treatment of secondary hyperparathyroidism in hemodialysis patients: a randomized crossover trial. Kidney Int. 2011 Oct;80(8):841-50. doi: 10.1038/ki.2011.226. Epub 2011 Aug 10.

[59] Kırış A, Erem C, Kırış G, Nuhoğlu I, Karaman K, Civan N, Örem C, Durmuş I, Kutlu M. The assessment of left ventricular systolic asynchrony in patients with primary hyperparathyroidism. Echocardiography. 2011 Oct;28(9):955-60. doi: 10.1111/j.1540-8175.2011.01468.x. Epub 2011 Aug 9.

[60] Maniero C, Fassina A, Guzzardo V, Lenzini L, Amadori G, Pelizzo MR, Gomez-Sanchez C, Rossi GP. Primary hyperparathyroidism with concurrent primary aldosteronism. Hypertension. 2011 Sep;58(3):341-6. Epub 2011 Aug 8.

[61] Islam MZ, Viljakainen HT, Kärkkäinen MU, Saarnio E, Laitinen K, Lamberg-Allardt C. Prevalence of vitamin D deficiency and secondary hyperparathyroidism during winter in pre-menopausal Bangladeshi and Somali immigrant and ethnic Finnish women: associations with forearm bone mineral density. Br J Nutr. 2012 Jan;107(2):277-83. Epub 2011 Aug 9.

[62] Padmanabhan H. Outpatient management of primary hyperparathyroidism. Am J Med. 2011 Oct;124(10):911-4. Epub 2011 Aug 3.

[63] Rudofsky G, Tsioga M, Reismann P, Leowardi C, Kopf S, Grafe IA, Nawroth PP, Isermann B. Transient hyperthyroidism after surgery for secondary hyperparathyroidism: a common problem. Eur J Med Res. 2011 Aug 8;16(8):375-80.

[64] Jain SK, Roy SP, Nagi ON. Alendronate induced femur fracture complicated with secondary hyperparathyroidism. Mymensingh Med J. 2011 Jul;20(3):501-6.

[65] Park JH, Kang SW, Jeong JJ, Nam KH, Chang HS, Chung WY, Park CS. Surgical treatment of tertiary hyperparathyroidism after renal transplantation: a 31-year experience in a single institution. Endocr J. 2011 Oct 29;58(10):827-33. Epub 2011 Jul 30.

[66] Isaksen T, Nielsen CS, Christensen SE, Nissen PH, Heickendorff L, Mosekilde L. Forearm bone mineral density in familial hypocalciuric hypercalcemia and primary hyperparathyroidism: a comparative study. Calcif Tissue Int. 2011 Oct;89(4):285-94. doi: 10.1007/s00223-011-9517-x. Epub 2011 Jul 22.

[67] Lieberman SM, Vouyiouklis M, Elangovan S, Morris LG. Image of the month. Tertiary hyperparathyroidism after parathyroidectomy with autotransplantation. Arch Surg. 2011 Jul;146(7):879-80.

[68] Bellavia M, Gioviale MC, Damiano G, Palumbo VD, Cacciabaudo F, Altomare R Buscemi G, Lo Monte AI. Is secondary hyperparathyroidism-related myelofibrosis a negative prognostic factor for kidney transplant outcome? Med Hypotheses. 2011 Oct;77(4):557-9. Epub 2011 Jul 16.

[69] Agorastos A, Weinas A, Agorastos AD, Wiedemann K. Psychosis-induced vitamin D deficiency with secondary hyperparathyroidism and osteoporotic fractures. Gen Hosp Psychiatry. 2011 Nov-Dec;33(6):641.e3-5. Epub 2011 Jul 16.

[70] Nagar S, Reid D, Czako P, Long G, Shanley C. Outcomes analysis of intraoperative adjuncts during minimally invasive parathyroidectomy for primary hyperparathyroidism. Am J Surg. 2012 Feb;203(2):177-81. Epub 2011 Jul 14.

[71] De Rosa A, Rinaldi C, Tucci T, Pappatà S, Rossi F, Morra VB, Faggiano A, Colao A, De Michele G. Co-existence of primary hyperparathyroidism and Parkinson's disease in three patients: an incidental finding? Parkinsonism Relat Disord. 2011 Dec;17(10):771-3. Epub 2011 Jul 5.

[72] Bargren AE, Repplinger D, Chen H, Sippel RS. Can biochemical abnormalities predict symptomatology in patients with primary hyperparathyroidism? J Am Coll Surg. 2011 Sep;213(3):410-4. Epub 2011 Jul 1.

[73] Meola M, Petrucci I, Colombini E, Barsotti G. Use of ultrasound to assess the response to therapy for secondary hyperparathyroidism. Am J Kidney Dis. 2011 Sep;58(3):485-91. Epub 2011 Jun 29.

[74] Schreinemakers JM, Pieterman CR, Scholten A, Vriens MR, Valk GD, Rinkes IH. The optimal surgical treatment for primary hyperparathyroidism in MEN1 patients: a systematic review. World J Surg. 2011 Sep;35(9):1993-2005.

[75] Alhefdhi A, Pinchot SN, Davis R, Sippel RS, Chen H. The necessity and reliability of intraoperative parathyroid hormone (PTH) testing in patients with mild hyperparathyroidism and PTH levels in the normal range. World J Surg. 2011 Sep;35(9):2006-9.

[76] Ikegami S, Kamimura M, Uchiyama S, Kato H. Women with insufficient 25-hydroxyvitamin D without secondary hyperparathyroidism have altered bone turnover and greater incidence of vertebral fractures. J Orthop Sci. 2011 Sep;16(5):573-80. Epub 2011 Jun 29.

[77] van Ginhoven TM, Morks AN, Schepers T, de Graaf PW, Smit PC. Surgeon-performed ultrasound as preoperative localization study in patients with primary hyperparathyroidism. Eur Surg Res. 2011;47(2):70-4. Epub 2011 Jun 23.

[78] Christensen MH, Dankel SN, Nordbø Y, Varhaug JE, Almås B, Lien EA, Mellgren G. Primary hyperparathyroidism influences the expression of inflammatory and metabolic genes in adipose tissue. PLoS One. 2011;6(6):e20481. Epub 2011 Jun 17.

[79] Stubbs JR, Wetmore JB. Does it matter how parathyroid hormone levels are suppressed in secondary hyperparathyroidism? Semin Dial. 2011 May-Jun;24(3):298-306. doi: 10.1111/j.1525-139X.2011.00935.x.

[80] Fujii T, Yamaguchi S, Yajima R, Tsutsumi S, Uchida N, Asao T, Oriuch N, Kuwano H. Use of a handheld, semiconductor (cadmium zinc telluride)-based gamma camera in navigation surgery for primary hyperparathyroidism. Am Surg. 2011 Jun;77(6):690-3.

[81] Kaji H, Imanishi Y, Sugimoto T, Seino S. Comparisons of serum sclerostin levels among patients with postmenopausal osteoporosis, primary hyperparathyroidism and osteomalacia. Exp Clin Endocrinol Diabetes. 2011 Jul;119(7):440-4. doi: 10.1055/s-0031-1275661. Epub 2011 Jun 10.

[82] Frank-Raue K, Haag C, Schulze E, Keuser R, Raue F, Dralle H, Lorenz K. CDC73-related hereditary hyperparathyroidism: five new mutations and the clinical spectrum. Eur J Endocrinol. 2011 Sep;165(3):477-83. Epub 2011 Jun 7.

[83] Rejnmark L, Vestergaard P, Mosekilde L. Nephrolithiasis and renal calcifications in primary hyperparathyroidism. J Clin Endocrinol Metab. 2011 Aug;96(8):2377-85. Epub 2011 Jun 6.

[84] Schillaci G, Pucci G, Pirro M, Monacelli M, Scarponi AM, Manfredelli MR, Rondelli F, Avenia N, Mannarino E. Large-artery stiffness: a reversible marker of cardiovascular risk in primary hyperparathyroidism. Atherosclerosis. 2011 Sep;218(1):96-101. Epub 2011 May 18.

[85] Mannstadt M, Holick E, Zhao W, Jüppner H. Mutational analysis of GCMB, a parathyroid-specific transcription factor, in parathyroid adenoma of primary hyperparathyroidism. J Endocrinol. 2011 Aug;210(2):165-71. Epub 2011 Jun 3.

8

Pulmonary Transplantation and Ischemia-Reperfusion Injury

Ashish K. Sharma, Matthew L. Stone,
Christine L. Lau and Victor E. Laubach
University of Virginia Health System, Charlottesville, VA,
USA

1. Introduction

Lung transplantation provides a curative hope for many with end-stage pulmonary disease. Since the first attempt at human lung transplantation in 1963, scientific and surgical advancements have supported improved survival and quality of life for lung transplant recipients (Hardy, et al., 1963). Significant contributions in cardiopulmonary bypass, pharmacologic immunosuppression, and donor-recipient risk stratification have increased the success and associated clinical adoption of this treatment strategy. Continued research efforts in novel methods for organ preservation, donor graft selection, and recipient risk stratification support a promising future for lung transplantation.

Improvements in surgical technique and perioperative care over the past two decades have led to a 30-fold increase in the number of lung transplant recipients worldwide to 2,769 patients in 2008 (Christie, et al., 2010). Since 1994, bilateral lung transplantation has supplanted single lung transplantation as the primary strategy for organ replacement to now account for 71% of lung transplants performed worldwide (Christie, et al., 2010). In 2010, the primary indications for lung transplantation included chronic obstructive pulmonary disease (35.5%), idiopathic pulmonary fibrosis (22.1%), and cystic fibrosis (16.0%) (Christie, et al., 2010). Despite this promising evolution and the increasing number of indications for lung transplantation, long-term survival has shown minimal improvement. Lung transplant outcomes remain the poorest of any solid organ transplant, with international survival estimates demonstrating a 21% one-year and 50% five-year mortality (Christie, et al., 2010).

Lung ischemia-reperfusion (IR) injury following transplantation imposes a significant threat to graft and recipient survival (Diamond & Christie, 2010). IR injury is the main cause of primary graft failure and significantly increases the risk for acute rejection and long-term graft dysfunction (de Perrot, et al., 2003). Multivariate analysis of long-term graft function has implicated IR injury as an independent predictor for bronchiolitis obliterans syndrome (BOS), the most common cause of long-term morbidity and mortality after lung transplantation (Fiser, et al., 2002). IR-induced lung injury is characterized by nonspecific alveolar damage, lung edema, and hypoxemia occurring within 72 hours after lung transplantation (de Perrot, et al., 2003). The estimated incidence of IR injury is 41% following lung transplantation with an associated 30-day mortality of 40%, compared to 7% for patients with no IR injury (Granton, 2006). Clinical studies have demonstrated increased in-hospital mortality and morbidity associated with IR injury resulting in prolonged ventilation, postoperative systolic pulmonary hypertension, longer intensive care unit stay, and increased cost of hospitalization (Cottini, et al., 2006; King, et al., 2000).

Currently no clinical therapies are available to prevent IR injury. The standard method used to help minimize IR injury for lung transplantation incorporates a universal cold crystalloid flush of the donor organ prior to explantation. Cold storage on ice during the preservation period limits metabolic activity, vasospasm, and thrombosis (Puri & Patterson, 2008). Reimplantation into the recipient restores warm perfusion to the allograft, initiating a characteristic inflammatory cascade leading to IR injury. Hypothermic organ storage is associated with oxidative stress, sodium pump inactivation, intracellular calcium overload, iron release, and cell death that induce cell surface expression patterns and proinflammatory mediators for leukocyte activation during the reperfusion period (de Perrot, et al., 2003). This inherent response mechanism implicates IR injury as a primary determinant of both immediate and long-term graft survival.

Quality of the donor allograft and nature of recipient pathophysiology are primary determinants for the severity of IR injury, with a defined spectrum from mild pulmonary infiltration to the most severe acute respiratory distress syndrome (King, et al., 2000). A significant research commitment in lung transplantation is focused on organ selection and preservation to limit the deleterious effects of IR injury. Currently a disparaging 10-30% of donor lungs are approved for transplantation based on predictive criteria incorporating donor history, arterial blood gas assessment, chest x-ray and bronchoscopic findings, and physical examination upon lung retrieval. Inherent limitations are present in the subjective assessment of the donor allograft, as evidenced in comparable outcomes with extended donor criteria with marginal donor organs (Sundaresan, et al., 1995). This finding supports continued research commitment to risk stratification and predictive modeling for IR injury in donor lung selection.

Allograft selection and donor pool expansion are primary aims for current lung transplantation research. Traditional organ procurements for lung transplantation involve donation following brain death, excluding donations after cardiac death as a result of the inherent extended period of ischemia. Study of systemic markers for inflammation in brain dead donors has established interleukin-8 as a predictive cytokine marker for primary graft failure after reperfusion (Fisher, et al., 2001). This foundational research exemplifies the potential role for systemic markers of inflammation in the predictive modeling of graft survival.

A recent study on lung donation after controlled cardiac death has demonstrated comparable early- and medium-term outcomes in contrast to donation after brain death (de Vleeschauwer, et al., 2011). These promising results introduce a potential for donor pool expansion in coordination with lung rehabilitation strategies prior to recipient lung implantation. A multicenter study has demonstrated a close relationship between graft ischemic time and both early gas exchange and long-term survival following single and double lung transplantation. The coordinated aim to increase the donor pool with donation after cardiac death and the principle strategy to minimize periods of warm and cold ischemia have inspired novel *ex-vivo* perfusion methods for the donor lung prior to recipient implantation (Cypel, et al., 2011a). An international commitment to technologic advancement and scientific understanding promises to support improved outcomes and needed expansion of the donor pool for future generations. The focus of this chapter is to define the principle immunologic and inflammatory mediators of IR injury, providing a mechanistic understanding for the multi-factorial pathogenesis of this clinical condition. Novel treatment strategies and current clinical methods for donor allograft treatment are reviewed as a foundational discussion for future research initiatives in the prevention of IR injury.

2. Cellular mediators of lung IR injury

A major complication after lung transplantation is IR injury. After the ischemic insult, reperfusion of the lungs is critical to maintain organ viability; however, reperfusion can also cause a wide variety of complex pathophysiological changes to the lung leading to inflammation and injury. IR causes a multi-faceted cascade of signal transduction events involving a milieu of pro-inflammatory cytokines and chemokines and the generation of reactive oxygen species (ROS) by a myriad of cells in the lung. The crosstalk between these cells via a plethora of molecules leads to the initiation and amplification of a signaling cascade that ultimately culminates in pulmonary injury and dysfunction. Many studies have now established that cells of the innate immune system (bone marrow-derived cells such as T cells, macrophages, dendritic cells and neutrophils) play an important role in lung IR injury. In addition, resident pulmonary cells, such as alveolar epithelial cells and endothelial cells, are also critical mediators of lung IR injury. These cell populations will be discussed below.

2.1 Neutrophils

One of the effector cells responsible for causing lung inflammation and injury are known to be neutrophils. Lung injury can be manifested by the multi-faceted role of infiltrating neutrophils to the site of injury, which adhere to and cross the endothelium upon activation. Although neutrophils play an important role in perpetuating lung IR injury, the role of neutrophils in the early phase is less predominant. Studies from Deeb and colleagues have shown that during the first few hours of IR injury, it is the neutrophil-independent events that play a major role and that neutrophil-dependent events exert their effects after several hours of reperfusion (Deeb, et al., 1990). Other studies have confirmed this biphasic cellular response and have suggested that T cells and macrophages have a more prominent role in the early phase of IR injury while neutrophils play a late, effector role in the execution of lung IR injury (Eppinger, et al., 1995; Fiser, et al., 2001). The infiltration and activation of neutrophils causes lung injury via release of oxygen free radicals and disruption of capillary-epithelial barrier which leads to increased microvascular permeability and pulmonary edema causing irreversible tissue damage.

2.2 Macrophages and dendritic cells

The role of antigen presenting cells such as macrophages and dendritic cells has been implicated in lung IR injury. Several studies suggest that lung IR injury is biphasic, with distinct acute macrophage-mediated injury followed later by neutrophil-dependent injury (Eppinger, et al., 1995, 1997; Fiser, et al., 2001a, 2001b). Abundant evidence suggests that alveolar macrophages in the donor lung are quickly activated by IR to subsequently release pro-inflammatory chemokines and cytokines, and it has been demonstrated that depletion of alveolar macrophages attenuates lung IR injury (Naidu, et al., 2003; Zhao, et al., 2006). This acute pulmonary damage is followed by a cascade of events leading to activation of the recipient inflammatory system against the already damaged vascular endothelium and airway epithelium. A number of studies have strengthened a position for alveolar macrophages and TNF-α in acute IR injury (Eppinger, et al., 1997; Maxey, et al., 2004; Zhao, et al., 2006). One possible mechanism for decreased injury after suppression of macrophage function involves the attenuation of TNF-α or IFN-γ in respiratory burst activity and other inflammatory functions of macrophages (Arenzana-Seisdedos, et al., 1985; Eden & Turino, 1986; Issekutz & Issekutz, 1993; Mayer, et al., 1993; Phillips, et al., 1990). These studies indicate that IR injury is in part initiated by activated macrophages whereas delayed injury is mediated by activated neutrophils.

Recent studies have implicated a contributory role for dendritic cells in organ injury after transplantation including lung IR injury (He, et al., 2007; Saemann, et al., 2009). The cross-talk between antigen presenting cells like macrophages or dendritic cells and T lymphocytes has been postulated to play an important role in the initiation of lung IR injury. A detailed role for dendritic cells in lung IR injury, however, remains to be defined.

2.3 T lymphocytes

Involvement of T cells in IR injury until recently has not been considered; however, it has been demonstrated that T cells can be activated by antigen-independent mechanisms including oxygen radicals and cytokines such as TNF-α, IFN-γ, IL-23, IL-6, and RANTES (Bacon, et al., 1995). It is well known that the lung harbors a substantial reservoir of lymphocytes, and various subsets of T cells such as CD4+ T cells, CD8+ T cells, iNKT cells and γδT cells, have been implicated in lung IR injury. Yang et al. have recently demonstrated a key role for CD4+ T cells in an in vivo hilar clamp model of lung IR injury (Yang, et al., 2009). In the microcirculation, T cells may amplify inflammation by simultaneously binding to endothelial cells, macrophages, platelets and neutrophils. Several studies describe lung, renal and hepatic protection from IR injury in either null mice or T cell-depleted mice (Le Moine, et al., 2000; Rabb, et al., 2000; Sharma, et al., 2008; Zwacka, et al., 1997). These studies demonstrate significantly reduced neutrophil recruitment and inflammation in T cell-deficient mice after IR injury and suggest a role for T cells in the amplification of innate inflammatory signals. Clavien et al. described the activation of T cells by ROS during rat liver IR (Clavien, et al., 1993), and it appears that CD4+ T cells, but not CD8+ T cells, play a key role in the initiation of lung IR injury in mice (Sharma, et al., 2008). It has also been shown that acute lymphocyte-mediated lung IR injury involves CD40-CD40L signaling mechanisms (Moore, et al., 2002). CD4+ T cells play an important role in the initiation of immune responses by providing help to other cells and by taking on a variety of effector functions during immune reactions. CD4+ T cell priming results in the differentiation of various T cell subsets distinguished by the production of particular cytokines and effector functions.

Classically, CD4+ effector cells were viewed in the context of the Th1-Th2 cell paradigm, but other subsets have recently emerged including IL-17-producing T cells (Th17 cells), T cells with regulatory function (Treg cells) and invariant natural killer T (iNKT) cells (Larosa & Orange, 2008). There is also evidence that IL-23, IL-6, and TGF-β are proximal regulators of

IL-17 production by Th17 cells (Kolls & Linden, 2004) and iNKT cells (Rachitskaya, et al., 2008). iNKT cells are typically CD4+ T cells that share receptor structure with conventional T and NK cells and are characterized by their ability to rapidly produce immunoregulatory cytokines such as IL-4 and/or IFN-γ. NKT cells also constitutively express IL-23R and RORγt which can be rapidly activated during a variety of infections and inflammatory responses, and are recruited to produce IL-17 under emergency conditions. In the setting of renal IR, iNKT cell activation mediates neutrophil infiltration, IFN-γ production, and renal IR injury (Li, et al., 2007). Accumulating evidence suggest that Th17 cells are highly pro-inflammatory in that IL-17 is a key cytokine for the recruitment, activation and migration of neutrophils (Kolls & Linden, 2004), and Th17 cell-produced IL-17 is implicated in the pathogenesis of autoimmunity in various animal models (Bettelli, et al., 2007). However, the acute time frame of IL-17 production in lung IR injury is not consistent with a role for Th17 cells, which are not normally present in the lung and which require differentiation from naïve CD4+ T cells. Recent studies have revealed a critical role for the IL-23/IL-17 axis in various models of inflammation including IR injury (Edgerton, et al., 2008; Hanschen, et al., 2008; Wu, et al., 2007; Yen, et al., 2006). A critical role for iNKT cells and their rapid production of IL-17A in lung IR injury and neutrophil infiltration has been recently demonstrated using a mouse lung IR model (Sharma, et al., 2011). These studies support the concept that T lymphocytes can and do mediate IR injury.

2.4 Alveolar epithelial cells
The role of alveolar type II epithelial cells in lung IR injury has been described in recent studies (Sharma, et al., 2007). Alveolar type II epithelial cells contribute to lung IR injury via release of pro-inflammatory cytokines and chemokines. For example, it is well known that KC mediates lung injury by promoting infiltration of neutrophils. The crosstalk between macrophages and type II epithelial cells also contributes to the exacerbation of lung injury after IR. Sharma *et al.* showed that TNF-α production by alveolar macrophages mediates alveolar type II epithelial cell activation and KC production in an *in vitro* hypoxia-reoxygenation model (Sharma, et al., 2007). Recent studies also implicate alveolar type I cell-released mediators such as soluble receptor for advanced glycation end products (sRAGE) as a potential biomarker and indicator of lung injury after lung transplantation (Calfee, et al., 2007). This new marker may be useful given the recent discovery of the role of alveolar type I cells in alveolar fluid clearance (Johnson, et al., 2006). However, the exact role of alveolar type I cells in lung transplant biology remains less understood.

2.5 Endothelial cells
Increased endothelial permeability has been postulated to be the primary cause of IR-induced pulmonary edema (Hidalgo, et al., 1996). In a syngeneic rat lung transplantation model, it has been reported that the destruction of endothelial cell barrier promotes pulmonary edema and lymphocyte migration and that sphingosine 1-phosphate, a G protein coupled receptor agonist, reduces endothelial cell permeability and protects lung function and injury after IR (Okazaki, et al., 2007). Lung endothelial cells also mediate lung injury by contributing to oxidative stress (Balyasnikova, et al., 2005; Shuvaev & Muzykantov, 2011). Free radical production in endothelial cells via NADPH oxidase- or xanthine oxidase-dependent pathways results in elevated lung oxidant burden during

reperfusion (Al-Mehdi, et al., 1998). However, other cells such as leukocytes also contribute to free radical-mediated lung damage during IR injury (Shimoyama, et al., 2005). The prevention of the disruption of endothelial cell barrier is crucial for attenuation of lung injury after IR.

3. Reactive oxygen species (ROS) in lung IR injury

Lung IR injury is a complex pathological phenomenon encompassing various cellular, biochemical and molecular mechanisms. One of the key signaling pathways involving multiple cell types includes oxidative stress due to the generation of reactive oxygen species (ROS). Several groups have demonstrated that inhibition of enzymes involved in ROS generation can dramatically reduce the pro-inflammatory profile after IR.

3.1 ROS generation

A burst of ROS production occurs immediately upon reperfusion of hypoxic cells including leukocytes, epithelial cells and endothelial cells. The antioxidant defense capabilities of the lung are unable to cope with this ROS burst leading to altered cellular metabolic functions and redox signaling. Oxidative stress due to ROS generation causes pro-inflammatory cytokine release and enhanced transcription of numerous genes resulting in inflammation, cell injury, and neutrophil recruitment and activation in the lung after IR. Reperfusion of ischemic tissue results in generation of ROS such as superoxide ($\bullet O_2^-$), hydrogen peroxide (H_2O_2), and the hydroxyl radical ($\bullet OH$), which leads to oxidative damage to lung tissue (Al-Mehdi, et al., 1994; Al-Mehdi, et al., 1997; Ayene, et al., 1992; Eckenhoff, et al., 1992; Fisher, et al., 1991; Zhao, et al., 1997). This oxidative burst begins to directly increase the adherence of neutrophils to the endothelium (McIntyre, et al., 1995). The release of ROS not only induces cellular lipid membrane peroxidation and the production of inflammatory cytokines, but also plays a role in regulating the activity of several antioxidant enzymes (e.g. glutathione peroxidase, catalase and superoxide dismutase) as well as key transcription factors such as NF-κB and activator protein-1 (AP-1) (Cho, et al., 2006; Morimoto, 1993; Schreck, et al., 1992). Fisher et al. demonstrated oxygen-dependent lipid peroxidation during rat lung ischemia (Fisher, et al., 1991). Two key mechanisms of ROS generation in the lung include the NADPH oxidase system and activated xanthine oxidase, as discussed further below.

3.2 NADPH oxidase

Recent studies have demonstrated a key role of the NADPH-oxidase enzyme complex in ROS generation after IR (Goyal, et al., 2004; Jackson, et al., 2004; van der Vliet, 2008; Yang, et al., 2008; Yao, et al., 2007). NADPH oxidase, which is present in epithelial cells, endothelial cells, macrophages, T cells and neutrophils, among others, utilizes NADPH as a substrate to generate superoxide from molecular oxygen. Superoxide is usually rapidly converted to hydrogen peroxide (H_2O_2) or can react with nitric oxide ($NO\bullet$) to generate peroxynitrite ($ONOO^-$). Thus NADPH oxidase activity is a major source of ROS in the lung after IR. The upregulation of NADPH oxidase-generated ROS can contribute to IR injury through important redox signaling pathways such as the activation of MAP kinases, NF-κB and AP-1, which stimulates the production of proinflammatory cytokines. Pharmacological antagonism of NADPH oxidase by apocynin has been shown to protect against lung IR injury (Pearse & Dodd, 1999; Zhu, et al., 2008).

3.3 Xanthine and xanthine oxidase

Xanthine oxidase-dependent superoxide generation after IR is also a possible mechanism of lung injury (Kennedy, et al., 1989; Lynch, et al., 1988). Under ischemic conditions, xanthine dehydrogenase is converted to xanthine oxidase, which in turn converts hypoxanthine to xanthine and then further catalyzes the oxidation of xanthine to uric acid. In lung endothelium and alveolar type II epithelial cells, this conversion changes the normal degradation of hypoxanthine to uric acid into a source of oxygen radicals. The xanthine oxidase-generated free radicals damage endothelial cells as well as aid the sequestration of neutrophils thereby leading to further injury after IR. Treatment with xanthine oxidase inhibitors, such as allopurinol or iodoxamide, has been shown to attenuate superoxide generation and lung IR injury in rabbit and mouse models of lung IR injury (Adkins & Taylor, 1990; Kennedy, et al., 1989; Lynch, et al., 1988). These investigations suggest an important role for xanthine oxidase in the production of ROS during lung IR.

4. Cytokines and transcription factors

A multitude of experimental studies have shown that IR injury entails a rapid release of pro-inflammatory cytokines and chemokines. Additionally, measurable amounts of pro- and anti-inflammatory cytokines have been reported in lung tissue after lung transplantation in humans (de Perrot, et al., 2002). Important roles for TNF-α, IL-8 (KC in mice), IL-10 and IL-17 in the initiation and progression of lung IR injury have now been demonstrated. Gene modulation of transcription factors like NF-κB and AP-1 has also been correlated to the sequential events involved in lung IR injury.

4.1 Cytokines and chemokines

Cytokines and chemokines are immunomodulating protein molecules secreted by bone marrow derived cells as well as resident lung cells after IR injury. Pro-inflammatory cytokines and chemokines are known to play roles in IR injury of the heart, kidney, small bowel, skin, and liver; however, until recently less was known about their role in lung IR. The C-C family of cytokines and chemokines includes many putative mediators of macrophages, lymphocytes, and granulocyte-derived responses in IR injury (Oppenheim, et al., 1991; Strieter & Kunkel, 1993). This family includes MCP-1 (CCL2), MIP-1α (CCL3), MIP-1β (CCL4), RANTES (CCL5), MCP-3 (CCL7), MCP-2 (CCL8), as well as others. In addition to serving as chemotactic factors, C-C chemokines can modulate cytokine production, adhesion molecule expression, and mononuclear cell proliferation. Krishnadasan et al. demonstrated that TNF-α and IL-1β promote lung IR injury likely by altering the expression of other pro-inflammatory cytokines and by influencing neutrophil recruitment (Krishnadasan, et al., 2003). Antibodies to TNF-α, IFN-γ, and MCP-1 have been utilized to demonstrate the importance of these mediators in lung IR injury (Eppinger, et al., 1997). A prominent role for TNF-α was demonstrated both in the acute (30 min) and delayed (4 hr) phases of IR injury, while IFN-γ and MCP-1 appear to have roles only in the acute phase (Eppinger, et al., 1997). Not only is TNF-α produced by stimulated alveolar macrophages, it can also have significant effects on the macrophage respiratory burst, which may lead to oxidative tissue injury (Phillips, et al., 1990). In human lung transplantation, cytokines such as TNF-α, IFN-γ, IL-8, IL-10, IL-12 and IL-18 have been detected in lung tissue (de Perrot, et al., 2002). Mal et al. showed that early failure of lung transplants is associated with massive release of pro-inflammatory cytokines including TNF-α, IL-1β, IL-6 and IL-8 (Mal, et al., 1998).

Recent evidence has demonstrated a crucial role of IL-17 produced by iNKT cells in the initiation of lung IR injury via modulation of neutrophil infiltration and activation in an *in vivo* mouse model (Sharma, et al., 2011). On the other hand, a potent role for IL-10 as an anti-inflammatory molecule, promoting the abrogation of lung IR injury, has been shown in experimental lung IR models (Boehler, et al., 1998; de Perrot, et al., 2003; Fischer, et al., 2001; Martins, et al., 2004; McRae, et al., 2001). The cytotoxic and immunomodulatory effects of cytokines and chemokines are critical in the progression of lung IR injury. Taken together, the balance between pro- and anti-inflammatory cytokines is key to the outcome of lung injury after IR, and pharmacological modulation of these specific cytokine targets offers therapeutic potential for patients with primary graft dysfunction after lung transplantation.

4.2 Transcription factors

The activation of several aforementioned cytokines has been linked to the increased expression of key transcription factors like NF-κB and AP-1 after lung IR. A prominent role of gene regulation via these transcription factors in lung IR injury has been summarized by a number of previous studies.

4.2.1 NF-κB

In the cytoplasm, NF-κB is normally inhibited by IκB. Thus, a decrease in NF-κB activity, due to prevention of IκB degradation by pharmacological agents, leads to the attenuation of pro-inflammatory cytokine activation thereby leading to protection after lung IR. Inhibition of NF-κB via pharmacological agents like cyclosporine A or tacrolimus has been shown to offer protection from lung IR injury (Krishnadasan, et al., 2002). Treatment with pyrrolidine dithiocarbonate (another NF-κB inhibitor) has also been shown to improve lung function and attenuate lung IR injury in a porcine lung transplantation model (Ross, et al., 2000). Naidu *et al.* reported that simvastatin treatment attenuates lung IR injury via inhibition of NF-κB activity (Naidu, et al., 2003). Prevention of lung IR injury by pharmacological agents that inhibit NF-κB may offer a therapeutic strategy for patients with primary graft dysfunction after lung transplantation.

4.2.2 AP-1

The JNK/AP-1 pathway involves regulation of AP-1 by c-Jun kinase (JNK). Like NF-κB, AP-1 is also involved in the activation of several pro-inflammatory cytokines including TNF-α (Zhang, et al., 2002). For example, in a rat lung transplantation model, inhibition of AP-1 leads to decreased TNF-α expression in bronchoalveolar lavage fluid and a significant decrease in protein leakage resulting in decreased lung injury (Ishii, et al., 2004). Inhibition of the JNK/AP-1 pathway may also offer a potential therapeutic target to reduce lung IR injury.

5. Role of endogenous receptors in lung IR injury

Improving outcomes after lung transplantation and extending the donor pool and recipient criteria are predicated on the ability to minimize the deleterious inflammatory responses that occur with lung IR. Cellular receptor-mediated signaling is critical for the initiation and modulation of inflammation and injury after IR. Using pharmacological agents that regulate receptor activation or antagonism, several ubiquitous cellular receptors like adenosine receptors, toll like receptors (TLRs) and receptor for advanced glycation end products (RAGE) have been shown to orchestrate lung IR injury.

5.1 Adenosine receptors

Adenosine is an endogenous mediator that generally serves as a cytoprotective modulator in response to various stress stimuli, and the protective effects of adenosine in the setting of organ IR injury have been shown in various studies (Day, et al., 2005, 2006; Reece, et al., 2008; Rork, et al., 2008). Adenosine signals through 4 subtypes of the G protein-coupled receptors, A_1R, $A_{2A}R$, $A_{2B}R$, and A_3R, all of which are expressed in the lung. Protective effects of adenosine receptor signaling classically occur through second messenger pathways such as the cAMP/PKA or phospholipase C pathways. Most studies have provided evidence that A_1R, $A_{2A}R$ and A_3R may primarily be involved in anti-inflammatory actions whereas the $A_{2B}R$ may have more pro-inflammatory actions in the lung (Anvari, et al., 2010; Ellman, et al., 2008; Gazoni, et al., 2010; Reece, et al., 2005, 2008; Rivo, et al., 2004; Sharma, et al., 2009, 2010; Sun, et al., 2006). However, the role of the $A_{2B}R$ in IR injury remains less understood. $A_{2A}R$ activation has shown remarkable attenuation of lung inflammation, decreased neutrophil infiltration, decreased vascular permeability and improved lung function in rabbit, rat and murine models of lung IR injury (Ellman, et al., 2008; Gazoni, et al., 2008; Lau, et al., 2009; Sharma, et al., 2009) as well as in a pig lung transplant model (Reece, et al., 2005). The anti-inflammatory effects of $A_{2A}R$ activation on CD4+ T cells has been shown to attenuate lung IR injury (Sharma, et al., 2010). In recent literature involving lung IR injury, pharmacological compounds modulating adenosine receptor agonism or antagonism have shown tremendous potential as possible therapeutic strategies for clinical applications to prevent or treat primary graft dysfunction after lung transplantation.

5.2 Toll-like receptors (TLRs)

TLRs are transmembrane receptors that play a crucial role in the innate immune response to a variety of trigger factors including IR injury (Marshak-Rothstein & Rifkin, 2007). TLR-2 and TLR-4 have been implicated in various models of IR injury (Arslan, et al., 2010; Leemans, et al., 2005; Oyama, et al., 2004). Lung biopsies of patients after lung transplantation showed elevated expression of mRNA for multiple TLRs (Andrade, et al., 2006), and lungs from TLR-4 knockout mice showed marked protection from lung IR injury (Shimamoto, et al., 2006; Zanotti, et al., 2009). Shimamoto *et al.* reported that TLR-4-mediated injury appears to occur through activation of c-Jun NH_2-terminal kinase (JNK) and translocation of NF-κβ.

5.3 Receptor for advanced glycation end products (RAGE)

RAGE is a multi-ligand receptor of the immunoglobulin superfamily expressed in most tissues and present on a wide range of cells where it plays a key role in inflammatory processes, especially at sites where its ligands accumulate. High-mobility group box 1 (HMGB1) is an intracellular protein, readily released from necrotic or damaged cells, that can signal through RAGE, TLR-2 or TLR-4, initiating an inflammatory response to further damage viable cells (Scaffidi, et al., 2002). Prior studies suggest that HMGB1 can interact with both TLR-2 and TLR-4 to induce an inflammatory response during liver IR injury (Park, et al., 2006). Similarly, recent reports suggest a predominant role of RAGE and its ligand HMGB1 in the initiation of lung IR injury (Sternberg, et al., 2008). In a multi-center study, Christie *et al.* reported that an elevated plasma level of soluble RAGE (a truncated form of RAGE) was associated with primary graft dysfunction in patients undergoing lung transplantation (Christie, et al., 2009). An in depth characterization of the role of HMGB1, TLRs and RAGE remains to be elucidated in pulmonary injury after IR and transplantation.

5.4 Complement and fibrinolytic pathways

The complement system encompasses a collective term used for plasma and cell membrane proteins that play a role in cell defense processes. In lung IR injury, it has been shown that activation of the complement system leads to cellular injury through direct or indirect mechanisms (Bishop, et al., 1991; Naka, et al., 1997). In a swine single-lung transplantation model, the administration of soluble complement receptor 1, a potent inhibitor of complement activation, significantly reduces lung edema and improves lung function (Pierre, et al., 1998; Schmid, et al., 1998). In a clinical study, it was shown that complement inhibition by TP-10, a soluble complement receptor 1, significantly decreases the duration of mechanical ventilation in lung transplant recipients (Keshavjee, et al., 2005). This suggests that complement inhibition may offer additional therapeutic strategies for lung transplant patients. Further research is required to elucidate the specific pathways of the complement-mediated inflammation in lung IR pathophysiology.

The interplay between the fibrinolytic cascade and the inflammatory process in acute lung injury has been shown to be involved in lung IR injury. Tissue plasminogen activator (tPA), a member of the serine proteinase family, is expressed by vascular endothelial cells and functions to convert zymogen plasminogen to the active protease plasmin, thus initiating a potent fibrinolytic process. tPA knockout mice have attenuated lung inflammation by decreased neutrophil extravasation in a mouse model of lung IR (Zhao, et al., 2011). In the same study, it was shown that deletion of tPA leads to the concomitant downregulation of PECAM-1 expression via tPA/LRP/NF-κB signaling pathway and upregulation of P-selectin expression in small pulmonary vessels as well as to decreased MMP-9 expression. It has also been demonstrated that increased fibrinolysis through depletion of plasminogen activator inhibitor-1 (PAI-1), the endogenous tPA inhibitor, attenuated lung IR injury (Lau, et al., 2009). The complex molecular mechanisms involved in the fibrinolytic pathway and its potential role in clinical primary graft dysfunction remains to be further investigated.

6. Therapeutic strategies

Advancements in our understanding of molecular and pathophysiologic mechanisms for lung IR injury have supported significant research contributions aimed at improved allograft function. While no standardized treatment strategies specifically targeting IR injury exist, promising early results have demonstrated a potential role for *ex vivo* allograft treatment, nitric oxide therapy, and ischemic preconditioning in the prevention of IR injury.

6.1 Lung preservation strategies

A significant research commitment over the past decade has been invested in the creation of an ideal preservation and flush solution for lung transplantation. Intracellular solutions with high potassium and low sodium are the current standard for kidney and liver transplantation, while extracellular solutions such as Perfadex® (Vitrolife, Gothenburg, Sweden) with low potassium, high sodium and dextran have emerged as the superior method for lung preservation (de Perrot, et al., 2003; Fischer, et al., 2001). Dextran induces erythrocyte deformation and prevents aggregation, preserving the pulmonary microcirculation and endothelial-epithelial barrier (Keshavjee, et al., 1992). This inherent quality may limit ischemia in regions of microcirculation thrombosis while creating an osmotic gradient that reduces protein and water extravasation during the reperfusion period (de Perrot, et al., 2003). In a clinical study, the absence of dextrose in extracellular solutions has been associated with an increased incidence of primary graft dysfunction and mortality (Marasco, et al., 2011; Oto, et al., 2006). While long-term outcomes remain the focus of future investigation, these findings support the clinical adoption of low-potassium dextran solutions as the primary method for lung allograft preservation.

6.2 Ex vivo lung perfusion (EVLP)

EVLP is an emerging technique for normothermic donor lung perfusion during the preservation period. EVLP with warm acellular Steen Solution™ (Vitrolife, Gothenburg, Sweden) following a period of cold storage is a promising modality for lung preservation with a demonstrated efficacy in the maintenance of lung function (Cypel, et al., 2008). This novel treatment strategy prevents ongoing injury and accelerates lung recovery (Cypel, et al., 2009). Recent prospective clinical data has demonstrated the successful transplantation of high-risk donor lungs following EVLP with comparable physiology to lungs transplanted under conventional methods of selection and transplantation (Cypel, et al., 2011b). These studies promote EVLP as a potential strategy for donor pool expansion and pre-implantation pulmonary function testing. In addition, this promising treatment strategy for lung rehabilitation may serve as a vehicle for future therapeutic treatment of the donor allograft during the inherent ischemic period.

6.3 Nitric oxide (NO)

NO is a messenger gas molecule with potent vasoregulatory and immunomodulatory properties (de Perrot, et al., 2003; Meyer, et al., 1998). NO inhibits xanthine oxidase as well as neutrophil chemotaxis and activation (de Perrot, et al., 2003; Meyer, et al., 1998). This mechanism of action establishes therapeutic potential for inhaled NO in the prevention of lung IR injury. NO ventilation during ischemia and following graft implantation in experimental models with *ex vivo* perfusion has demonstrated a reduction in pulmonary edema, improvement in oxygenation capacity, reduction in pulmonary vascular resistance, and decreased TNF-α with treatment (Dong, et al., 2009). Treatment of experimental recipient lungs with inhalational NO during reperfusion improved the ventilation-perfusion mismatch and decreased pulmonary artery pressures associated with IR injury (Adatia, et al., 1994). Unfortunately, this promising experimental data for inhalational NO has had limited translation to the clinical prevention of human lung IR injury. In a randomized clinical trial to evaluate the use of inhaled NO treatment, no significant differences in immediate oxygenation, time to extubation, length of intensive care unit stay or 30-day mortality were demonstrated (Meade, et al., 2001). While experimental data supports improved gas exchange with inhaled NO treatment, clinical lung transplantation data has not yet demonstrated significant improvements in outcomes for lung transplantation recipients with inhaled NO treatment (de Perrot, et al., 2003) .

6.4 Preconditioning

Ischemic preconditioning enhances the ability of organs to withstand a sustained IR injury through repeated exposure to short periods of ischemia prior to the primary ischemic insult (Jun, et al., 2011). Ischemic preconditioning has demonstrated an ability to alter gene expression profiles within 6 hours of ischemia which is sustained until 24 hours following insult (Jun, et al., 2011). The proposed mechanism for ischemic preconditioning in the lung involves anti-inflammatory mediators, antioxidant stress, and the regulation of cellular energy metabolism (Jun, et al., 2011). Further experimental studies have suggested a role for adenosine A_1 receptor activation in the modulation of protective ischemic preconditioning (Yildiz, et al., 2007). Additional potential therapeutic preconditioning methods include hyperthermic and pharmacologic administration to improve the allograft response to the period of ischemia and subsequent reperfusion (Hiratsuka, et al., 1998; Schutte, et al., 2001). The role of preconditioning in clinical lung transplantation remains undefined (de Perrot, et al., 2003). Future application and study of preconditioning methods in the lung may demonstrate parallel beneficial effects to other organ systems, establishing this strategy for lung IR injury prevention.

7. Conclusions

Lung IR injury involves many cellular and molecular mechanisms making it a complex pathological process. Improvements in the technique of lung preservation and better understanding of the molecular mechanisms of IR injury are needed to prevent the occurrence of primary graft dysfunction after lung transplantation. The development of new strategies to improve the number of donor lungs available for transplantation could have a significant impact on the number of transplants performed and thus reduce the number of patients on the transplant waiting list. Additionally, improvements in lung preservation solution can help attenuate acute lung IR injury as well as chronic graft dysfunction. It is imperative that further experimental studies and multicenter clinical trials continue to be performed to reduce the morbidity and mortality associated with lung IR injury.

Research commitment to further define cellular responses to IR within the lung promises to support therapeutic advancement. Novel *ex vivo* treatment strategies may provide a therapeutic bridge for treatment of the donor allograft prior to recipient implantation. The combination of pharmacologic mechanistic inhibition and innovative approaches to sustained allograft perfusion support a promising future for lung transplantation. A dedicated and multidisciplinary approach to IR injury prevention is critical. Therapeutic advancement to ameliorate IR injury will increase the number of available donor grafts and improve lung transplantation outcomes for the increasing number of potential transplant recipients with end-stage pulmonary disease.

8. References

Adatia, I., Lillehei, C., Arnold, J. H., Thompson, J. E., Palazzo, R., Fackler, J. C. & Wessel, D. L. (1994). Inhaled nitric oxide in the treatment of postoperative graft dysfunction after lung transplantation. *Ann Thorac Surg*, Vol.57, No.5, (May), pp. 1311-1318, ISSN 0003-4975

Adkins, W. K. & Taylor, A. E. (1990). Role of xanthine oxidase and neutrophils in ischemia-reperfusion injury in rabbit lung. *J Appl Physiol*, Vol.69, No.6, (Dec), pp. 2012-2018, ISSN 8750-7587

Al-Mehdi, A., Shuman, H. & Fisher, A. B. (1994). Fluorescence microtopography of oxidative stress in lung ischemia-reperfusion. *Lab Invest*, Vol.70, No.4, (Apr), pp. 579-587, ISSN 0023-6837

Al-Mehdi, A. B., Shuman, H. & Fisher, A. B. (1997). Intracellular generation of reactive oxygen species during nonhypoxic lung ischemia. *Am J Physiol*, Vol.272, No.2 Pt 1, (Feb), pp. L294-300, ISSN 0002-9513

Al-Mehdi, A. B., Zhao, G., Dodia, C., Tozawa, K., Costa, K., Muzykantov, V., Ross, C., Blecha, F., Dinauer, M. & Fisher, A. B. (1998). Endothelial NADPH oxidase as the source of oxidants in lungs exposed to ischemia or high K+. *Circ Res*, Vol.83, No.7, (Oct 5), pp. 730-737, ISSN 0009-7330

Andrade, C. F., Kaneda, H., Der, S., Tsang, M., Lodyga, M., Chimisso Dos Santos, C., Keshavjee, S. & Liu, M. (2006). Toll-like receptor and cytokine gene expression in the early phase of human lung transplantation. *J Heart Lung Transplant*, Vol.25, No.11, (Nov), pp. 1317-1323, ISSN 1053-2498

Anvari, F., Sharma, A. K., Fernandez, L. G., Hranjec, T., Ravid, K., Kron, I. L. & Laubach, V. E. (2010). Tissue-derived proinflammatory effect of adenosine A2B receptor in lung ischemia-reperfusion injury. *J Thorac Cardiovasc Surg*, Vol.140, No.4, (Oct), pp. 871-877, ISSN 0022-5223

Arenzana-Seisdedos, F., Virelizier, J. L. & Fiers, W. (1985). Interferons as macrophage-activating factors. III. Preferential effects of interferon-gamma on the interleukin 1 secretory potential of fresh or aged human monocytes. *J Immunol*, Vol.134, No.4, (Apr), pp. 2444-2448, ISSN 0022-1767

Arslan, F., Keogh, B., McGuirk, P. & Parker, A. E. (2010). TLR2 and TLR4 in ischemia reperfusion injury. *Mediators Inflamm*, Vol.2010, pp. 704202, ISSN 0962-9351

Ayene, I. S., Dodia, C. & Fisher, A. B. (1992). Role of oxygen in oxidation of lipid and protein during ischemia/reperfusion in isolated perfused rat lung. *Arch Biochem Biophys*, Vol.296, No.1, (Jul), pp. 183-189, ISSN 0003-9861

Bacon, K. B., Premack, B. A., Gardner, P. & Schall, T. J. (1995). Activation of dual T cell signaling pathways by the chemokine RANTES. *Science*, Vol.269, No.5231, (Sep 22), pp. 1727-1730, ISSN 0036-8075

Balyasnikova, I. V., Visintine, D. J., Gunnerson, H. B., Paisansathan, C., Baughman, V. L., Minshall, R. D. & Danilov, S. M. (2005). Propofol attenuates lung endothelial injury induced by ischemia-reperfusion and oxidative stress. *Anesth Analg*, Vol.100, No.4, (Apr), pp. 929-936, ISSN 0003-2999

Bettelli, E., Korn, T. & Kuchroo, V. K. (2007). Th17: the third member of the effector T cell trilogy. *Curr Opin Immunol*, Vol.19, No.6, (Dec), pp. 652-657, ISSN 0952-7915

Bishop, M. J., Giclas, P. C., Guidotti, S. M., Su, M. L. & Chi, E. Y. (1991). Complement activation is a secondary rather than a causative factor in rabbit pulmonary artery ischemia/reperfusion injury. *Am Rev Respir Dis*, Vol.143, No.2, (Feb), pp. 386-390, ISSN 0003-0805

Boehler, A., Chamberlain, D., Xing, Z., Slutsky, A. S., Jordana, M., Gauldie, J., Liu, M. & Keshavjee, S. (1998). Adenovirus-mediated interleukin-10 gene transfer inhibits post-transplant fibrous airway obliteration in an animal model of bronchiolitis obliterans. *Hum Gene Ther*, Vol.9, No.4, (Mar 1), pp. 541-551, ISSN 1043-0342

Calfee, C. S., Budev, M. M., Matthay, M. A., Church, G., Brady, S., Uchida, T., Ishizaka, A., Lara, A., Ranes, J. L., deCamp, M. M. & Arroliga, A. C. (2007). Plasma receptor for advanced glycation end-products predicts duration of ICU stay and mechanical ventilation in patients after lung transplantation. *J Heart Lung Transplant*, Vol.26, No.7, (Jul), pp. 675-680, ISSN 1053-2498

Cho, H. Y., Reddy, S. P. & Kleeberger, S. R. (2006). Nrf2 defends the lung from oxidative stress. *Antioxid Redox Signal*, Vol.8, No.1-2, (Jan-Feb), pp. 76-87, ISSN 1523-0864

Christie, J. D., Shah, C. V., Kawut, S. M., Mangalmurti, N., Lederer, D. J., Sonett, J. R., Ahya, V. N., Palmer, S. M., Wille, K., Lama, V., Shah, P. D., Shah, A., Weinacker, A., Deutschman, C. S., Kohl, B. A., Demissie, E., Bellamy, S. & Ware, L. B. (2009). Plasma levels of receptor for advanced glycation end products, blood transfusion, and risk of primary graft dysfunction. *Am J Respir Crit Care Med*, Vol.180, No.10, (Nov 15), pp. 1010-1015, ISSN 1073-449X

Christie, J. D., Edwards, L. B., Kucheryavaya, A. Y., Aurora, P., Dobbels, F., Kirk, R., Rahmel, A. O., Stehlik, J. & Hertz, M. I. (2010). The Registry of the International Society for Heart and Lung Transplantation: twenty-seventh official adult lung and heart-lung transplant report--2010. *J Heart Lung Transplant*, Vol.29, No.10, (Oct), pp. 1104-1118, ISSN 1053-2498

Clavien, P. A., Harvey, P. R., Sanabria, J. R., Cywes, R., Levy, G. A. & Strasberg, S. M. (1993). Lymphocyte adherence in the reperfused rat liver: mechanisms and effects. *Hepatology*, Vol.17, No.1, (Jan), pp. 131-142, ISSN 0270-9139

Cottini, S. R., Lerch, N., de Perrot, M., Treggiari, M. M., Spiliopoulos, A., Nicod, L. & Ricou, B. (2006). Risk factors for reperfusion injury after lung transplantation. *Intensive Care Med*, Vol.32, No.4, (Apr), pp. 557-563, ISSN 0342-4642

Cypel, M., Yeung, J. C., Hirayama, S., Rubacha, M., Fischer, S., Anraku, M., Sato, M., Harwood, S., Pierre, A., Waddell, T. K., de Perrot, M., Liu, M. & Keshavjee, S. (2008). Technique for prolonged normothermic ex vivo lung perfusion. *J Heart Lung Transplant*, Vol.27, No.12, (Dec), pp. 1319-1325, ISSN 1053-2498

Cypel, M., Rubacha, M., Yeung, J., Hirayama, S., Torbicki, K., Madonik, M., Fischer, S., Hwang, D., Pierre, A., Waddell, T. K., de Perrot, M., Liu, M. & Keshavjee, S. (2009). Normothermic ex vivo perfusion prevents lung injury compared to extended cold preservation for transplantation. *Am J Transplant*, Vol.9, No.10, (Oct), pp. 2262-2269, ISSN 1600-6135

Cypel, M., Yeung, J. C. & Keshavjee, S. (2011a). Novel approaches to expanding the lung donor pool: donation after cardiac death and ex vivo conditioning. *Clin Chest Med*, Vol.32, No.2, (Jun), pp. 233-244, ISSN 0272-5231

Cypel, M., Yeung, J. C., Liu, M., Anraku, M., Chen, F., Karolak, W., Sato, M., Laratta, J., Azad, S., Madonik, M., Chow, C. W., Chaparro, C., Hutcheon, M., Singer, L. G.,

Slutsky, A. S., Yasufuku, K., de Perrot, M., Pierre, A. F., Waddell, T. K. & Keshavjee, S. (2011b). Normothermic ex vivo lung perfusion in clinical lung transplantation. *N Engl J Med*, Vol.364, No.15, (Apr 14), pp. 1431-1440, ISSN 0028-4793

Day, Y. J., Li, Y., Rieger, J. M., Ramos, S. I., Okusa, M. D. & Linden, J. (2005). A2A adenosine receptors on bone marrow-derived cells protect liver from ischemia-reperfusion injury. *J Immunol*, Vol.174, No.8, (Apr 15), pp. 5040-5046, ISSN 0022-1767

Day, Y. J., Huang, L., Ye, H., Li, L., Linden, J. & Okusa, M. D. (2006). Renal ischemia-reperfusion injury and adenosine 2A receptor-mediated tissue protection: the role of CD4+ T cells and IFN-gamma. *J Immunol*, Vol.176, No.5, (Mar 1), pp. 3108-3114, ISSN 0022-1767

de Perrot, M., Sekine, Y., Fischer, S., Waddell, T. K., McRae, K., Liu, M., Wigle, D. A. & Keshavjee, S. (2002). Interleukin-8 release during early reperfusion predicts graft function in human lung transplantation. *Am J Respir Crit Care Med*, Vol.165, No.2, (Jan 15), pp. 211-215, ISSN 1073-449X

de Perrot, M., Fischer, S., Liu, M., Imai, Y., Martins, S., Sakiyama, S., Tabata, T., Bai, X. H., Waddell, T. K., Davidson, B. L. & Keshavjee, S. (2003). Impact of human interleukin-10 on vector-induced inflammation and early graft function in rat lung transplantation. *Am J Respir Cell Mol Biol*, Vol.28, No.5, (May), pp. 616-625, ISSN 1044-1549

de Perrot, M., Liu, M., Waddell, T. K. & Keshavjee, S. (2003). Ischemia-reperfusion-induced lung injury. *Am J Respir Crit Care Med*, Vol.167, No.4, (Feb 15), pp. 490-511, ISSN 1073-449X

de Vleeschauwer, S. I., Wauters, S., Dupont, L. J., Verleden, S. E., Willems-Widyastuti, A., Vanaudenaerde, B. M., Verleden, G. M. & Van Raemdonck, D. E. (2011). Medium-term outcome after lung transplantation is comparable between brain-dead and cardiac-dead donors. *J Heart Lung Transplant*, (Jun 10), pp. ISSN 1053-2498

Deeb, G. M., Grum, C. M., Lynch, M. J., Guynn, T. P., Gallagher, K. P., Ljungman, A. G., Bolling, S. F. & Morganroth, M. L. (1990). Neutrophils are not necessary for induction of ischemia-reperfusion lung injury. *J Appl Physiol*, Vol.68, No.1, (Jan), pp. 374-381, ISSN 0161-7567

Diamond, J. M. & Christie, J. D. (2010). The contribution of airway and lung tissue ischemia to primary graft dysfunction. *Curr Opin Organ Transplant*, Vol.15, No.5, (Oct), pp. 552-557, ISSN 1087-2418

Dong, B. M., Abano, J. B. & Egan, T. M. (2009). Nitric oxide ventilation of rat lungs from non-heart-beating donors improves posttransplant function. *Am J Transplant*, Vol.9, No.12, (Dec), pp. 2707-2715, ISSN 1600-6135

Eckenhoff, R. G., Dodia, C., Tan, Z. & Fisher, A. B. (1992). Oxygen-dependent reperfusion injury in the isolated rat lung. *J Appl Physiol*, Vol.72, No.4, (Apr), pp. 1454-1460, ISSN 0161-7567

Eden, E. & Turino, G. M. (1986). Interleukin-1 secretion by human alveolar macrophages stimulated with endotoxin is augmented by recombinant immune (gamma) interferon. *Am Rev Respir Dis*, Vol.133, No.3, (Mar), pp. 455-460, ISSN 0003-0805

Edgerton, C., Crispin, J. C., Moratz, C. M., Bettelli, E., Oukka, M., Simovic, M., Zacharia, A., Egan, R., Chen, J., Dalle Lucca, J. J., Juang, Y. T. & Tsokos, G. C. (2008). IL-17 producing CD4(+) T cells mediate accelerated ischemia/reperfusion-induced injury in autoimmunity-prone mice. *Clin Immunol*, (Dec 3), pp. ISSN 1521-7035

Ellman, P. I., Reece, T. B., Law, M. G., Gazoni, L. M., Singh, R., Laubach, V. E., Linden, J., Tribble, C. G. & Kron, I. L. (2008). Adenosine A2A activation attenuates nontransplantation lung reperfusion injury. *J Surg Res*, Vol.149, No.1, (Sep), pp. 3-8, ISSN 0022-4804

Eppinger, M. J., Jones, M. L., Deeb, G. M., Bolling, S. F. & Ward, P. A. (1995). Pattern of injury and the role of neutrophils in reperfusion injury of rat lung. *J Surg Res*, Vol.58, No.6, (Jun), pp. 713-718, ISSN 0022-4804

Eppinger, M. J., Deeb, G. M., Bolling, S. F. & Ward, P. A. (1997). Mediators of ischemia-reperfusion injury of rat lung. *Am J Pathol*, Vol.150, No.5, (May), pp. 1773-1784, ISSN 0002-9440

Fischer, S., Liu, M., Maclean, A. A., De Perrot, M., Bai, X., Cardella, J., Imai, Y. & Keshavjee, S. (2001). In vivo donor adenoviral-mediated transtracheal transfection of human IL-10 (HIL-10) gene ameliorates ischemia-reperfusion (IR) injury and enhances transplanted lung function. *J Heart Lung Transplant*, Vol.20, No.2, (Feb), pp. 152-153, ISSN 1053-2498

Fischer, S., Matte-Martyn, A., De Perrot, M., Waddell, T. K., Sekine, Y., Hutcheon, M. & Keshavjee, S. (2001). Low-potassium dextran preservation solution improves lung function after human lung transplantation. *J Thorac Cardiovasc Surg*, Vol.121, No.3, (Mar), pp. 594-596, ISSN 0022-5223

Fiser, S. M., Tribble, C. G., Long, S. M., Kaza, A. K., Cope, J. T., Laubach, V. E., Kern, J. A. & Kron, I. L. (2001a). Lung transplant reperfusion injury involves pulmonary macrophages and circulating leukocytes in a biphasic response. *J Thorac Cardiovasc Surg*, Vol.121, No.6, (Jun), pp. 1069-1075, ISSN 0022-5223

Fiser, S. M., Tribble, C. G., Long, S. M., Kaza, A. K., Kern, J. A. & Kron, I. L. (2001b). Pulmonary macrophages are involved in reperfusion injury after lung transplantation. *Ann Thorac Surg*, Vol.71, No.4, (Apr), pp. 1134-1138, ISSN 0003-4975

Fiser, S. M., Tribble, C. G., Long, S. M., Kaza, A. K., Kern, J. A., Jones, D. R., Robbins, M. K. & Kron, I. L. (2002). Ischemia-reperfusion injury after lung transplantation increases risk of late bronchiolitis obliterans syndrome. *Ann Thorac Surg*, Vol.73, No.4, (Apr), pp. 1041-1047; discussion 1047-1048, ISSN 0003-4975

Fisher, A. B., Dodia, C., Tan, Z. T., Ayene, I. & Eckenhoff, R. G. (1991). Oxygen-dependent lipid peroxidation during lung ischemia. *J Clin Invest*, Vol.88, No.2, (Aug), pp. 674-679, ISSN 0021-9738

Fisher, A. J., Donnelly, S. C., Hirani, N., Haslett, C., Strieter, R. M., Dark, J. H. & Corris, P. A. (2001). Elevated levels of interleukin-8 in donor lungs is associated with early graft failure after lung transplantation. *Am J Respir Crit Care Med*, Vol.163, No.1, (Jan), pp. 259-265, ISSN 1073-449X

Gazoni, L. M., Laubach, V. E., Mulloy, D. P., Bellizzi, A., Unger, E. B., Linden, J., Ellman, P. I., Lisle, T. C. & Kron, I. L. (2008). Additive protection against lung ischemia-reperfusion injury by adenosine A2A receptor activation before procurement and during reperfusion. *J Thorac Cardiovasc Surg*, Vol.135, No.1, (Jan), pp. 156-165, ISSN 0022-5223

Gazoni, L. M., Walters, D. M., Unger, E. B., Linden, J., Kron, I. L. & Laubach, V. E. (2010). Activation of A1, A2A, or A3 adenosine receptors attenuates lung ischemia-reperfusion injury. *J Thorac Cardiovasc Surg*, Vol.140, No.2, (Aug), pp. 440-446, ISSN 0022-5223

Goyal, P., Weissmann, N., Grimminger, F., Hegel, C., Bader, L., Rose, F., Fink, L., Ghofrani, H. A., Schermuly, R. T., Schmidt, H. H., Seeger, W. & Hanze, J. (2004). Upregulation of NAD(P)H oxidase 1 in hypoxia activates hypoxia-inducible factor 1 via increase in reactive oxygen species. *Free Radic Biol Med*, Vol.36, No.10, (May 15), pp. 1279-1288, ISSN 0891-5849

Granton, J. (2006). Update of early respiratory failure in the lung transplant recipient. *Curr Opin Crit Care*, Vol.12, No.1, (Feb), pp. 19-24, ISSN 1070-5295

Hanschen, M., Zahler, S., Krombach, F. & Khandoga, A. (2008). Reciprocal activation between CD4+ T cells and Kupffer cells during hepatic ischemia-reperfusion. *Transplantation*, Vol.86, No.5, (Sep 15), pp. 710-718, ISSN 1534-6080

Hardy, J. D., Webb, W. R., Dalton, M. L. J. & Walker, G. R. J. (1963). Lung homotransplantation in man. *JAMA*, Vol.186, (Dec), pp. 1065-1074, ISSN 0098-7484

He, X., Han, B. & Liu, M. (2007). Long pentraxin 3 in pulmonary infection and acute lung injury. *Am J Physiol Lung Cell Mol Physiol*, Vol.292, No.5, (May), pp. L1039-1049, ISSN 1040-0605

Hidalgo, M. A., Shah, K. A., Fuller, B. J. & Green, C. J. (1996). Cold ischemia-induced damage to vascular endothelium results in permeability alterations in transplanted lungs. *J Thorac Cardiovasc Surg*, Vol.112, No.4, (Oct), pp. 1027-1035, ISSN 0022-5223

Hiratsuka, M., Yano, M., Mora, B. N., Nagahiro, I., Cooper, J. D. & Patterson, G. A. (1998). Heat shock pretreatment protects pulmonary isografts from subsequent ischemia-reperfusion injury. *J Heart Lung Transplant*, Vol.17, No.12, (Dec), pp. 1238-1246, ISSN 1053-2498

Ishii, M., Suzuki, Y., Takeshita, K., Miyao, N., Kudo, H., Hiraoka, R., Nishio, K., Sato, N., Naoki, K., Aoki, T. & Yamaguchi, K. (2004). Inhibition of c-Jun NH2-terminal kinase activity improves ischemia/reperfusion injury in rat lungs. *J Immunol*, Vol.172, No.4, (Feb 15), pp. 2569-2577, ISSN 0022-1767

Issekutz, A. C. & Issekutz, T. B. (1993). Quantitation and kinetics of blood monocyte migration to acute inflammatory reactions, and IL-1 alpha, tumor necrosis factor-alpha, and IFN-gamma. *J Immunol*, Vol.151, No.4, (Aug 15), pp. 2105-2115, ISSN 0022-1767

Jackson, S. H., Devadas, S., Kwon, J., Pinto, L. A. & Williams, M. S. (2004). T cells express a phagocyte-type NADPH oxidase that is activated after T cell receptor stimulation. *Nat Immunol*, Vol.5, No.8, (Aug), pp. 818-827, ISSN 1529-2908

Johnson, M. D., Bao, H. F., Helms, M. N., Chen, X. J., Tigue, Z., Jain, L., Dobbs, L. G. & Eaton, D. C. (2006). Functional ion channels in pulmonary alveolar type I cells support a role for type I cells in lung ion transport. *Proc Natl Acad Sci U S A*, Vol.103, No.13, (Mar 28), pp. 4964-4969, ISSN 0027-8424

Jun, N., Ke, J., Gang, C., Lin, C., Jinsong, L. & Jianjun, W. (2011). The protective effect of ischemic preconditioning associated with altered gene expression profiles in rat lung after reperfusion. *J Surg Res*, Vol.168, No.2, (Jun 15), pp. 281-293, ISSN 0022-4804

Kennedy, T. P., Rao, N. V., Hopkins, C., Pennington, L., Tolley, E. & Hoidal, J. R. (1989). Role of reactive oxygen species in reperfusion injury of the rabbit lung. *J Clin Invest*, Vol.83, No.4, (Apr), pp. 1326-1335, ISSN 0021-9738

Keshavjee, S., Davis, R. D., Zamora, M. R., de Perrot, M. & Patterson, G. A. (2005). A randomized, placebo-controlled trial of complement inhibition in ischemia-reperfusion injury after lung transplantation in human beings. *J Thorac Cardiovasc Surg*, Vol.129, No.2, (Feb), pp. 423-428, ISSN 0022-5223

Keshavjee, S. H., Yamazaki, F., Yokomise, H., Cardoso, P. F., Mullen, J. B., Slutsky, A. S. & Patterson, G. A. (1992). The role of dextran 40 and potassium in extended hypothermic lung preservation for transplantation. *J Thorac Cardiovasc Surg*, Vol.103, No.2, (Feb), pp. 314-325, ISSN 0022-5223

King, R. C., Binns, O. A., Rodriguez, F., Kanithanon, R. C., Daniel, T. M., Spotnitz, W. D., Tribble, C. G. & Kron, I. L. (2000). Reperfusion injury significantly impacts clinical outcome after pulmonary transplantation. *Ann Thorac Surg*, Vol.69, No.6, (Jun), pp. 1681-1685, ISSN 0003-4975

Kolls, J. K. & Linden, A. (2004). Interleukin-17 family members and inflammation. *Immunity*, Vol.21, No.4, (Oct), pp. 467-476, ISSN 1074-7613

Krishnadasan, B., Naidu, B., Rosengart, M., Farr, A. L., Barnes, A., Verrier, E. D. & Mulligan, M. S. (2002). Decreased lung ischemia-reperfusion injury in rats after preoperative administration of cyclosporine and tacrolimus. *J Thorac Cardiovasc Surg*, Vol.123, No.4, (Apr), pp. 756-767, ISSN 0022-5223

Krishnadasan, B., Naidu, B. V., Byrne, K., Fraga, C., Verrier, E. D. & Mulligan, M. S. (2003). The role of proinflammatory cytokines in lung ischemia-reperfusion injury. *J Thorac Cardiovasc Surg*, Vol.125, No.2, (Feb), pp. 261-272, ISSN 0022-5223

Larosa, D. F. & Orange, J. S. (2008). Lymphocytes. *J Allergy Clin Immunol*, Vol.121, No.2 Suppl, (Feb), pp. S364-369, ISSN 1097-6825

Lau, C. L., Zhao, Y., Kim, J., Kron, I. L., Sharma, A., Yang, Z., Laubach, V. E., Linden, J., Ailawadi, G. & Pinsky, D. J. (2009). Enhanced fibrinolysis protects against lung ischemia-reperfusion injury. *J Thorac Cardiovasc Surg*, Vol.137, No.5, (May), pp. 1241-1248, ISSN 0022-5223

Lau, C. L., Zhao, Y., Kron, I. L., Stoler, M. H., Laubach, V. E., Ailawadi, G. & Linden, J. (2009). The role of adenosine A2A receptor signaling in bronchiolitis obliterans. *Ann Thorac Surg*, Vol.88, No.4, (Oct), pp. 1071-1078, ISSN 1552-6259

Le Moine, O., Louis, H., Demols, A., Desalle, F., Demoor, F., Quertinmont, E., Goldman, M. & Deviere, J. (2000). Cold liver ischemia-reperfusion injury critically depends on liver T cells and is improved by donor pretreatment with interleukin 10 in mice. *Hepatology*, Vol.31, No.6, (Jun), pp. 1266-1274, ISSN 0270-9139

Leemans, J. C., Stokman, G., Claessen, N., Rouschop, K. M., Teske, G. J., Kirschning, C. J., Akira, S., van der Poll, T., Weening, J. J. & Florquin, S. (2005). Renal-associated

TLR2 mediates ischemia/reperfusion injury in the kidney. *J Clin Invest*, Vol.115, No.10, (Oct), pp. 2894-2903, ISSN 0021-9738

Li, L., Huang, L., Sung, S. S., Lobo, P. I., Brown, M. G., Gregg, R. K., Engelhard, V. H. & Okusa, M. D. (2007). NKT cell activation mediates neutrophil IFN-gamma production and renal ischemia-reperfusion injury. *J Immunol*, Vol.178, No.9, (May 1), pp. 5899-5911, ISSN 0022-1767

Lynch, M. J., Grum, C. M., Gallagher, K. P., Bolling, S. F., Deeb, G. M. & Morganroth, M. L. (1988). Xanthine oxidase inhibition attenuates ischemic-reperfusion lung injury. *J Surg Res*, Vol.44, No.5, (May), pp. 538-544, ISSN 0022-4804

Mal, H., Dehoux, M., Sleiman, C., Boczkowski, J., Leseche, G., Pariente, R. & Fournier, M. (1998). Early release of proinflammatory cytokines after lung transplantation. *Chest*, Vol.113, No.3, (Mar), pp. 645-651, ISSN 0012-3692

Marasco, S. F., Bailey, M., McGlade, D., Snell, G., Westall, G., Oto, T. & Pilcher, D. (2011). Effect of donor preservation solution and survival in lung transplantation. *J Heart Lung Transplant*, Vol.30, No.4, (Apr), pp. 414-419, ISSN 1557-3117

Marshak-Rothstein, A. & Rifkin, I. R. (2007). Immunologically active autoantigens: the role of toll-like receptors in the development of chronic inflammatory disease. *Annu Rev Immunol*, Vol.25, pp. 419-441, ISSN 0732-0582

Martins, S., de Perrot, M., Imai, Y., Yamane, M., Quadri, S. M., Segall, L., Dutly, A., Sakiyama, S., Chaparro, A., Davidson, B. L., Waddell, T. K., Liu, M. & Keshavjee, S. (2004). Transbronchial administration of adenoviral-mediated interleukin-10 gene to the donor improves function in a pig lung transplant model. *Gene Ther*, Vol.11, No.24, (Dec), pp. 1786-1796, ISSN 0969-7128

Maxey, T. S., Enelow, R. I., Gaston, B., Kron, I. L., Laubach, V. E. & Doctor, A. (2004). Tumor necrosis factor-alpha from resident lung cells is a key initiating factor in pulmonary ischemia-reperfusion injury. *J Thorac Cardiovasc Surg*, Vol.127, No.2, (Feb), pp. 541-547, ISSN 0022-5223

Mayer, A. M., Pittner, R. A., Lipscomb, G. E. & Spitzer, J. A. (1993). Effect of in vivo TNF administration on superoxide production and PKC activity of rat alveolar macrophages. *Am J Physiol*, Vol.264, No.1 Pt 1, (Jan), pp. L43-52, ISSN 0002-9513

McRae, K., De Perrot, M., Fischer, S., Waddell, T. K., Liu, M. & Keshavjee, S. (2001). Detection of IL-10 in the exhaled breath condensate, plasma and tissue during ischemia-reperfusion injury in experimental lung transplantation. *J Heart Lung Transplant*, Vol.20, No.2, (Feb), pp. 184, ISSN 1557-3117

Meade, M., Granton, J. T., Matte-Martyn, A., McRae, K., Cripps, P. M., Weaver, B. & Keshavjee, S. H. (2001). A randomized trial of inhaled nitric oxide to prevent reperfusion injury following lung transplantation. *J Heart Lung Transplant*, Vol.20, No.2, (Feb), pp. 254-255, ISSN 1557-3117

Meyer, K. C., Love, R. B. & Zimmerman, J. J. (1998). The therapeutic potential of nitric oxide in lung transplantation. *Chest*, Vol.113, No.5, (May), pp. 1360-1371, ISSN 0012-3692

Moore, T. M., Shirah, W. B., Khimenko, P. L., Paisley, P., Lausch, R. N. & Taylor, A. E. (2002). Involvement of CD40-CD40L signaling in postischemic lung injury. *Am J Physiol Lung Cell Mol Physiol*, Vol.283, No.6, (Dec), pp. L1255-1262, ISSN 1040-0605

Morimoto, R. I. (1993). Cells in stress: transcriptional activation of heat shock genes. *Science*, Vol.259, No.5100, (Mar 5), pp. 1409-1410, ISSN 0036-8075

Naidu, B. V., Woolley, S. M., Farivar, A. S., Thomas, R., Fraga, C. & Mulligan, M. S. (2003). Simvastatin ameliorates injury in an experimental model of lung ischemia-reperfusion. *J Thorac Cardiovasc Surg*, Vol.126, No.2, (Aug), pp. 482-489, ISSN 0022-5223

Naka, Y., Marsh, H. C., Scesney, S. M., Oz, M. C. & Pinsky, D. J. (1997). Complement activation as a cause for primary graft failure in an isogeneic rat model of hypothermic lung preservation and transplantation. *Transplantation*, Vol.64, No.9, (Nov 15), pp. 1248-1255, ISSN 0041-1337

Okazaki, M., Kreisel, F., Richardson, S. B., Kreisel, D., Krupnick, A. S., Patterson, G. A. & Gelman, A. E. (2007). Sphingosine 1-phosphate inhibits ischemia reperfusion injury following experimental lung transplantation. *Am J Transplant*, Vol.7, No.4, (Apr), pp. 751-758, ISSN 1600-6135

Oppenheim, J. J., Zachariae, C. O., Mukaida, N. & Matsushima, K. (1991). Properties of the novel proinflammatory supergene "intercrine" cytokine family. *Annu Rev Immunol*, Vol.9, pp. 617-648, ISSN 0732-0582

Oto, T., Griffiths, A. P., Rosenfeldt, F., Levvey, B. J., Williams, T. J. & Snell, G. I. (2006). Early outcomes comparing Perfadex, Euro-Collins, and Papworth solutions in lung transplantation. *Ann Thorac Surg*, Vol.82, No.5, (Nov), pp. 1842-1848, ISSN 1552-6259

Oyama, J., Blais, C., Jr., Liu, X., Pu, M., Kobzik, L., Kelly, R. A. & Bourcier, T. (2004). Reduced myocardial ischemia-reperfusion injury in toll-like receptor 4-deficient mice. *Circulation*, Vol.109, No.6, (Feb 17), pp. 784-789, ISSN 1524-4539

Park, J. S., Gamboni-Robertson, F., He, Q., Svetkauskaite, D., Kim, J. Y., Strassheim, D., Sohn, J. W., Yamada, S., Maruyama, I., Banerjee, A., Ishizaka, A. & Abraham, E. (2006). High mobility group box 1 protein interacts with multiple Toll-like receptors. *Am J Physiol Cell Physiol*, Vol.290, No.3, (Mar), pp. C917-924, ISSN 0363-6143

Pearse, D. B. & Dodd, J. M. (1999). Ischemia-reperfusion lung injury is prevented by apocynin, a novel inhibitor of leukocyte NADPH oxidase. *Chest*, Vol.116, No.1 Suppl, (Jul), pp. 55S-56S, ISSN 0012-3692

Phillips, W. A., Croatto, M. & Hamilton, J. A. (1990). Priming the macrophage respiratory burst with IL-4: enhancement with TNF-alpha but inhibition by IFN-gamma. *Immunology*, Vol.70, No.4, (Aug), pp. 498-503, ISSN 0019-2805

Pierre, A. F., Xavier, A. M., Liu, M., Cassivi, S. D., Lindsay, T. F., Marsh, H. C., Slutsky, A. S. & Keshavjee, S. H. (1998). Effect of complement inhibition with soluble complement receptor 1 on pig allotransplant lung function. *Transplantation*, Vol.66, No.6, (Sep 27), pp. 723-732, ISSN 0041-1337

Puri, V. & Patterson, G. A. (2008). Adult lung transplantation: technical considerations. *Semin Thorac Cardiovasc Surg*, Vol.20, No.2, (Summer), pp. 152-164, ISSN 1043-0679

Rabb, H., Daniels, F., O'Donnell, M., Haq, M., Saba, S. R., Keane, W. & Tang, W. W. (2000). Pathophysiological role of T lymphocytes in renal ischemia-reperfusion injury in mice. *Am J Physiol Renal Physiol*, Vol.279, No.3, (Sep), pp. F525-531, ISSN 1931-857X

Rachitskaya, A. V., Hansen, A. M., Horai, R., Li, Z., Villasmil, R., Luger, D., Nussenblatt, R. B. & Caspi, R. R. (2008). Cutting edge: NKT cells constitutively express IL-23 receptor and RORgammat and rapidly produce IL-17 upon receptor ligation in an IL-6-independent fashion. *J Immunol*, Vol.180, No.8, (Apr 15), pp. 5167-5171, ISSN 0022-1767

Reece, T. B., Laubach, V. E., Tribble, C. G., Maxey, T. S., Ellman, P. I., Warren, P. S., Schulman, A. M., Linden, J., Kern, J. A. & Kron, I. L. (2005). Adenosine A2A receptor agonist improves cardiac dysfunction from pulmonary ischemia-reperfusion injury. *Ann Thorac Surg*, Vol.79, No.4, (Apr), pp. 1189-1195, ISSN 1552-6259

Reece, T. B., Tribble, C. G., Okonkwo, D. O., Davis, J. D., Maxey, T. S., Gazoni, L. M., Linden, J., Kron, I. L. & Kern, J. A. (2008). Early adenosine receptor activation ameliorates spinal cord reperfusion injury. *J Cardiovasc Med (Hagerstown)*, Vol.9, No.4, (Apr), pp. 363-367, ISSN 1558-2027

Rivo, J., Zeira, E., Galun, E. & Matot, I. (2004). Activation of A3 adenosine receptor provides lung protection against ischemia-reperfusion injury associated with reduction in apoptosis. *Am J Transplant*, Vol.4, No.12, (Dec), pp. 1941-1948, ISSN 1600-6135

Rork, T. H., Wallace, K. L., Kennedy, D. P., Marshall, M. A., Lankford, A. R. & Linden, J. (2008). Adenosine A2A receptor activation reduces infarct size in the isolated, perfused mouse heart by inhibiting resident cardiac mast cell degranulation. *Am J Physiol Heart Circ Physiol*, Vol.295, No.5, (Nov), pp. H1825-1833, ISSN 0363-6135

Ross, S. D., Kron, I. L., Gangemi, J. J., Shockey, K. S., Stoler, M., Kern, J. A., Tribble, C. G. & Laubach, V. E. (2000). Attenuation of lung reperfusion injury after transplantation using an inhibitor of nuclear factor-kappaB. *Am J Physiol Lung Cell Mol Physiol*, Vol.279, No.3, (Sep), pp. L528-536, ISSN 1040-0605

Saemann, M. D., Haidinger, M., Hecking, M., Horl, W. H. & Weichhart, T. (2009). The multifunctional role of mTOR in innate immunity: implications for transplant immunity. *Am J Transplant*, Vol.9, No.12, (Dec), pp. 2655-2661, ISSN 1600-6143

Scaffidi, P., Misteli, T. & Bianchi, M. E. (2002). Release of chromatin protein HMGB1 by necrotic cells triggers inflammation. *Nature*, Vol.418, No.6894, (Jul 11), pp. 191-195, ISSN 0028-0836

Schmid, R. A., Zollinger, A., Singer, T., Hillinger, S., Leon-Wyss, J. R., Schob, O. M., Hogasen, K., Zund, G., Patterson, G. A. & Weder, W. (1998). Effect of soluble complement receptor type 1 on reperfusion edema and neutrophil migration after lung allotransplantation in swine. *J Thorac Cardiovasc Surg*, Vol.116, No.1, (Jul), pp. 90-97, ISSN 0022-5223

Schreck, R., Albermann, K. & Baeuerle, P. A. (1992). Nuclear factor kappa B: an oxidative stress-responsive transcription factor of eukaryotic cells (a review). *Free Radic Res Commun*, Vol.17, No.4, pp. 221-237, ISSN 8755-0199

Schutte, H., Witzenrath, M., Mayer, K., Rosseau, S., Seeger, W. & Grimminger, F. (2001). Short-term "preconditioning" with inhaled nitric oxide protects rabbit lungs against ischemia-reperfusion injury. *Transplantation*, Vol.72, No.8, (Oct 27), pp. 1363-1370, ISSN 0041-1337

Sharma, A. K., Fernandez, L. G., Awad, A. S., Kron, I. L. & Laubach, V. E. (2007). Proinflammatory response of alveolar epithelial cells is enhanced by alveolar macrophage-produced TNF-alpha during pulmonary ischemia-reperfusion injury. *Am J Physiol Lung Cell Mol Physiol*, Vol.293, No.1, (Jul), pp. L105-113, ISSN 1040-0605

Sharma, A. K., Yang, Z., Linden, J., Kron, I. L. & Laubach, V. E. (2008). Pulmonary ischemia-reperfusion injury is mediated by CD4+ T lymphocytes. *Am J Resp Crit Care Med*, Vol.177, No.Abstract Issue, pp. A38, ISSN

Sharma, A. K., Linden, J., Kron, I. L. & Laubach, V. E. (2009). Protection from pulmonary ischemia-reperfusion injury by adenosine A2A receptor activation. *Respir Res*, Vol.10, pp. 58, ISSN 1465-993X

Sharma, A. K., Laubach, V. E., Ramos, S. I., Zhao, Y., Stukenborg, G., Linden, J., Kron, I. L. & Yang, Z. (2010). Adenosine A2A receptor activation on CD4+ T lymphocytes and neutrophils attenuates lung ischemia-reperfusion injury. *J Thorac Cardiovasc Surg*, Vol.139, No.2, (Feb), pp. 474-482, ISSN 1097-685X

Sharma, A. K., Lapar, D. J., Zhao, Y., Li, L., Lau, C. L., Kron, I. L., Iwakura, Y., Okusa, M. D. & Laubach, V. E. (2011). Natural Killer T Cell-derived IL-17 Mediates Lung Ischemia-Reperfusion Injury. *Am J Respir Crit Care Med*, Vol.183, No.11, (Jun 1), pp. 1539-1549, ISSN 1535-4970

Shimamoto, A., Pohlman, T. H., Shomura, S., Tarukawa, T., Takao, M. & Shimpo, H. (2006). Toll-like receptor 4 mediates lung ischemia-reperfusion injury. *Ann Thorac Surg*, Vol.82, No.6, (Dec), pp. 2017-2023, ISSN 1552-6259

Shimoyama, T., Tabuchi, N., Kojima, K., Akamatsu, H., Arai, H., Tanaka, H. & Sunamori, M. (2005). Aprotinin attenuated ischemia-reperfusion injury in an isolated rat lung model after 18-hours preservation. *Eur J Cardiothorac Surg*, Vol.28, No.4, (Oct), pp. 581-587, ISSN 1010-7940

Shuvaev, V. V. & Muzykantov, V. R. (2011). Targeted modulation of reactive oxygen species in the vascular endothelium. *J Control Release*, (Mar 30), pp. ISSN 1873-4995

Sternberg, D. I., Gowda, R., Mehra, D., Qu, W., Weinberg, A., Twaddell, W., Sarkar, J., Wallace, A., Hudson, B., D'Ovidio, F., Arcasoy, S., Ramasamy, R., D'Armiento, J., Schmidt, A. M. & Sonett, J. R. (2008). Blockade of receptor for advanced glycation end product attenuates pulmonary reperfusion injury in mice. *J Thorac Cardiovasc Surg*, Vol.136, No.6, (Dec), pp. 1576-1585, ISSN 1097-685X

Strieter, R. M. & Kunkel, S. L. (1993). The immunopathology of chemotactic cytokines. *Adv Exp Med Biol*, Vol.351, pp. 19-28, ISSN 0065-2598

Sun, C. X., Zhong, H., Mohsenin, A., Morschl, E., Chunn, J. L., Molina, J. G., Belardinelli, L., Zeng, D. & Blackburn, M. R. (2006). Role of A2B adenosine receptor signaling in adenosine-dependent pulmonary inflammation and injury. *J Clin Invest*, Vol.116, No.8, (Aug), pp. 2173-2182, ISSN 0021-9738

Sundaresan, S., Semenkovich, J., Ochoa, L., Richardson, G., Trulock, E. P., Cooper, J. D. & Patterson, G. A. (1995). Successful outcome of lung transplantation is not compromised by the use of marginal donor lungs. *J Thorac Cardiovasc Surg*, Vol.109, No.6, (Jun), pp. 1075-1079, ISSN 0022-5223 van der Vliet, A. (2008). NADPH oxidases in lung biology and pathology: host defense enzymes, and more. *Free Radic Biol Med*, Vol.44, No.6, (Mar 15), pp. 938-955, ISSN 0891-5849

Wu, Q., Martin, R. J., Rino, J. G., Breed, R., Torres, R. M. & Chu, H. W. (2007). IL-23-dependent IL-17 production is essential in neutrophil recruitment and activity in mouse lung defense against respiratory Mycoplasma pneumoniae infection. *Microbes Infect*, Vol.9, No.1, (Jan), pp. 78-86, ISSN 1286-4579

Yang, Z., Sharma, A. K., Marshall, M., Kron, I. L. & Laubach, V. E. (2008). NADPH oxidase in bone marrow-derived cells mediates pulmonary ischemia-reperfusion injury. *Am J Respir Cell Mol Biol*, (Sep 11), pp. ISSN 1535-4989

Yang, Z., Sharma, A. K., Linden, J., Kron, I. L. & Laubach, V. E. (2009). CD4+ T lymphocytes mediate acute pulmonary ischemia-reperfusion injury. *J Thorac Cardiovasc Surg*, Vol.137, No.3, (Mar), pp. 695-702; discussion 702, ISSN 1097-685X

Yao, H., Yang, S. R., Kode, A., Rajendrasozhan, S., Caito, S., Adenuga, D., Henry, R., Edirisinghe, I. & Rahman, I. (2007). Redox regulation of lung inflammation: role of NADPH oxidase and NF-kappaB signalling. *Biochem Soc Trans*, Vol.35, No.Pt 5, (Nov), pp. 1151-1155, ISSN 0300-5127

Yen, D., Cheung, J., Scheerens, H., Poulet, F., McClanahan, T., McKenzie, B., Kleinschek, M. A., Owyang, A., Mattson, J., Blumenschein, W., Murphy, E., Sathe, M., Cua, D. J., Kastelein, R. A. & Rennick, D. (2006). IL-23 is essential for T cell-mediated colitis and promotes inflammation via IL-17 and IL-6. *J Clin Invest*, Vol.116, No.5, (May), pp. 1310-1316, ISSN 0021-9738

Yildiz, G., Demiryurek, A. T., Gumusel, B. & Lippton, H. (2007). Ischemic preconditioning modulates ischemia-reperfusion injury in the rat lung: role of adenosine receptors. *Eur J Pharmacol*, Vol.556, No.1-3, (Feb 5), pp. 144-150, ISSN 0014-2999

Zanotti, G., Casiraghi, M., Abano, J. B., Tatreau, J. R., Sevala, M., Berlin, H., Smyth, S., Funkhouser, W. K., Burridge, K., Randell, S. H. & Egan, T. M. (2009). Novel critical role of Toll-like receptor 4 in lung ischemia-reperfusion injury and edema. *Am J Physiol Lung Cell Mol Physiol*, Vol.297, No.1, (Jul), pp. L52-63, ISSN 1522-1504

Zhang, X., Bedard, E. L., Potter, R., Zhong, R., Alam, J., Choi, A. M. & Lee, P. J. (2002). Mitogen-activated protein kinases regulate HO-1 gene transcription after ischemia-reperfusion lung injury. *Am J Physiol Lung Cell Mol Physiol*, Vol.283, No.4, (Oct), pp. L815-829, ISSN 1040-0605

Zhao, G., al-Mehdi, A. B. & Fisher, A. B. (1997). Anoxia-reoxygenation versus ischemia in isolated rat lungs. *Am J Physiol*, Vol.273, No.6 Pt 1, (Dec), pp. L1112-1117, ISSN 0002-9513

Zhao, M., Fernandez, L. G., Doctor, A., Sharma, A. K., Zarbock, A., Tribble, C. G., Kron, I. L. & Laubach, V. E. (2006). Alveolar macrophage activation is a key initiation signal for acute lung ischemia-reperfusion injury. *Am J Physiol Lung Cell Mol Physiol*, Vol.291, No.5, (Nov), pp. L1018-1026, ISSN 1040-0605

Zhao, Y., Sharma, A. K., LaPar, D. J., Kron, I. L., Ailawadi, G., Liu, Y., Jones, D. R., Laubach, V. E. & Lau, C. L. (2011). Depletion of tissue plasminogen activator attenuates lung ischemia-reperfusion injury via inhibition of neutrophil extravasation. *Am J Physiol Lung Cell Mol Physiol*, Vol.300, No.5, (May), pp. L718-729, ISSN 1522-1504

Zhu, C., Bilali, A., Georgieva, G. S., Kurata, S., Mitaka, C. & Imai, T. (2008). Salvage of
    nonischemic control lung from injury by unilateral ischemic lung with apocynin, a
    nicotinamide adenine dinucleotide phosphate (NADPH) oxidase inhibitor, in
    isolated perfused rat lung. *Transl Res*, Vol.152, No.6, (Dec), pp. 273-282, ISSN 1878-
    1810

Zwacka, R. M., Zhang, Y., Halldorson, J., Schlossberg, H., Dudus, L. & Engelhardt, J. F.
    (1997).   CD4(+)   T-lymphocytes   mediate   ischemia/reperfusion-induced
    inflammatory responses in mouse liver. *J Clin Invest*, Vol.100, No.2, (Jul 15), pp.
    279-289, ISSN 0021-9738

9

Compensatory Lung Growth After Pneumonectomy

Lucas G. Fernández, James M. Isbell,
David R. Jones and Victor E. Laubach
University of Virginia Health System, Charlottesville, VA,
USA

1. Introduction

Pneumonectomy, the surgical removal of a lung, elicits a number of anatomical changes within the thoracic cavity that augments the diffusion capacity of the remaining lung. Pneumonectomy directs the entire cardiac output into the remaining lung and creates an empty hemithorax that results in a shift of the mediastinum toward the vacated thoracic compartment. In a number of experimental animal models, pneumonectomy initiates compensatory, regenerative growth of the remaining lung tissue that restores normal mass, structure and function. This growth process, called compensatory lung growth (CLG), is qualitatively similar across species, but differs with gender, age and hormonal status. CLG involves unique structure-function interactions not seen in solid organs. Little is known about the regenerative potential of human lungs. Although CLG has been reported in children after major lung resection, CLG in adults rarely occurs and remains a significant challenge. Mechanical feedback between the lung and thorax constitutes a major signal that sustains both post-natal lung development as well as post-pneumonectomy CLG. After pneumonectomy, increased mechanical stress and strain on the remaining lung induce adaptive responses to augment oxygen transport, including 1) recruitment of alveolar-capillary reserves, 2) remodeling of existing tissue, and 3) regenerative growth of acinar tissue when strain exceeds a critical threshold. This chapter will discuss the clinical aspects of pneumonectomy and will primarily review cellular and molecular mechanisms of CLG via experimental pneumonectomy models, which offers powerful insights into regenerative organ growth.

2. Clinical pneumonectomy

2.1 Historical perspective

Before the 1930s, all pneumonectomies in humans were fatal due primarily to complications such as hemorrhage and sepsis. Another major challenge was to perform lung surgery with an open pneumothorax. A significant step to solve this problem was taken in 1903 by Ferdinand Sauerbruch, who designed a negative pressure chamber that allowed a team of surgeons to operate within the open chest without collapse of the lung (Sauerbruch, 1953). Sauerbruch brought his machine to New York in 1908, where Willy

Meyer modified it to work with positive and negative pressure. Meyer successfully performed pulmonary resections in dogs in 1909 using suture closure of the bronchus and individual vessel ligation (Meyer, 1909), but he did not attempt his technique in humans. Years later, Quinby and Morse used a modification of this technique in dogs and showed that after pneumonectomy, the hemithorax fills with fluid and the remaining lung will shift to this empty side (Quinby & Morse, 1911). After the experimental use of endotracheal delivery of oxygen and anesthetics (Meltzer & Auer, 1909), Howard Lilienthal performed the first thoracotomy under endotracheal anesthesia at Mount Sinai Hospital (Lilienthal, 1910). He also had the largest published series of lobectomies, which he considered dangerous, reaching a mortality rate of 70% if more than one lobe was removed (Lilienthal, 1922). The first successful case of total pneumonectomy was described in 1931 by Roudolph Nissen in Berlin. The patient was a 12 year-old girl with trauma injury of the left chest (Naef, 1987). She recovered completely after two months, and Nissen was quoted saying that the occlusion of the pulmonary artery did not cause cardiopulmonary collapse as predicted 20 years earlier by Quinby and Morse. A year later, Cameron Haight was the first surgeon to perform a successful pneumonectomy in the west at the University of Michigan, USA (Haight, 1934). This time, a 13 year-old girl developed pneumonia in the left lung and subsequent pyopneumothorax. After a small bronchial fistula, she recovered 3.5 months later. On April 1933, Evarts Graham performed the first successful pneumonectomy for cancer disease in a 48 year-old patient with a squamous cell cancer of the left upper lobe bronchus that survived almost 30 years after surgery (Graham & Berck, 1933). In his paper, Clarence Crawford standardized the pneumonectomy technique used for many years, including the use of periscapular incision, individual vessel ligation, suture closure of the bronchus and a new rhythmic ventilatory technique (O'Shaughnessy & Crawford, 1938). In 1950, the introduction of a new double lumen tube allowed the ventilatory exclusion of the operated side (Bjork & Carlens, 1950). By the 1970s, a new technique changed the surgical method with the design of surgical staplers for lung resection. The first successful thoracic surgery performed using video assisted thoracic surgery (VDATS) was for treatment of pneumothorax in 1990. Shortly thereafter the first descriptions of pulmonary lobectomies and pneumonectomies appeared (Davies & Panasuk, 1992). There has been steady progress in thoracic surgery and pneumonectomy in particular through the years, with advances in knowledge of respiratory physiology, anesthetics and ventilation techniques, as well as more sophisticated methods of lung resection. These advancements have transformed pneumonectomy surgery from a "dangerous procedure" to become a very useful treatment for both malignant and non malignant diseases of the lung and airways.

2.2 Indications and risk factors

Pneumonectomy is known to be associated with high morbidity and mortality. However, in certain instances, it offers the only chance for a cure. The indications for pneumonectomy are usually classified in two major groups: pneumonectomy for benign disease and pneumonectomy for malignant disease. Due to the improvement of antimicrobial therapies and better control of inflammatory diseases, pneumonectomy for benign diseases is not a routine procedure in our times. The conditions considered in this group belong to several categories including inflammatory, traumatic, congenital and other miscellaneous conditions (Conlan & Kopec, 1999). These conditions carry a high mortality rate in most cases, but some examples of non-malignant disease have an excellent cure rate. Indications for pneumonectomy in cases of bacterial or fungal infections include symptomatic patients with hemoptysis, productive cough or chronic empyema, as well as unilateral lung destruction documented by CT or bronchography (Blyth, 2000). In patients with pulmonary tuberculosis, pneumonectomy is indicated for either multidrug resistance disease or for complications or sequelae of tuberculosis infection. The most common fungal infection that requires pneumonectomy is produced by Aspergillum, which can produce severe infections with recurrent or massive hemoptysis in over 75% of patients (Conlan, et al., 1987). Pneumonectomy for trauma is uncommon, but is associated with high morbidity and mortality (66-75%). The most obvious indication of the procedure is the laceration of the lung and airways, which can produce massive hemorrhage and air leakage. Complications of congenital and other miscellaneous lung diseases, as well as completion pneumonectomy are rare indications for pneumonectomy, which can be associated with high mortality. Pneumonectomy for malignant disease has become the most common indication for lung resection today, which includes both primary lung tumors and metastatic lung disease. It is regarded as the only curative treatment for non small cell lung cancer (Shields, 1982) and also as an effective therapeutic option for pulmonary metastasis; however, these can be associated with high mortality (Spaggiari, et al., 1998).

2.3 Morbidity and mortality

Pneumonectomy is associated with a 38-59% rate of morbidity and a 30-day mortality ranging from 3-12%. Postoperative cardiac dysrhythmias (e.g., atrial fibrillation and supraventricular tachycardia) are relatively common complications occurring in approximately 20-40% of patients following pneumonectomy. Postpneumonectomy pulmonary edema (PPE) and acute respiratory distress syndrome (ARDS) occur in 4-7% of patients and are increasingly believed to be the same disease process. PPE/ARDS results in noncardiogenic pulmonary edema and is manifest by diffuse pulmonary infiltrates on chest radiograph combined with profound hypoxia and respiratory failure frequently requiring mechanical ventilation. One of the more devastating complications of pneumonectomy is an empyema involving the postpneumonectomy space. A postpneumonectomy empyema is usually associated with a bronchopleural fistula (BPF), which is a communication between the mainstem bronchial stump and the pleural cavity. The incidence of BPF and empyema ranges from 2-8%, but both complications are significantly more common in patients who undergo pneumonectomy for septic pulmonary disease (e.g., tuberculosis or fungal disease) (Deschamps, et al., 2001). Postpneumonectomy syndrome is a rare complication characterized by stridor, dyspnea and recurring pneumonia. Postpneumonectomy syndrome is more common following right pneumonectomy and results from severe shifting of the mediastinum and contralateral lung into the postpneumonectomy pleural space, which in turn leads to compression of the contralateral mainstem bronchus between the vertebral bodies and descending aorta (Kopec, et al., 1998).

2.4 Physiological changes

Pneumonectomy results in reduced lung function. Although residual volume (RV) declines after pneumonectomy, it decreases less than expected as a result of the hyperexpansion that occurs in the remaining lung. Forced expiratory volume in one second (FEV_1) and forced vital capacity (FVC) both typically decrease by 25-40%. Diffusion capacity usually decreases by less than 50% whereas PaO_2 and $PaCO_2$ typically remain unchanged from preoperative levels (Kopec, et al., 1998).

3. Experimental CLG following pneumonectomy

The removal of a lung entails profound mechanical, metabolic and vascular changes in response to the reduction in lung volume and the empty space in the hemithorax. These changes trigger a compensatory response in experimental models, known as CLG, which are directed toward reestablishing the normal rate of oxygen exchange capacity. This section describes a number of experimental animal models of CLG that are currently used to study this process, as well as a detailed evaluation of the CLG response in these models, including lung morphometry and imaging.

3.1 Animal models

In many animal models, pneumonectomy (or lobectomy) induces CLG of the remaining lung, resulting in rapid restoration of total lung volume, compliance, mass, DNA, protein, alveolar number, and normal lung cell populations. Pneumonectomy has proven to be a reliable model for characterizing the sources, mechanisms, and functional limits of the compensatory growth response after removal of lung tissue. Pulmonary resections in animals began in 1881 when it was documented that the remaining lung eventually expands to the same size as both lungs. Early animal studies established the basis for application of the procedure to humans, beginning in the 1900s. Cohn in 1939 first established mechanical forces as a major signal for the compensatory increase in lung mass following lobectomy. In the 1950s, Schilling detailed the well-preserved functional status in dogs that underwent removal in stages of up to nearly 70% of lung mass (Schilling, et al., 1958). The use of small animals (e.g. rabbit, rat, and mouse) from the 1960s to the current day has had a great impact in uncovering the hormonal, cellular, and molecular responses to pneumonectomy (Bennett, et al., 1985; Buhain & Brody, 1973; Rannels, et al., 1979; Romanova, et al., 1967). Significant progress in understanding the cellular and molecular pathways of tissue regeneration in vertebrates were achieved using both transgenic mice and molecular biology techniques (Leuwerke, et al., 2002; Sakamaki, et al., 2002; Sakuma, et al., 2002). Functional compensation to pneumonectomy has been described mainly in dogs to define the limits of such compensation (Ravikumar, et al., 2004; Takeda, et al., 1997).

3.2 Alveolar growth

Alveolar epithelial cells in pneumonectomized rats exhibit metabolic changes typical of accelerated cell growth. Studies in mice and rats indicate that type II epithelial cell hypertrophy, proliferation and differentiation into type I cells characterize CLG in a fashion similar to early postnatal lung growth and lung repair after injury (Kaza, et al., 2002).

The post-pneumonectomy CLG response is independent of the lobe or lobes removed in small animals; and all remaining lobes grow rapidly until normal total lung mass is restored. Increases in lung volume after pneumonectomy parallel accumulation of tissue growth. However, the increase of growth in the remaining lobes is not uniform (Fernandez, et al., 2007). Development of sophisticated morphometric methods has permitted accurate analysis of lung volume and alveolar number, and studies indicate that new alveoli are formed during post-pneumonectomy CLG (Kaza, et al., 2002; Sakamaki, et al., 2002). In dogs, however, it appears that the CLG response is initiated after a certain threshold is achieved (removal of >50% of total lung mass) (Hsia, et al., 1994). Bronchoalveolar stem cells (BASC) have also been implicated in CLG. Their proliferation and differentiation into alveolar epithelial cells type II and I, contribute between 0-25% to the regenerative lung growth process (Nolen-Walston, et al., 2008).

3.3 Vascular growth and angiogenesis

Vascular growth and angiogenesis during CLG has not been well characterized. Stimuli known to initiate angiogenesis include hypoxia, inflammation, and mechanical factors such as shear stress and stretch. Our laboratory has shown that angiogenesis is necessary for successful CLG by demonstrating that angiogenesis inhibitors such as fumagillin or thalidomide prevented increased lung weight and volume after pneumonectomy (Maxey, et al., 2003). We have also shown that pneumonectomy induces arterial growth including the increase in length and number of branches of pulmonary arteries and that these changes are proportional to the amount of tissue removed (Le Cras, et al., 2005). When a bilobectomy was performed in rats (24% of lung tissue removed), the arterial area of the remaining lung increased by 26% compared to sham animals. Furthermore, when lung resection was more extensive (trilobectomy, 52%) we found that the increase in arterial area increased by 47% (Le Cras, et al., 2005). Other researchers have shown the effects of exogenous angiogenic factors, such as vascular endothelial growth factor (VEGF) in the mouse model. Additional VEGF therapy accelerated the CLG response, which was completed in only 4 days compared to 10 days in the pneumonectomy control group (Sakurai, et al., 2007).

4. Initiation of CLG

Several general hypotheses have been advanced to account for events that initiate the cellular and molecular changes that lead to CLG. Mechanical signals, transient hypoxia associated with thoracotomy, and elevated blood flow have been considered; however, no single event has been proven to account for the growth response.

4.1 Mechanical forces

After resection of the lung, increased inflation of the remaining lung and increased blood flow will induce stretch in both alveolar and endothelial structures. The displacement of the lung to the empty hemithorax is also a feature of CLG. These mechanical forces have an important role in initiating and regulating CLG as it was demonstrated when lateral displacement of the lung was restricted by the use of an inflatable prosthesis. This prevention of the mediastinal shift significantly limited mechanical lung strain, and CLG was thus significantly impaired by 30-60% (Hsia, et al., 2001). Another factor, increased alveolar inflation, was also implicated when experiments using *in vitro* perfusion of lungs with or without constant positive pressure ventilation (CPAP) of 20 cmH$_2$O, demonstrated that lungs with increased inflation had cellular hyperplastic changes, such as elevated levels of cAMP and PKA activity, but perfusion alone did not account for these changes (Russo, et al., 1989). It is clear that CLG is very complex with multiple metabolic factors. Hyperinflation and stretch applied to the remaining lung after pneumonectomy are powerful signals to initiate CLG, and it is known that stretch of alveolar cells induces important changes associated with cell growth and septal formation, including signal transduction, protein turnover, growth factor production, proliferation, and apoptosis (Brody, 1975; Davies, et al., 1982; Fehrenbach, et al., 2008; Karl, et al., 1989). It appears that lung stress and strain generated after pneumonectomy, overlaid on a background of heightened developmental lung strain generated by the expanding thorax, intensifies the CLG responses. Importantly, minimizing post-pneumonectomy strain of the remaining lung with space-occupying, inert material blunts the CLG response.

4.2 Elevated blood flow
Post-pneumonectomy changes in pulmonary blood flow have been considered as possible signals for CLG. Increased perfusion, reflecting elevated cardiac output to the remaining lung, likely causes physical distention of the pulmonary vasculature, resulting in a mechanical signal for lung growth and a concurrent increase in the growth factor and/or nutrient availability to the lung. It has been described that, after banding of the left caudal pulmonary artery in ferrets that reduced blood flow to the lung by 25%, CLG still occurred after pneumonectomy. However, the caudal lobes in the banded animals were 17% smaller than those of non-banded animals and tended to have lower protein content (McBride, et al., 1992). In our laboratory, we have shown that after left pneumonectomy, increases in growth and proliferation were not uniform among the right lobes but were greater in the upper and cardiac lobes. These unequal changes coincided with a predominant vascular growth in the upper lobe, which received the highest fraction of relative blood flow (Fernandez, et al., 2007).

4.3 Hypoxia
Hypoxia has been shown to stimulate alveolar growth either directly or via interaction with other signals. The effects of hypoxia after pneumonectomy were initially described in the rat model, where pneumonectomized rats that recovered at hypoxic levels showed significant increases in lung weight and volume indices, increased alveolar surface area and total alveolar numbers compared to normoxic and hyperoxic rats (Sekhon, et al., 1993). Hypoxia-inducible factors (HIFs), which are activated in response to oxidative stress, hypoxia, injury, and physical forces, regulate transcription of genes involved in a wide array of functions including glycolysis, erythropoiesis, apoptosis, and angiogenesis. Most of these stressors are directly or indirectly associated with a change of intracellular oxygen tension, which leads to stabilization of the HIF-1α protein and increases the transcriptional activation of target genes. Elevated hypoxia-induced mitogenic factor (HIMF) and HIF-1α mRNA and protein expression has been documented during CLG, thus these pathways may play an important role in mediating CLG (Li, et al., 2005; Zhang, et al., 2006; Zhang, et al., 2007).

5. Molecular mediators of CLG

The molecular mediators of CLG remain poorly understood. CLG involves regulated pathways of cell cycle activity, cell differentiation, synthesis and organization of connective tissue components, tissue remodeling, and angiogenesis. Studies in animals have led to several hypotheses that various pathways play a role in the induction of CLG including post-operative release of hormones and growth factors, as well as changes in cellular behavior. This section describes several important aspects of post-pneumonectomy CLG regulatory mechanisms.

5.1 Hormones

The most substantial evidence for hormonal regulation of CLG stems from investigations that involved surgical ablation of the adrenal glands, or adrenalectomy, which alone does not stimulate lung growth. Adrenalectomy performed prior to pneumonectomy increases the rate and extent of CLG above that observed in rats after pneumonectomy alone. This stimulatory effect on lung growth was blocked by daily doses of hydrocortisone acetate, evidenced by parameters such as dry lung weigh and DNA content, which were similar to the pneumonectomy group (Bennett, et al., 1985). This blocking effect was found only if the therapy was used continuously for the entire period after surgery (Rannels, et al., 1987). A combination of dexamethasone, 8-bromo-3'-5'-cAMP and isobutylmethyl-xanthine (DCI) has been successfully used to accelerate CLG in mice, represented by an increase in lung dry weight index and an increased number of alveoli by morphometric analysis. The effect of a single airway dose was enough to maintain the effect for the entire 28-day period of study. This effect seems to be modulated by thyroid transcription factor 1 (TTF-1), since its transient inhibition attenuated CLG (Takahashi, et al., 2011). Adrenal glucocorticosteroids seem to have a role in the modulation of the accelerated CLG initiated by pneumonectomy. Several lines of evidence suggest a possible role of growth hormone in the regulation of CLG. Significantly higher serum levels of growth hormone were detected in pregnant rats 3 days after pneumonectomy when compared with sham and unoperated rats (Khadempour, et al., 1992). In diabetic rats, which normally have greater levels of growth hormone and adrenal corticosteroids, pneumonectomy was accompanied by an increased dry lung weight index as well as higher elastin and collagen content, when compared to control pneumonectomy and sham rats (Ofulue & Thurlbeck, 1995). Following pneumonectomy, rats implanted with a subcutaneous growth hormone-secreting tumor (MtTF4) underwent a CLG response similar to non-tumor-bearing controls; however, lung growth in MtTF4 rats was associated with a greater lung volume.

5.2 Growth factors

There is ample evidence that growth factors regulate CLG, and the production of many growth factors is known to be sensitive to mechanical strain. Each growth factor modulates different aspects of cellular growth, but any one growth factor cannot recapitulate the entire CLG response, and there is much functional overlap among growth factors. Our laboratory, among others, has demonstrated important roles for epidermal growth factor (EGF), hypoxia-induced mitogenic factor (HIMF), keratinocyte growth factor (KGF) and retinoic acid in CLG. Other growth factor signaling pathways have been found to be activated after PNX including insulin-like growth factor-1 (IGF-1), hepatocyte growth factor (HGF), erythropoietin receptor, and hypoxia-inducible factor-1α (HIF-1α). These growth factors will be discussed below.

5.2.1 Epidermal growth factor (EGF)

It is been shown that EGF via its receptor (EGFR) plays a role in prenatal and postnatal lung development. Its actions involve the synthesis of surfactant precursors and the differentiation of type 2 epithelial cells. Using a pig lobectomy model, our laboratory demonstrated an upregulation of EGFR expression two weeks after lobectomy, which coincided with an increased alveolar cell proliferation index of the remaining lung. At 3 months after surgery, there was an increase in the lung protein/DNA ratio in the lobectomy group compared to controls (Kaza, et al., 2001; Kaza, et al., 2002). We also have documented the effects of EGF in CLG using a rodent pneumonectomy model. When exogenous EGF was administered to rats after pneumonectomy, it caused significantly higher lung weight and volume indices when compared to pneumonectomy control animals. We also detected an upregulation of EGFR after exogenous EGF supplementation (Kaza, et al., 2000), suggesting that the upregulation of EGF signaling is a feature of this process and is capable of modulating post-pneumonectomy GLG.

5.2.2 Erythropoietin (EPO)

Erythropoietin (EPO) actions have been classically associated with the induction of erythropoiesis; however, organ specific EPO receptor (EPOR) signaling is also involved in development, angiogenesis and organ growth. Researchers have shown that EPOR is upregulated both during postnatal lung maturation and during CLG in adult dogs (Foster, et al., 2004). Furthermore, they demonstrated an upregulation of one of its upstream activators, HIF-1α, during the same processes. Using an *in vitro* system, the same group showed that upregulation of HIF-1α in cultured HEK-293 cells also caused the upregulation of endogenous EPOR expression (Zhang, et al., 2006). This also provided evidence of a possible role of EPOR in CLG after pneumonectomy.

5.2.3 Hepatocyte growth factor (HGF)

HGF is known to selectively stimulate epithelial and endothelial cells, and the major sources for HGF in the lung are macrophages, fibroblasts, and endothelial cells. The increase of serum HGF during the first week after major lung resections in humans has been documented (Dikmen, et al., 2006; Sugahara, et al., 1998). A more comprehensive study of the role of HGF in CLG was performed using a mouse pneumonectomy model (Sakamaki, et al., 2002). In this study, the authors demonstrated an increased level of both lung mRNA and protein expression of HGF after pneumonectomy, and serum HGF levels were also higher when compared to sham operated animals. These findings were accompanied by an increased proliferation index of alveolar and airway epithelial cells, which peaked at day 5 after surgery. They also detected an upregulation of the HGF receptor (c-Met) at day 3 post-pneumonectomy. In addition, injections of HGF twice daily enhanced the proliferative response of these cells as well as increased lung weight index at day 3 when compared to controls. Use of a neutralizing antibody against HGF resulted in the inhibition, although incomplete, of the increase in lung weight and DNA synthesis observed. Another interesting study evaluated the effects of CLG in a rat model of elastase-induced emphysema, with transfection of the human HGF cDNA into the lung (Shigemura, et al., 2005) or implantation of adipose tissue-derived stromal cells (ASCs), which produce a large amount of angiogenic factors including HGF (Shigemura, et al., 2006). Therapy with gene transfection was performed using the hemagglutinating virus of Japan (HVJ) envelope-plasmid complex. In the HGF- and ASC-treated animals, increased levels of both exogenous and endogenous HGF were detected; and furthermore, HGF enhanced the CLG response by increasing lung cell proliferation and improving functional parameters. Taken together, these studies provide strong evidence for a role of HGF in the proliferative responses during CLG.

5.2.4 Hypoxia-induced mitogenic factor (HIMF)

In a collaborative study, we demonstrated the role of HIMF in the context of CLG (Li, et al., 2005). The mRNA and protein expression of HIMF, which is known by its mitogenic and angiogenic properties, was upregulated after pneumonectomy (days 3-14) when compared to sham operated mice. The elevated HIMF expression also coincided with an increase in cell proliferation index in lungs of these animals. HIMF expression after pneumonectomy was mainly detected in airway epithelial, endothelial and type 2 epithelial cells. Intratracheal instillation of exogenous HIMF increased the proliferative activity in these cells, documenting its mitogenic properties and establishing its role in CLG.

5.2.5 Hypoxia-inducible factor-1α (HIF-1α)

Researchers have shown that HIF-1α expression is upregulated both during postnatal lung maturation and during adult CLG in dogs and that this coincides with the upregulation of one of its downstream targets, EPOR. *In vitro* experiments also provided evidence that upregulation of HIF-1α in cultured HEK-293 cells triggers the upregulation of endogenous EPOR expression (Zhang, et al., 2006). Another study found that lung expansion is a major contributor to the activation and stabilization of HIF-1α. Acute deflation of prosthesis in the chest cavity of pneumonectomized dogs triggered the increase of both HIF-1 and several HIF-1 targets including EPOR and VEGF compared to non-deflated animals. They concluded that these increases did not depend on hypoxia but instead were due to stretch-related signals after lung resection (Zhang, et al., 2007).

5.2.6 Insulin-like growth factor-I (IGF-I)

IGF-1, its receptor and binding proteins are naturally expressed in the lung during development, and IGF-1 is known to contribute to the regulation of postnatal lung cell proliferation. Researchers have shown that 2 and 6 days after pneumonectomy in rats, the bronchoalveolar lavage fluid from these animals demonstrated significantly increased mitogenic activity when applied *in vitro* to fibroblasts compared with controls. Importantly, such activity was partially inhibited by the use of neutralizing antibody against IGF-1, and the levels of IGF-1 were elevated by 100% at day 2 after pneumonectomy (McAnulty, et al., 1992). In a separate study, IGF-1 mRNA expression was again significantly increased after 21 days post-pneumonectomy in a model of neonatal CLG in lambs (Nobuhara, et al., 1998).

5.2.7 Keratinocyte growth factor-I (KGF)

KGF has been shown to play an important role in alveolar epithelial cell proliferation and lung development. In our laboratory, exogenous KGF administered to rats after pneumonectomy further enhanced several parameters of CLG compared to control animals. Changes in lung weight index, lung volume index as well as morphometric parameters were accompanied by a significant increase in pulmonary cell proliferation index, providing the first evidence for a role of KGF in CLG (Kaza, et al., 2002). A more recent study corroborated our findings where epithelial cell proliferation was further enhanced after *in vivo* transfection of a KGF cDNA vector in a model of CLG in rats, confirming KGF as an important lung mitogenic factor (Matsumoto, et al., 2009).

5.2.8 Retinoic acid

Retinoic acid, a metabolite of vitamin A, has been implicated in normal lung development and cell proliferation. Our laboratory described the effects of exogenous retinoic acid during CLG in a rat model (Kaza, et al., 2001). At 10 and 21 days after pneumonectomy, lung weight, lung volume and cellular proliferation indices were all significantly augmented in rats that received exogenous retinoic acid versus vehicle controls. Interestingly, we also found that pulmonary expression of EGFR was upregulated in lungs after retinoic acid treatment, uncovering a possible relationship between these two important growth factors in CLG. Another similarly designed study corroborated our results several years later (Karapolat, et al., 2008); however, these effects did not translate into functional recovery according to studies developed using the dog model (Dane, et al., 2004).

5.2.9 Vascular endothelial growth factor (VEGF)

Angiogenesis, the formation of new blood vessels, is a critical step in normal organ development and in abnormal processes such as tumor growth and metastasis. In the lung, alveolar growth and angiogenesis should occur concurrently in order to result in normal organ development or regeneration. One of the most important angiogenic growth factors, VEGF has been studied in CLG, revealing its importance in this regenerative process. Researchers described the effects of exogenous VEGF in the mouse model, showing that exogenous VEGF therapy accelerated the CLG response, which was completed in only 4 days compared to 10 days in control animals. However, these effects could not be blocked by the use of either VEGF receptor inhibitors or neutralizing antibodies (Sakurai, et al., 2007). Another study associated lung expansion and other signaling pathways to VEGF. The acute deflation of prosthesis in the chest cavity of pneumonectomized dogs triggered the increase of HIF-1α and its targets EPOR and VEGF compared to non-deflated animals, showing the interaction between these signals in the regulation of CLG (Zhang, et al., 2007). A recent paper studied the modulation of different VEGF isoforms along with its receptor during CLG, where VEGF 188 mRNA expression was decreased compared to sham animals and VEGF 164 and VEGF 120 mRNAs increased during days 1 and 3 respectively, describing what they believe is the recapitulation of the pattern of expression for these isoforms in the fetal lung (Jancelewicz, et al., 2010). A brief summary of evidence for the role of growth factors in CLG is shown in Table 1.

Growth Factor	Evidence	Species
EGF	• Pneumonectomy increased EGFR lung expression.	Rat, pig
	• Exogenous EGF enhances CLG.	Rat
EPOR	• Pneumonectomy increased EPOR lung expression.	Dog
HGF	• Pneumonectomy increased serum HGF, along with expression of HGF and its receptor (c-Met) in lung.	Mouse Mouse,
	• Exogenous HGF enhances CLG.	rat
	• Neutralizing antibody against HGF attenuate CLG.	Mouse
HIMF	• Pneumonectomy increased lung HIMF mRNA and protein expression.	Mouse
	• Exogenous HIMF enhances proliferation.	
HIF-1α	• Pneumonectomy increased lung HIF-1α mRNA and protein expression.	Dog
	• Lung expansion modulates HIF-1α expression.	
IGF-1	• Pneumonectomy increased lung IGF-1 mRNA and protein expression.	Lamb, rat
	• Neutralizing antibody against IGF-1 attenuate mitogenic *in vitro* effects.	Rat
KGF	• Pneumonectomy increased lung KGF mRNA.	Rat
	• Exogenous KGF enhances CLG.	
Retinoic Acid	• Exogenous retinoic acid enhances CLG.	Rat
	• Exogenous retinoic acid induces EGFR.	
VEGF	• Pneumonectomy increased lung VEGF 164 and 120 mRNA expressions.	Mouse
	• Exogenous VEGF accelerates CLG.	

Table 1. Summary of potential roles of growth factors in CLG.

5.3 Transcription factors

Pneumonectomy induces shear stress in the lung, and several key transcription factors provide links between shear-mediated signaling and CLG. Mitogen-activated protein kinases (MAPKs), composed of extracellular signal-regulated kinases (ERKs), c-jun NH2-terminal kinases (JNKs), and p38 MAPKs, play a critical role in cell differentiation, growth and apoptosis and the regulation of various transcription factors and gene expression. One of the first reports about stretch-induced early gene expression demonstrated that in as early as 30 minutes post-pneumonectomy in rats, c-fos and JunB are significantly increased. These results were also reproduced when *in vitro* ventilation-perfusion was used (Gilbert & Rannels, 1998). Using array technology, researchers have also shown significant increases in six different transcription factors as early as 6 hours after pneumonectomy in mice including Erg-1 and Nur77, all of which have important roles in vascular biology, development and stress response (Landesberg, et al., 2001). In addition, a more recent paper found an important role for thyroid transcription factor 1 (TTF-1) in CLG (Takahashi, et al., 2010). These investigators detected a significant increase of TTF-1 expression 12 hours after pneumonectomy with TTF-1 expression primarily observed in cells of the alveolar ducts. When TTF-1 was repressed using small inhibitory RNAs (siRNAs), the CLG response was also temporally delayed.

5.4 Telomerase

Telomerase is an important enzyme for DNA repair and contributes to cell maintenance. Telomerase prevents the excess shortening of telomeres, and it has been demonstrated that telomerase is active in proliferating cells in a number of organs, including the lung. In humans, mutations of the telomerase gene results in a pathological condition known as idiopathic pulmonary fibrosis (IPF). Its role in preserving lung epithelial integrity was demonstrated in an experimental model in mice, where telomerase deficiency resulted in a reduction in the number and integrity of type 2 alveolar epithelial cells (AEC2) (Lee, et al., 2009). It is important to know that this defect may not be apparent in early generations, but after progressive inbreeding, it was possible to establish the deficiency in AEC2s as well as in bronchoalveolar stem cell (BASC) populations in the lung, due to shortening of the telomeres. In a recent study, the importance of telomerase was demonstrated for CLG after pneumonectomy using telomerase deficient mice from second (F2), third (F3) and fourth (F4) generation animals (Jackson, et al., 2011). In wild-type mice, the activity of telomerase was found to increase in isolated AEC2s up to 3.5-fold during post-pneumonectomy days 3 and 7. In addition, the total number of AEC2s and BASCs also increased at day 3 after pneumonectomy. However, pneumonectomy resulted in diminished CLG in F3 telomerase null animals, expressed as failure to induce an increase in lung mass by day 7 after pneumonectomy. In addition, the number of AEC2s and BASCs did not increase during the initial period after pneumonectomy when compared to wild-type mice. The normal CLG, both in lung mass and AEC2 numbers, in wild-type mice was also accompanied by an elevation in the proliferation marker Ki-67, early growth response gene (Egr-1) and repair transcription factors such as ERK 1/2, which were not observed in telomerase null mice. The authors concluded that telomerase deletion produces an attenuated CLG response after pneumonectomy by arresting cell growth and inducing DNA damage.

6. Conclusion

The extent of CLG in humans following pneumonectomy or lobectomy is incompletely investigated, but a number of long-term physiological studies suggest, however, that some degree of CLG may occur, especially in children (Nakajima, et al., 1998; Nonoyama, et al., 1986). The ability to manipulate the gain/loss of function for a particular gene in experimental animals has begun to provide a more detailed understanding of the molecular mediators and the pathologic consequences of CLG. Also, recent developments in cell therapy of diseased lungs with the use of adipose stem cells are indeed promising (Shigemura, et al., 2006). An important long-term goal of research into mechanisms of CLG is to generate knowledge that will allow the induction of alveolar regeneration or that rescues failed alveologenesis in humans. Such understanding will facilitate the development of therapies for the management of end-stage lung disease, lung volume reduction surgery, and transplantation. The potential clinical applications of this research are great. Specific examples of patients who would clearly benefit from lung regenerative therapies include chronic obstructive pulmonary disease (COPD), emphysema, pulmonary hypertension, bronchopulmonary dysplasia (BPD), as well as premature infants whose lungs are too underdeveloped to support life.

7. References

Bennett, R. A., Colony, P. C., Addison, J. L. & Rannels, D. E. (1985). Effects of prior adrenalectomy on postpneumonectomy lung growth in the rat. *Am J Physiol*, Vol.248, No.1 Pt 1, (Jan), pp. E70-74, ISSN 0002-9513

Bjork, V. O. & Carlens, E. (1950). The prevention of spread during pulmonary resection by the use of a double-lumen catheter. *J Thorac Surg*, Vol.20, No.1, (Jul), pp. 151-157, ISSN 0096-5588

Blyth, D. F. (2000). Pneumonectomy for inflammatory lung disease. *Eur J Cardiothorac Surg*, Vol.18, No.4, (Oct), pp. 429-434, ISSN 1010-7940

Brody, J. S. (1975). Time course of and stimuli to compensatory growth of the lung after pneumonectomy. *J Clin Invest*, Vol.56, No.4, (Oct), pp. 897-904, ISSN 0021-9738

Buhain, W. J. & Brody, J. S. (1973). Compensatory growth of the lung following pneumonectomy. *J Appl Physiol*, Vol.35, No.6, (Dec), pp. 898-902, ISSN 0021-8987

Conlan, A. A., Abramor, E. & Moyes, D. G. (1987). Pulmonary aspergilloma--indications for surgical intervention. An analysis of 22 cases. *S Afr Med J*, Vol.71, No.5, (Mar 7), pp. 285-288, ISSN 0256-9574

Conlan, A. A. & Kopec, S. E. (1999). Indications for pneumonectomy. Pneumonectomy for benign disease. *Chest Surg Clin N Am*, Vol.9, No.2, (May), pp. 311-326, ISSN 1052-3359

Dane, D. M., Yan, X., Tamhane, R. M., Johnson, R. L., Jr., Estrera, A. S., Hogg, D. C., Hogg, R. T. & Hsia, C. C. (2004). Retinoic acid-induced alveolar cellular growth does not improve function after right pneumonectomy. *J Appl Physiol*, Vol.96, No.3, (Mar), pp. 1090-1096, ISSN 8750-7587

Davies, A. L. & Panasuk, D. B. (1992). Video-assisted thoracic surgery: our first 20 cases. *Del Med J*, Vol.64, No.4, (Apr), pp. 267-272, ISSN 0011-7781

Davies, P., McBride, J., Murray, G. F., Wilcox, B. R., Shallal, J. A. & Reid, L. (1982). Structural changes in the canine lung and pulmonary arteries after pneumonectomy. *J Appl Physiol*, Vol.53, No.4, (Oct), pp. 859-864, ISSN 0161-7567

Deschamps, C., Bernard, A., Nichols, F. C., 3rd, Allen, M. S., Miller, D. L., Trastek, V. F., Jenkins, G. D. & Pairolero, P. C. (2001). Empyema and bronchopleural fistula after pneumonectomy: factors affecting incidence. *Ann Thorac Surg*, Vol.72, No.1, (Jul), pp. 243-247; ISSN 0003-4975

Dikmen, E., Kara, M., Kisa, U., Atinkaya, C., Han, S. & Sakinci, U. (2006). Human hepatocyte growth factor levels in patients undergoing thoracic operations. *Eur Respir J*, Vol.27, No.1, (Jan), pp. 73-76, ISSN 0903-1936

Fehrenbach, H., Voswinckel, R., Michl, V., Mehling, T., Fehrenbach, A., Seeger, W. & Nyengaard, J. R. (2008). Neoalveolarisation contributes to compensatory lung growth following pneumonectomy in mice. *Eur Respir J*, Vol.31, No.3, (Mar), pp. 515-522, ISSN 1399-3003

Fernandez, L. G., Le Cras, T. D., Ruiz, M., Glover, D. K., Kron, I. L. & Laubach, V. E. (2007). Differential vascular growth in postpneumonectomy compensatory lung growth. *J Thorac Cardiovasc Surg*, Vol.133, No.2, (Feb), pp. 309-316, ISSN 1097-685X

Foster, D. J., Moe, O. W. & Hsia, C. C. (2004). Upregulation of erythropoietin receptor during postnatal and postpneumonectomy lung growth. *Am J Physiol Lung Cell Mol Physiol*, Vol.287, No.6, (Dec), pp. L1107-1115, ISSN 1040-0605

Gilbert, K. A. & Rannels, D. E. (1998). Increased lung inflation induces gene expression after pneumonectomy. *Am J Physiol*, Vol.275, No.1 Pt 1, (Jul), pp. L21-29, ISSN 0002-9513

Graham, E. A. & Berck, M. (1933). Principle versus details in the treatment of acute empyema. *Ann Surg*, Vol.98, No.4, (Oct), pp. 520-527, ISSN 0003-4932

Haight, C. (1934). Total removal of the lung for bronchiectasis. *Surgery, Gynecology and Obstetrics*, Vol.58, pp. ISSN

Hsia, C. C., Herazo, L. F., Fryder-Doffey, F. & Weibel, E. R. (1994). Compensatory lung growth occurs in adult dogs after right pneumonectomy. *J Clin Invest*, Vol.94, No.1, (Jul), pp. 405-412, ISSN 0021-9738

Hsia, C. C., Wu, E. Y., Wagner, E. & Weibel, E. R. (2001). Preventing mediastinal shift after pneumonectomy impairs regenerative alveolar tissue growth. *Am J Physiol Lung Cell Mol Physiol*, Vol.281, No.5, (Nov), pp. L1279-1287, ISSN 1040-0605

Jackson, S. R., Lee, J., Reddy, R., Williams, G. N., Kikuchi, A., Freiberg, Y., Warburton, D. & Driscoll, B. (2011). Partial pneumonectomy of telomerase null mice carrying shortened telomeres initiates cell growth arrest resulting in a limited compensatory growth response. *Am J Physiol Lung Cell Mol Physiol*, Vol.300, No.6, (Jun), pp. L898-909, ISSN 1522-1504

Jancelewicz, T., Grethel, E. J., Chapin, C. J., Clifton, M. S. & Nobuhara, K. K. (2010). Vascular endothelial growth factor isoform and receptor expression during compensatory lung growth. *J Surg Res*, Vol.160, No.1, (May 1), pp. 107-113, ISSN 1095-8673

Karapolat, S., Sanli, A., Onen, A., Acikel, U. & Sivrikoz, O. (2008). Effects of retinoic acid on compensatory lung growth. *J Cardiothorac Surg*, Vol.3, pp. 37, ISSN 1749-8090

Karl, H. W., Russo, L. A. & Rannels, D. E. (1989). Inflation-associated increases in lung polyamine uptake: role of altered pulmonary vascular flow. *Am J Physiol*, Vol.257, No.5 Pt 1, (Nov), pp. E729-735, ISSN 0002-9513

Kaza, A. K., Laubach, V. E., Kern, J. A., Long, S. M., Fiser, S. M., Tepper, J. A., Nguyen, R. P., Shockey, K. S., Tribble, C. G. & Kron, I. L. (2000). Epidermal growth factor augments postpneumonectomy lung growth. *J Thorac Cardiovasc Surg*, Vol.120, No.5, (Nov), pp. 916-921, ISSN 0022-5223

Kaza, A. K., Kron, I. L., Kern, J. A., Long, S. M., Fiser, S. M., Nguyen, R. P., Tribble, C. G. & Laubach, V. E. (2001). Retinoic acid enhances lung growth after pneumonectomy. *Ann Thorac Surg*, Vol.71, No.5, (May), pp. 1645-1650, ISSN 0003-4975

Kaza, A. K., Kron, I. L., Long, S. M., Fiser, S. M., Stevens, P. M., Kern, J. A., Tribble, C. G. & Laubach, V. E. (2001). Epidermal growth factor receptor up-regulation is associated with lung growth after lobectomy. *Ann Thorac Surg*, Vol.72, No.2, (Aug), pp. 380-385, ISSN 0003-4975

Kaza, A. K., Cope, J. T., Fiser, S. M., Long, S. M., Kern, J. A., Tribble, C. G., Kron, I. L. & Laubach, V. E. (2002). Contrasting natures of lung growth after transplantation and lobectomy. *J Thorac Cardiovasc Surg*, Vol.123, No.2, (Feb), pp. 288-294, ISSN 0022-5223

Kaza, A. K., Kron, I. L., Leuwerke, S. M., Tribble, C. G. & Laubach, V. E. (2002). Keratinocyte growth factor enhances post-pneumonectomy lung growth by alveolar proliferation. *Circulation*, Vol.106, No.12 Suppl 1, (Sep 24), pp. I120-124, ISSN 1524-4539

Khadempour, M. H., Ofulue, A. F., Sekhon, H. S., Cherukupalli, K. M. & Thurlbeck, W. M. (1992). Changes of growth hormone, somatomedin C, and bombesin following pneumonectomy. *Exp Lung Res*, Vol.18, No.3, (May-Jun), pp. 421-432, ISSN 0190-2148

Kopec, S. E., Irwin, R. S., Umali-Torres, C. B., Balikian, J. P. & Conlan, A. A. (1998). The postpneumonectomy state. *Chest*, Vol.114, No.4, (Oct), pp. 1158-1184, ISSN 0012-3692

Landesberg, L. J., Ramalingam, R., Lee, K., Rosengart, T. K. & Crystal, R. G. (2001). Upregulation of transcription factors in lung in the early phase of postpneumonectomy lung growth. *Am J Physiol Lung Cell Mol Physiol*, Vol.281, No.5, (Nov), pp. L1138-1149, ISSN 1040-0605

Le Cras, T. D., Fernandez, L. G., Pastura, P. A. & Laubach, V. E. (2005). Vascular growth and remodeling in compensatory lung growth following right lobectomy. *J Appl Physiol*, Vol.98, No.3, (Mar), pp. 1140-1148, ISSN 8750-7587

Lee, J., Reddy, R., Barsky, L., Scholes, J., Chen, H., Shi, W. & Driscoll, B. (2009). Lung alveolar integrity is compromised by telomere shortening in telomerase-null mice. *Am J Physiol Lung Cell Mol Physiol*, Vol.296, No.1, (Jan), pp. L57-70, ISSN 1040-0605

Leuwerke, S. M., Kaza, A. K., Tribble, C. G., Kron, I. L. & Laubach, V. E. (2002). Inhibition of compensatory lung growth in endothelial nitric oxide synthase-deficient mice. *Am J Physiol Lung Cell Mol Physiol*, Vol.282, No.6, (Jun), pp. L1272-1278, ISSN 1040-0605

Li, D., Fernandez, L. G., Dodd-o, J., Langer, J., Wang, D. & Laubach, V. E. (2005). Upregulation of hypoxia-induced mitogenic factor in compensatory lung growth after pneumonectomy. *Am J Respir Cell Mol Biol*, Vol.32, No.3, (Mar), pp. 185-191, ISSN 1044-1549

Lilienthal, H. (1910). IV. The First Case of Thoracotomy in a Human Being under Anaesthesia by Intratracheal Insufflation. *Ann Surg*, Vol.52, No.1, (Jul), pp. 30-33, ISSN 0003-4932

Lilienthal, H. (1922). Resection of the Lung for Suppurative Infections with a Report Based on 31 Operative Cases in Which Resection Was Done or Intended. *Ann Surg*, Vol.75, No.3, (Mar), pp. 257-320, ISSN 0003-4932

Matsumoto, K., Nagayasu, T., Hishikawa, Y., Tagawa, T., Yamayoshi, T., Abo, T., Tobinaga, S., Furukawa, K. & Koji, T. (2009). Keratinocyte growth factor accelerates compensatory growth in the remaining lung after trilobectomy in rats. *J Thorac Cardiovasc Surg*, Vol.137, No.6, (Jun), pp. 1499-1507, ISSN 1097-685X

Maxey, T. S., Reece, T. B., Dimling, G. M., Tribble, C. G., Kron, I. L. & Laubach, V. E. (2003). Inhibition of angiogenesis prevents post-pneumonectomy compensatory lung growth. *Am J Respir Crit Care Med*, Vol.167, No.7, (April), pp. A575, ISSN 1073-449X

McAnulty, R. J., Guerreiro, D., Cambrey, A. D. & Laurent, G. J. (1992). Growth factor activity in the lung during compensatory growth after pneumonectomy: evidence of a role for IGF-1. *Eur Respir J*, Vol.5, No.6, (Jun), pp. 739-747, ISSN 0903-1936

McBride, J. T., Kirchner, K. K., Russ, G. & Finkelstein, J. (1992). Role of pulmonary blood flow in postpneumonectomy lung growth. *J Appl Physiol*, Vol.73, No.6, (Dec), pp. 2448-2451, ISSN 8750-7587

Meltzer, S. J. & Auer, J. (1909). Continuous Respiration without Respiratory Movements. *J Exp Med*, Vol.11, No.4, (Jul 17), pp. 622-625, ISSN 0022-1007

Meyer, W. (1909). Pneumonectomy with the aid of differential air pressure: an experimental study. *J Amer Acad Med*, Vol.53, pp. ISSN

Naef, A. P. (1987). [Development of thoracic surgery from 1880 to the present]. *Rev Med Suisse Romande*, Vol.107, No.11, (Nov), pp. 949-957, ISSN 0035-3655

Nakajima, C., Kijimoto, C., Yokoyama, Y., Miyakawa, T., Tsuchiya, Y., Kuroda, T., Nakano, M. & Saeki, M. (1998). Longitudinal follow-up of pulmonary function after lobectomy in childhood - factors affecting lung growth. *Pediatr Surg Int*, Vol.13, No.5-6, (Jul), pp. 341-345, ISSN 0179-0358

Nobuhara, K. K., DiFiore, J. W., Ibla, J. C., Siddiqui, A. M., Ferretti, M. L., Fauza, D. O., Schnitzer, J. J. & Wilson, J. M. (1998). Insulin-like growth factor-I gene expression in three models of accelerated lung growth. *J Pediatr Surg*, Vol.33, No.7, (Jul), pp. 1057-1060; discussion 1061, ISSN 0022-3468

Nolen-Walston, R. D., Kim, C. F., Mazan, M. R., Ingenito, E. P., Gruntman, A. M., Tsai, L., Boston, R., Woolfenden, A. E., Jacks, T. & Hoffman, A. M. (2008). Cellular kinetics and modeling of bronchioalveolar stem cell response during lung regeneration. *Am J Physiol Lung Cell Mol Physiol*, Vol.294, No.6, (Jun), pp. L1158-1165, ISSN 1040-0605

Nonoyama, A., Tanaka, K., Osako, T., Saito, Y., Umemoto, M., Masuda, A. & Kagawa, T. (1986). Pulmonary function after lobectomy in children under ten years of age. *Jpn J Surg*, Vol.16, No.6, (Nov), pp. 425-434, ISSN 0047-1909

O'Shaughnessy, L. & Crawford, J. H. (1938). The Surgical Treatment of Pulmonary Tuberculosis. *Postgrad Med J*, Vol.14, No.148, (Feb), pp. 38-48, ISSN 0032-5473

Ofulue, A. F. & Thurlbeck, W. M. (1995). Effects of streptozotocin-induced diabetes on postpneumonectomy lung growth and connective tissue levels. *Pediatr Pulmonol*, Vol.19, No.6, (Jun), pp. 365-370, ISSN 8755-6863

Quinby, W. & Morse, J. (1911). Experimental pneumonectomy, the implication of data obtained to surgery of the thorax. *Boston Medical and Surgical Journal*, Vol.165, pp. 121, ISSN

Rannels, D. E., White, D. M. & Watkins, C. A. (1979). Rapidity of compensatory lung growth following pneumonectomy in adult rats. *J Appl Physiol*, Vol.46, No.2, (Feb), pp. 326-333, ISSN 0161-7567

Rannels, D. E., Karl, H. W. & Bennett, R. A. (1987). Control of compensatory lung growth by adrenal hormones. *Am J Physiol*, Vol.253, No.4 Pt 1, (Oct), pp. E343-348, ISSN 0002-9513

Ravikumar, P., Yilmaz, C., Dane, D. M., Johnson, R. L., Jr., Estrera, A. S. & Hsia, C. C. (2004). Regional lung growth following pneumonectomy assessed by computed tomography. *J Appl Physiol*, Vol.97, No.4, (Oct), pp. 1567-1574; discussion 1549, ISSN 8750-7587

Romanova, L. K., Leikina, E. M. & Antipova, K. K. (1967). [Nucleic acid synthesis and mitotic activity during the development of compensatory pulmonary hypertrophy in rats]. *Biull Eksp Biol Med*, Vol.63, No.3, (Mar), pp. 96-100, ISSN 0365-9615

Russo, L. A., Rannels, S. R., Laslow, K. S. & Rannels, D. E. (1989). Stretch-related changes in lung cAMP after partial pneumonectomy. *Am J Physiol*, Vol.257, No.2 Pt 1, (Aug), pp. E261-268, ISSN 0002-9513

Sakamaki, Y., Matsumoto, K., Mizuno, S., Miyoshi, S., Matsuda, H. & Nakamura, T. (2002). Hepatocyte growth factor stimulates proliferation of respiratory epithelial cells during postpneumonectomy compensatory lung growth in mice. *Am J Respir Cell Mol Biol*, Vol.26, No.5, (May), pp. 525-533, ISSN 1044-1549

Sakuma, T., Sagawa, M., Hida, M., Nambu, Y., Osanai, K., Toga, H., Takahashi, K., Ohya, N. & Matthay, M. A. (2002). Time-dependent effect of pneumonectomy on alveolar epithelial fluid clearance in rat lungs. *J Thorac Cardiovasc Surg*, Vol.124, No.4, (Oct), pp. 668-674, ISSN 0022-5223

Sakurai, M. K., Lee, S., Arsenault, D. A., Nose, V., Wilson, J. M., Heymach, J. V. & Puder, M. (2007). Vascular endothelial growth factor accelerates compensatory lung growth after unilateral pneumonectomy. *Am J Physiol Lung Cell Mol Physiol*, Vol.292, No.3, (Mar), pp. L742-747, ISSN 1040-0605

Schilling, J. A., Lategola, M. T. & Massion, W. H. (1958). Physiologic effects of lung resection in dogs; mechanics of breathing, gas exchange, pulmonary arterial pressure, compliance, and lung weights. *Bull Soc Int Chir*, Vol.17, No.5-6, (Dec), pp. 310-319, ISSN 0037-945X

Sekhon, H. S., Smith, C. & Thurlbeck, W. M. (1993). Effect of hypoxia and hyperoxia on postpneumonectomy compensatory lung growth. *Exp Lung Res*, Vol.19, No.5, (Sep-Oct), pp. 519-532, ISSN 0190-2148

Shields, T. W. (1982). Surgical therapy for carcinoma of the lung. *Clin Chest Med*, Vol.3, No.2, (May), pp. 369-387, ISSN 0272-5231

Shigemura, N., Sawa, Y., Mizuno, S., Ono, M., Minami, M., Okumura, M., Nakamura, T., Kaneda, Y. & Matsuda, H. (2005). Induction of compensatory lung growth in pulmonary emphysema improves surgical outcomes in rats. *Am J Respir Crit Care Med*, Vol.171, No.11, (Jun 1), pp. 1237-1245, ISSN 1073-449X

Shigemura, N., Okumura, M., Mizuno, S., Imanishi, Y., Matsuyama, A., Shiono, H., Nakamura, T. & Sawa, Y. (2006). Lung tissue engineering technique with adipose stromal cells improves surgical outcome for pulmonary emphysema. *Am J Respir Crit Care Med*, Vol.174, No.11, (Dec 1), pp. 1199-1205, ISSN 1073-449X

Spaggiari, L., Grunenwald, D. H., Girard, P., Solli, P. & Le Chevalier, T. (1998). Pneumonectomy for lung metastases: indications, risks, and outcome. *Ann Thorac Surg*, Vol.66, No.6, (Dec), pp. 1930-1933, ISSN 0003-4975

Sugahara, K., Matsumoto, M., Baba, T., Nakamura, T. & Kawamoto, T. (1998). Elevation of serum human hepatocyte growth factor (HGF) level in patients with pneumonectomy during a perioperative period. *Intensive Care Med*, Vol.24, No.5, (May), pp. 434-437, ISSN 0342-4642

Takahashi, Y., Izumi, Y., Kohno, M., Kimura, T., Kawamura, M., Okada, Y., Nomori, H. & Ikeda, E. (2010). Thyroid transcription factor-1 influences the early phase of compensatory lung growth in adult mice. *Am J Respir Crit Care Med*, Vol.181, No.12, (Jun 15), pp. 1397-1406, ISSN 1535-4970

Takahashi, Y., Izumi, Y., Kohno, M., Kawamura, M., Ikeda, E. & Nomori, H. (2011). Airway administration of dexamethasone, 3'-5'-cyclic adenosine monophosphate, and isobutylmethylxanthine facilitates compensatory lung growth in adult mice. *Am J Physiol Lung Cell Mol Physiol*, Vol.300, No.3, (Mar), pp. L453-461, ISSN 1522-1504

Takeda, S., Wu, E. Y., Epstein, R. H., Estrera, A. S. & Hsia, C. C. (1997). In vivo assessment of changes in air and tissue volumes after pneumonectomy. *J Appl Physiol*, Vol.82, No.4, (Apr), pp. 1340-1348, ISSN 8750-7587

Zhang, Q., Moe, O. W., Garcia, J. A. & Hsia, C. C. (2006). Regulated expression of hypoxia-inducible factors during postnatal and postpneumonectomy lung growth. *Am J Physiol Lung Cell Mol Physiol*, Vol.290, No.5, (May), pp. L880-889, ISSN 1040-0605
Zhang, Q., Bellotto, D. J., Ravikumar, P., Moe, O. W., Hogg, R. T., Hogg, D. C., Estrera, A. S., Johnson, R. L., Jr. & Hsia, C. C. (2007). Postpneumonectomy lung expansion elicits hypoxia-inducible factor-1alpha signaling. *Am J Physiol Lung Cell Mol Physiol*, Vol.293, No.2, (Aug), pp. L497-504, ISSN 1040-0605

10

Superior Vena Cava Syndrome

Francesco Puma and Jacopo Vannucci
University of Perugia Medical School,
Thoracic Surgery Unit,
Italy

1. Introduction

1.1 Anatomy

The superior vena cava (SVC) originates in the chest, behind the first right sternocostal articulation, from the confluence of two main collector vessels: the right and left brachiocephalic veins which receive the ipsilateral internal jugular and subclavian veins. It is located in the anterior mediastinum, on the right side.

The internal jugular vein collects the blood from head and deep sections of the neck while the subclavian vein, from the superior limbs, superior chest and superficial head and neck.

Several other veins from the cervical region, chest wall and mediastinum are directly received by the brachiocephalic veins.

After the brachiocephalic convergence, the SVC follows the right lateral margin of the sternum in an inferoposterior direction. It displays a mild internal concavity due to the adjacent ascending aorta. Finally, it enters the pericardium superiorly and flows into the right atrium; no valve divides the SVC from right atrium.

The SVC's length ranges from 6 to 8 cm. Its diameter is usually 20-22 mm. The total diameters of both brachiocephalic veins are wider than the SVC's caliber. The blood pressure ranges from -5 to 5 mmHg and the flow is discontinuous depending on the heart pulse cycle.

The SVC can be classified anatomically in two sections: extrapericardial and intrapericardial. The extrapericardial segment is contiguous to the sternum, ribs, right lobe of the thymus, connective tissue, right mediastinal pleura, trachea, right bronchus, lymphnodes and ascending aorta. In the intrapericardial segment, the SVC enters the right atrium on the upper right face of the heart; in front it is close to the right main pulmonary artery. On the right side, the lung is in its proximity, separated only by mediastinal pleura. The right phrenic nerve runs next to the SVC for its entire course [1] (Figure 1).

The SVC receives a single affluent vein: the azygos vein. The azygos vein joins the SVC from the right side, at its mid length, above the right bronchus. The Azygos vein constantly receives the superior intercostal vein, a large vessel which drains blood from the upper two or three right intercostal spaces. In the case of SVC obstruction, the azygos vein is responsible for the most important collateral circulation. According to the expected collateral pathways, the SVC can be divided into two segments: the supra-azygos or preazygos and the infra-azygos or postazygos SVC. There are four possible collateral systems which were first described in 1949 by McIntire and Sykes. They are represented by the azygos venous system, the internal thoracic venous system, the vertebral venous system and the external thoracic venous system [2]. The azygos venous system is the only direct path into the SVC. The internal thoracic vein is the collector between SVC and inferior vena cava (IVC) via epigastric and iliac veins. The vertebral veins with intercostals, lumbar and sacral veins, represent the posterior network between SVC and IVC. The external thoracic vein system is the most superficial and it is represented by axillary, lateral thoracic and superficial epigastric veins.

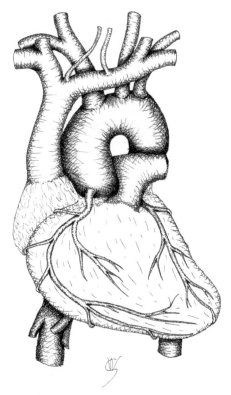

Fig. 1.

The SVC is a constituent part of the right paratracheal space (also called "Barety's space"), containing the main lymphatic route of the mediastinum, i.e. the right lateral tracheal chain. Barety's space is bounded laterally by the SVC, posteriorly by the tracheal wall, and medially by the ascending aorta. The nodes of the right paratracheal space are frequently involved in malignant growths: the SVC is undoubtedly the anatomical structure of this space which offers less resistance to compression, due to its thin wall and low internal pressure.

Anatomical anomalies are rare. The most frequent is the double SVC which has an embryologic etiology [1].

2. Etiology

SVC syndrome (SVCS) may be related to various etiological factors. Malignancies are predominant (95%) while, in the past, infectious diseases used to be common. During the last century, progression in anti-bacterial therapies and improvement in social conditions have led to a consistent decrease in the benign origin of this condition. The incidence of iatrogenic SVCS is currently increasing [3,4].

SVCS etiology is summarized as follows:

- Malignant

  - Lung cancer
  - Lymphomas
  - Thymoma
  - Mediastinal germ cell tumors
  - Mediastinal metastases
  - Mesothelioma
  - Leiomyosarcoma and angiosarcoma
  - Neoplastic thrombi
  - Anaplastic thyroid cancer

- Benign

  - Fibrosing mediastinitis (idiopathic or radiation-induced)
  - Infectious diseases (tubercolosis, histoplasmosis, echinococcosis, syphilis, aspergillosis, blastomycosis, filariasis, nocardiosis...)
  - Thrombosis (non-neoplastic)
  - Lymphadenopaties (sarcoidosis, Behçet's syndrome, Castelman's disease...)
  - Aortic aneurysm
  - Substernal goiter
  - Pericardial, thymic, bronchogenic cysts

- Iatrogenic

  - Pacemaker and defibrillator placement
  - Central venous catheters

3. Pathophysiology

The pathogenetic basis of SVCS is obstruction to the blood flow. It can result from intrinsic or extrinsic obstacles. The former are uncommon and are represented by thrombosis or invading tissue. Extrinsic factors develop from compression or stricture of the vein.

In physiologic conditions, blood return to the right atrium is facilitated by the pressure gradient between the right atrium and venae cavae. When obstruction of the SVC occurs, the vascular resistances rise and the venous return decreases. SVC pressure may increase consistently [4].

When SVC shows a significant stenosis (3/5 of the lumen or more), blood flow is redirected through the collateral circulation in order to bypass the obstruction and restore the venous return [5]. The timing of the obstruction development is important for its clinical implications. In acute impairments, the blood flow is not rapidly distributed through the collateral network so symptoms arise markedly. In the case of slow-growing diseases, the collateral venous network has enough time to expand in order to receive the circulating volume. For this reason, long-lasting, severe SVC obstruction can sometimes be found without significant related signs and symptoms [3,6].

4. Clinical presentation

The SVC wall does not offer resistance to compression. When SVC lumen reduction is greater than 60%, hemodynamic changes occur: proximal dilatation, congestion and flow slowdown. The clinical signs of this condition are mainly represented by cyanosis (due to venous stasis with normal arterial oxygenation) and edema of the upper chest, arms, neck and face (periorbital initially). Swelling is usually more important on the right side, because of the better possibility of collateral circulation in the left brachiocephalic vein compared to the contralateral (Figure 2). Vein varicosities of the proximal tongue and dark purple ears are also typical. Other signs or symptoms are: coughing, epistaxis, hemoptysis, dysphagia, dysphonia and hoarseness (caused by vocal cord congestion), esophageal, retinal and conjuntival bleeding. In the case of significant cephalic venous stasis, headache, dizziness, buzzing, drowsiness, stupor, lethargy and even coma may be encountered. Headache is a common symptom and it is usually continuous and pressing, exacerbated by coughing. Epilepsy has been occasionally reported as well as psychosis, probably due to carbon dioxide accumulation [3,4,7-14]. Dyspnea can be directly related to the mediastinal mass or be caused by pleural effusion or cardiocirculatory impairment. Supine position may worsen the clinical scenarios.

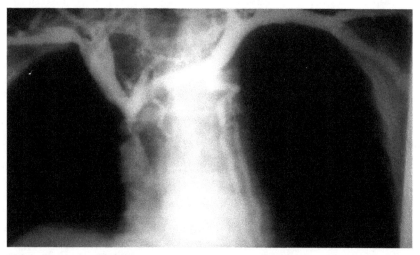

Fig. 2. Phlebogram showing obstruction of the SVC with azygos involvement. Blood return is distributed through a collateral circulation, mainly sustained by branches of the left brachiocephalic vein. Edema in this patient was more severe in the right arm than the left.

The clinical seriousness of the syndrome is related to several factors:
- Level of obstruction and rapidity of development, determining the effectiveness of collateral circulation
- Impairment of lymphatic drainage (pulmonary interstitial edema or pleural effusion)
- Involvement of other mediastinal structures (compression or invasion of heart, pulmonary artery and central airways, phrenic nerve paralysis…)

Intolerance of the supine position is always linked to a severe prognostic significance for patients with mediastinal syndromes [15]. The variation in decubitus may worsen the already existing signs and symptoms: in the supine position, an anterior mediastinal mass may compress the trachea or the heart by means of gravity, with possible cardiorespiratory problems. Direct compression of the common trunk of the pulmonary artery is also possible, although this is not as likely to happen, given that such structure is cranially protected by the aortic arch [16].

The presence of dyspnea at rest, especially in the sitting position, carries a severe prognostic significance in patients with mediastinal syndromes. Dyspnea at rest can be caused by either cardiovascular or respiratory problems:
- pulmonary congestion caused by lymphatic stasis
- combination with pulmonary atelectasis
- pleural effusion
- pericardial effusion
- direct compression of the mass on the airways, on the heart, or on the pulmonary artery
- laryngeal edema

Dyspnea at rest is not uncommon in the natural evolution of SVCS and it should always be considered as a high risk factor for invasive procedures under general anesthesia. If the shortness of breath is related to laryngeal edema, the patient should not be presented for general anesthesia and surgery.

Superficial dilated vascular routes are the main sign of collateral circulation and appear swollen and non-pulsating. In the case of marked obesity, superficial veins can be missing at inspection. The variety of collateral circulation and the differences in the venous re-arrangement are expression of the SVC obstruction site (Figure 3,4,5).

The anatomic classification includes three levels of obstruction:
1. Obstruction of the upper SVC, proximal to the azygos entry point.
2. Obstruction with azygos involvement.
3. Obstruction of the lower SVC, distal to the azygos entry point.
1. In this situation, there is no impediment to normal blood flow through the azygos vein which opens into the patent tract of the SVC. Venous drainage coming from the head neck, shoulders and arms cannot directly reach the right atrium. A longer but effective way is provided by several veins, the most important being the right superior intercostal vein. From the superior tract of the SVC, blood flow is reversed and directed to the azygos, mainly through the right superior intercostal vein. The azygos collateral system is eminently deep; therefore the presence of superficial vessels is usually lacking, even if possible in the area of the internal thoracic vein's superficial tributaries. The volumetric increase of the vessels can be consistent and capacity may increase up to eight times. The efficiency of this collateral route is reliable, thus the clinical compensation is unbalanced only in the case of a rapid development of the obstruction or if the stenosis is more than 90% (Figure 3).

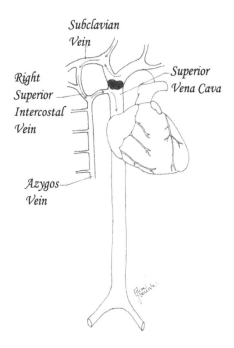

Fig. 3. Obstruction of the upper SVC, proximal to the azygos entry point. Collateral pathways.

2. In this case, the azygos vein cannot be available as collateral pathway and the only viable blood return is carried by minor vessels to IVC (cava-cava or anazygotic circulation). From the internal thoracic veins, blood is forced to the intercostal veins, then to azygos and emiazygos veins. The flow is thus reversed into the ascending lumbar veins to the iliac veins. Direct anastomosis between the azygos' origin and the IVC and between emiazygos and left renal vein are also active. In addition, the internal thoracic veins can flow into the superior epigastric veins. From the superior epigastric veins, blood is carried to the inferior epigastric veins across the superficial system of the cutaneous abdominal veins and finally to the iliac veins. Another course is between the thoraco-epigastric vein (collateral of the axillary vein) and the external iliac vein.

    In these conditions, the collateral circulation is partly deep and partly superficial. The physical examination often reveals SVC obstruction. The reversed circulation through the described pathways, remains less efficient than the azygos system and venous hypertension is usually more severe. For this reason, this kind of SVC obstruction is often related to important symptoms, dyspnea and pleural effusion. The ensuing slow blood flow may be responsible for superimposed thrombosis. In the disease progression, renal impairment can evolve as the SVC obstruction affects the lumbar plexus (mostly the ascending lumbar veins, left side) which congests the renal vein (Figure 4).

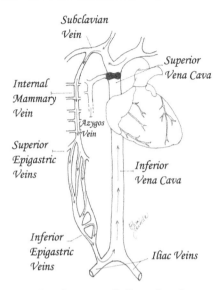

Fig. 4. Obstruction with azygos involvement. Collateral pathways.

3. In this condition, the obstruction is just below the azygos arch. The blood flow is distributed from the superior body into the azygos and emiazygos veins, in which the flow is inverted, to the IVC tributaries. In this type of case, the superficial collateral system is not always evident but the azygos and emiazygos congestion and dilatation are usually important. The hemodynamic changes lead to edema and cyanosis of the upper chest and pleural effusion. Pleural effusion is often slowly-growing and right-sided, probably due to anatomical reasons: there is a wider anastomosis between emiazygos and IVC than between azygos and IVC [17] (Figure 5).

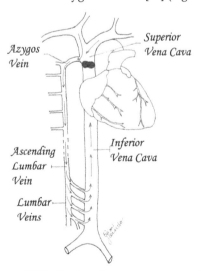

Fig. 5. Obstruction of the lower SVC, distal to the azygos entry point. Collateral pathways.

5. Classification of SVCS

Several classifications of SVCS have been proposed even though further investigations are required to achieve a definitive staging system. There are three main classification proposals which follow different methods of categorization [18-20].

1. Doty and Standford's classification (anatomical)

    - Type I: stenosis of up to 90% of the supra-azygos SVC
    - Type II: stenosis of more than 90% of the supra-azygos SVC
    - Type III: complete occlusion of SVC with azygos reverse blood flow
    - Type IV: complete occlusion of SVC with the involvement of the major tributaries and azygos vein

2. Yu's classification (clinical)

    - Grade 0: asymptomatic (imaging evidence of SVC obstruction)
    - Grade 1: mild (plethora, cyanosis, head and neck edema)
    - Grade 2: moderate (grade 1 evidence + functional impairment)
    - Grade 3: severe (mild/moderate cerebral or laryngeal edema, limited cardiac reserve)
    - Grade 4: life-threatening (significant cerebral or laryngeal edema, cardiac failure)
    - Grade 5: fatal

3. Bigsby's classification (operative risk)

    - Low risk
    - High risk

The authors proposed an algorithm for SVCS to assess the operative risk in order to submit the patient to invasive diagnostic procedures. The low risk patients present: no dyspnea at rest, no facial cyanosis in the upright position, no change of dyspnea and no worsening of facial edema and cyanosis, during the supine position. The high risk patients present facial cyanosis or dyspnea at rest in the sitting position.

6. Diagnosis

Physical examination is often crucial: the presence of edema and superficial venous network of the upper chest may support the clinical diagnosis. Imaging studies are however required. Most cases are suspected at the standard chest X-ray and the most common radiological findings are right mediastinal widening and pleural effusion [3].

Computed tomography (CT) with multislice detector is the most useful tool in the evaluation of the mediastinal syndromes. CT imaging is widely employed in SVCS assessment because of its large availability and short acquisition time. Intravenous contrast should be administered, in order to provide high-quality vascular imaging. Contrast enhanced multidetector CT may show the site of the obstruction, some aspects of the primary disease and eventual intraluminal thrombi. Multiplanar and 3D reconstructions may provide better image detection and definition. The contrast flow can also help to distinguish the extent of the collateral network (Figure 6) [21].

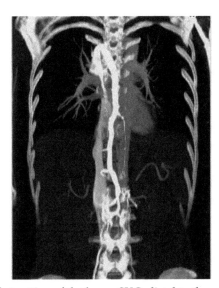

Fig. 6. Angio-CT scan: Obstruction of the lower SVC, distal to the azygos entry point. Collateral pathways: in the azygos vein system the blood flow is inverted and venous return occurs by means of IVC.

Magnetic resonance imaging (MRI) plays a side role; it is indicated when CT cannot be performed (e.g. pregnancy, endovenous contrast intollerance). The long acquisition times of MRI limit its use in critically ill patients.

Invasive venography is now rarely used due to the huge improvement in vascular CT imaging. It is currently performed only as a preliminary to operative procedures such as stent placement.

Once the thoracic imaging is obtained, the work-up should include brain, abdominal and bone studies in view of the probable malignant nature of the primary lesion. Recently Fluorodeoxyglucose-Positron Emission Tomography has gained an important role in oncology [22].

The histological definition remains the key factor for the causative treatment, in the case of neoplastic etiology. Superficial adenopathies have to be carefully investigated in order to find a possible source of tissue and the easiest target for biopsy. The invasive diagnostic procedure varies largely depending on the suspected malignancy and its site. The biopsy can be obtained through traditional bronchoscopy or echo-guided endoscopy, superficial node biopsy, mediastinoscopy, mediastinotomy, transthoracic needle biopsy, thoracoscopy, cervical or supraclavicular biopsies; thoracotomy and sternotomy are rarely indicated. Operative endoscopy has gained a new significance in the evaluation of SVCS since echography has been introduced but the best diagnostic result is still obtained by the mediastinoscopy. Venous hypertension may increase the procedure-related risk [23-27].

7. Treatment

Therapy should be causative. Syndrome management recognizes different levels of priority depending on the severity of symptoms, etiology and prognosis. SVCS needs a multidisciplinary approach and symptoms relief is often the first objective of complex care.

The therapeutic plan is usually targeted to clinical palliation. In fact, most cases are diagnosed as advanced-stage malignancies.

The patient must immediately assume an orthostatic position. Other supportive treatments are usually promptly established; oxygen, diuretics, and steroids are also suggested. The risk of an overlying thrombosis is particularly high and anticoagulant therapy should be introduced.

In case of malignancy, the treatment can have palliative or, rarely, curative intent. Chemotherapy is usually employed in lymphomas, small-cell lung cancer and germ cell tumors. Besides chemotherapy, radiotherapy is widely used in the treatment of non-small cell lung cancer. Radiation therapy can obtain good results but can also produce an initial inflammatory response with a possible temporary worsening [28,29]. Some cases must be approached as an emergency. In this type of situation, the treatment of choice is usually endovascular with the aim of restoring blood flow as soon as possible. The acute life-threatening presentation is the only situation in which radiotherapy before histological diagnosis can be considered. However, this approach should be avoided, whenever possible.

Endovascular stenting provides fast functional relief. It is the best option in an emergency and sometimes the clinical benefit is immediate. It is also advocated in the case of chemo-radiotherapy non-responders [3].

Surgery has a central role in the diagnosis but rarely in the therapy. A SVC resection and reconstruction is not often recommended and is a demanding procedure. The main proposal for SVC resection is direct infiltration in thymomas or in N0-N1 non-small cell lung cancer. In the case of infiltration of less than 30% of the SVC circumference, direct suture is favored (Figure 7). Larger involvements require a prosthetic repair. Different methods of SVC repair have been investigated using different materials (Figures 8, 9, 10a-b). Armoured PTFE grafts and biologic material are the preferred choices. Morbidity after SVC surgical procedures is high and the post-operative care must be intensive [4]. Long-term patency of a SVC by-pass graft is uncertain but, usually, the slow onset of the graft thrombosis favors the development of effective collateral circulation.

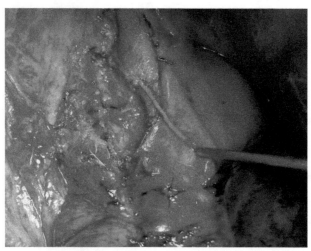

Fig. 7. SVC resection for limited infiltration by a right upper lobe NSCLC. The moderate stenosis following the direct SVC suture did not have hemodynamic consequences, in this patient.

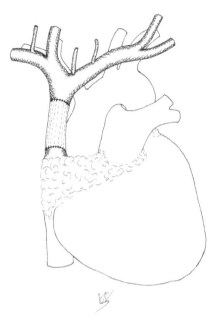

Fig. 8. Graft reconstruction by end-to-end anastomosis between proximal and distal SVC.

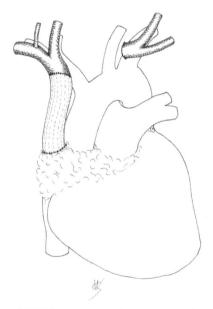

Fig. 9. Graft reconstruction of SVC by end-to-end anastomosis between the right brachiocephalic vein and the SVC.

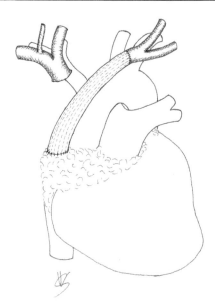

Fig. 10a. Graft reconstruction of SVC by end-to-end anastomosis between the left brachiocephalic vein and the SVC.

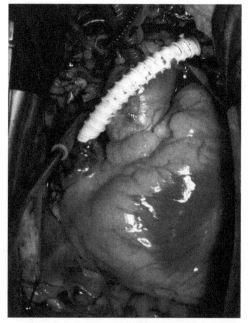

Fig. 10b. Armoured PTFE reconstruction of SVC by end-to-end anastomosis between the left brachiocephalic vein and the SVC.

Artworks by Walter Santilli R.N. and Elisa Scarnecchia M.D.

8. References

[1] Testut L, Latarjet A. Trattato di Anatomia Umana. 4th edition, Unione tipografica – Editrice Torinese. 1971. pp. 918-921

[2] McIntire FT, Sykes EM jr. Obstruction of the superior vena cava: A review of the literature and report of two personal cases. Ann Intern Med 1949; 30:925.

[3] Wan JF, Bezjak A. Superior vena cava syndrome. Hematol Oncol Clin North Am. 2010; 24:501-13

[4] Macchiarini P. Superior vena cava obstruction. In: Patterson GA, Cooper JD, Deslauriers J, Lerut AEM, Luketic JD, Rive TW, editors. Pearson's thoracic & esophageal surgery. 3rd edition, Philadelphia, PA: Churchill Livingstone, Elsevier; 2008. pp. 1684-96

[5] Sy WM, Lao RS. Collateral pathways in superior vena cava obstruction as seen on gamma images. Br J Radiol 1982; 55:294-300

[6] Rice TW, Rodriguez RM, Light RW. The superior vena cava syndrome: clinical characteristics and evolving etiology. Medicine (Baltimore) 2006; 85:37-42

[7] Ahmann FR. A reassessment of the clinical implications of the superior vena caval syndrome. J Clin Oncol 1984; 2:961-969

[8] Ganeshan A, Hon LQ, Warakaulle DR, Morgan R, Uberoi R. Superior vena caval stenting for SVC obstruction: current status. Eur J Radiol. 2009; 71:343-9

[9] Armstrong BA, Perez CA, Simpson JR, Hederman MA. Role of irradiation in the management of superior vena cava syndrome. Int J Radiat Oncol Biol Phys 1987; 13:531-539

[10] Yelling A, Rosen A, Reichert N, Lieberman Y. Superior vena cava syndrome: the Myth-the facts. Am Rev Respir Dis 1990; 141:1114-18

[11] Schraufnagel DE, Hill R, Leech JA, Pare JAP. Superior vena caval obstruction: is it a medical emergency? Am J Med 1981; 70:1169-74

[12] Chen JC, Bongard F, Klein SR. A contemporary perspective on superior vena cava syndrome. Am J Surg 1990; 160:207-11

[13] Rice TW, Rodriguez RM, Barnette R, Light RW. Prevalence and characteristics of pleural effusions in superior vena cava syndrome. Respirology 2006; 11:299-305

[14] Urruticoechea A, Mesía R, Domínguez J, Falo C, Escalante E, Montes A, Sancho C, Cardenal F, Majem M, Germà JR. Treatment of malignant superior vena cava syndrome by endovascular stent insertion. Experience on 52 patients with lung cancer. Lung Cancer 2004; 43:209-14

[15] Northrip DR, Bohman BK, Tsueda K. Total airway occlusion and superior vena cava syndrome in a child with an anterior mediastinal tumor. Anesth Analg 1986; 65:1079-82

[16] Levin H, Bursztein S, Haifetz M. Cardiac arrest in a child with an anterior mediastinal mass. Anesth Analg 1985; 64:1129-30

[17] Introzzi P. Trattato Italiano di Medicina Interna, parte quinta. 2nd edition, Industria grafica "l'impronta". 1974. pp.1514-25

[18] Stanford W, Doty DB. The role of venography and surgery in the management of patients with superior vena cava obstruction. Ann Thorac Surg 1986; 41:158

[19] Yu JB, Wilson LD, Detterbeck FC. Superior vena cava syndrome--a proposed classification system and algorithm for management. J Thorac Oncol 2008; 3:811-4

[20] Bigsby R, Greengrass R, Unruh H. Diagnostic algorithm for acute superior vena caval obstruction (SVCO). J Cardiovasc Surg 1993; 34:347-50

[21] Sheth S, Ebert MD, Fishman EK. Superior vena cava obstruction evaluation with MDCT. Am J Roentgenol 2010; 194:336-46

[22] Abner A: Approach to the patient who presents with superior vena cava obstruction. Chest 1993; 103:394-397

[23] Mineo TC, Ambrogi V, Nofroni I, Pistolese C. Mediastinoscopy in superior vena cava obstruction: analysis of 80 consecutive patients. Ann Thorac Surg 1999; 68:223-6

[24] Porte H, Metois D, Finzi L, Lebuffe G, Guidat A, Conti M, Wurtz A. Superior vena cava syndrome of malignant origin. Which surgical procedure for which diagnosis? Eur J Cardiothorac Surg 2000; 17:384-8

[25] Trinkle JK, Bryant LR, Malette WG, Playforth RH, Wood RC. Mediastinoscopy-- diagnostic value compared to bronchoscopy: scalene biopsy and sputum cytology in 155 patients. Am Surg 1968; 34:740-3

[26] Jahangiri M, Taggart DP, Goldstraw P. Role of mediastinoscopy in superior vena cava obstruction. Cancer 1993; 71:3006-8

[27] Callejas MA, Rami R, Catalán M, Mainer A, Sánchez-Lloret J. Mediastinoscopy as an emergency diagnostic procedure in superior vena cava syndrome. Scand J Thorac Cardiovasc Surg 1991; 25:137-9

[28] Sculier JP, Evans WK, Feld R, DeBoer G, Payne DG, Shepherd FA, Pringle JF, Yeoh JL, Quirt IC, Curtis JE, et al. Superior vena caval obstruction syndrome in small cell lung cancer. Cancer 1986; 57:847-51

[29] Lonardi F, Gioga G, Agus G, Coeli M, Campostrini F. Double-flash, large-fraction radiation therapy as palliative treatment of malignant superior vena cava syndrome in the elderly. Support Care Cancer 2002; 10:156-60

11

The Role of PET-CT in the Clinical Management of Oesophageal Cancer

Reubendra Jeganathan, Jim McGuigan and Tom Lynch
Royal Victoria Hospital, Belfast,
United Kingdom

1. Introduction

Oesophageal cancer, once a relatively rare form of cancer, with a non-uniform geographical distribution, is the sixth most common cause of cancer related death in UK for 2005 (1-3). By the time of presentation, only 24-31% of patients are suitable for curative surgical resection and the overall 5-year survival is 20-30% (2, 4). PET-CT, a new staging modality is said to improve patient selection, by the detection of metastatic disease, which is not readily identifiable by other imaging modalities.

Recent published literature demonstrates an ever-evolving role for PET-CT in the management of various cancer types. PET-CT is not only used as a staging tool but can be used to assess early response to chemotherapy and radiotherapy (5). PET-CT can also be employed to identify disease recurrence, often detecting sites of relapse, before any other imaging modality (6). Additionally, metabolic parameters determined from the PET-CT study can provide prognostic information for individual patients (7).

The aim of this chapter is to provide the reader with an introduction to PET-CT, covering cellular metabolism, imaging of glucose metabolism, imaging protocols and the utility of standard uptake value. Following this, we will provide a pertinent review of the current published literature on the prognostic potential of standard uptake value of PET-CT in the management of oesophageal cancer and its ability to supplement the TNM classification. Finally, we will include future applications of PET-CT, including its role as a measure of tumour response following neo-adjuvant chemotherapy, and other de novo techniques currently being considered in the field of PET-CT.

2. Positron emission tomography and computed tomography

Positron Emission Tomography or PET involves an intravenous injection of a radioactive tracer, attached to a biological substance, which then distributes within the body in a recognised pattern. The radiation emitted from this injected substance can then be imaged to reveal the pattern of distribution within the body and abnormal areas of tracer accumulation, can therefore be identified. This creates a functional image. There are many radioactive tracers used, but in the context of this chapter, we will only consider fluourodeoxyglucose, FDG. FDG is a glucose analogue, which has a distribution, similar to simple glucose molecules within the body.

A CT scan uses X-rays to provide an anatomical image of the patient and a PET scan gives an image revealing the distribution of glucose like, metabolic function. Each on its own is a powerful tool but when combined they start to revolutionise cancer imaging. A PET-CT scanner is a single device that combines both modalities to produce an image that contains the metabolic functional information from the PET image and the anatomical information from the CT scan, displaying the resultant data as a fused PET-CT image.

2.1 Cellular metabolism

Cancer cells share similar traits to normal cells, in that they divide and multiply, but do so at a faster rate. Cancer cells also have an inherent tendency to metastasise, once they have overcome the body immunological defence. In order to achieve this objective the cancer cells must have an energy source capable of fuelling this division and growth. Otto Warburg, a German biochemist, noted over 80 years ago that many cancers use glucose as their primary energy substrate for this process (8). As the cancer cells grow, they often become starved of oxygen and therefore anaerobic metabolism of glucose becomes easier to sustain than aerobic metabolism, within the tricarboxylic acid cycle. The result of this is an increase in utilization of glucose within cancer cells, relative to most normal cells. Thus, a cancer cell will tend to have a much greater metabolic rate than the average normal cell.

Some cells within the body can use several different energy sources to fulfill their metabolic needs. Cardiac muscle, for example, preferentially uses free fatty acids as an energy source, but can also use glucose, lipids or amino acids if required. As a result the glucose uptake within the heart varies between people and can change considerably within an individual over a short period, in relation to the blood glucose at the time. Brain cells do not have the ability to use any fuel other than glucose and consequently the glucose activity within the normal brain is always high. In a fasting state, most body tissues, with the exception of the brain, actually use free fatty acids as their preferred energy source. After a glucose-rich meal, these cells may temporarily switch from free fatty acid to glucose metabolism, under the influence of rising insulin levels.

Transmembrane proteins, called glucose transporters, facilitate glucose uptake into the cell. At least 12 different glucose transporters have been identified and are known as GLUT 1, GLUT 2, and so forth.

When the glucose molecule enters the cell, it usually becomes phosphorylated by the enzyme hexokinase. The resultant compound is glucose-6-phosphate. Under normal circumstances the glucose-6-phosphate will undergo further enzymatic change to be converted into other smaller compounds thereby releasing energy, a process called 'glycolysis'. Alternatively the glucose-6-phosphate may be stored as a future energy reserve in the form of glycogen by the glyconeogenesis pathway, or it can be converted into either lipid or protein by other pathways.

The increased energy demands of a growing cancer cell necessitate a more rapid efficient delivery of glucose. As cellular division and growth proceed, a cancer cell uses some ingenious ways of meeting its energy requirements. First the cell can increase the number of transmembrane GLUT transporters to aid glucose delivery. If this is still not sufficient to meet demand, the cell can then increase the rate of phosphorylation, by up-regulating hexokinase activity. The resultant effect is that many cancer cells demonstrate a marked increase in glucose metabolism when compared to normal cells.

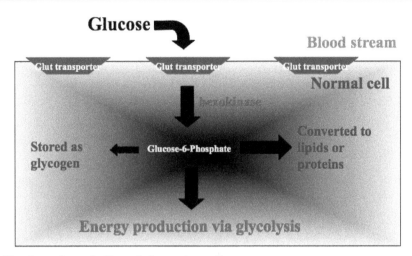

Fig. 1. Uptake and metabolism of glucose in a cell

2.2 Imaging glucose metabolism

FDG is produced in a device called a cyclotron. FDG is a radioactive positron emitter and decays with a half-life of approximately two hours. Due to the relatively long half-life of the FDG, a PET scanner can be located within a 2-hour drive from the cyclotron site. Other positron emitters such as Carbon-11 and Nitrogen-13 have much shorter half-lives and can only be used for PET scanners located in close proximity to a cyclotron.

FDG is injected intravenously and is taken up by normal and cancer cells alike. Cancer cells and normal cells compete with each other for cellular uptake using the GLUT transporters. Within a cell, FDG will be converted into FDG-6-phosphate by the action of hexokinase, just like normal glucose. Beyond this point, the fate of FDG and glucose are different. Due to the isomeric constitution of FDG, it cannot undergo further enzymatic change, unlike the glucose molecule. As a result, their pathways diverge; glucose is converted into either energy or stored as glycogen, whereas FDG undergoes no further metabolism and mostly remains trapped in the cell.

The distribution of radioactivity within the body can be imaged using a specialized camera called a PET scanner. An image gives a picture of the areas of the body that have FDG and therefore glucose uptake. The intense accumulation of FDG within many cancer cells allows those cells to be identified, compared to the less intense uptake in normal cells. Patients are imaged in the fasting state since most normal cells will more likely be using free fatty acids as their energy substrate. Figure 2 is a PET scan showing the normal distribution of glucose as identified by FDG uptake.

This image is called the maximum intensity projection image or MIP and is the two-dimensional representation of the accumulation of FDG uptake in the body as a whole. We can see that the brain has intense uptake, with less marked uptake in the heart, liver and spleen. We also see intense uptake in the renal system. Individuals, under normal circumstances, do not excrete glucose through the urinary system. Although FDG is an analogue of glucose, it behaves differently in this regard and is excreted in large amounts through the renal system. Whereas most normal glucose is freely filtered within the renal glomeruli and rapidly reabsorbed by the nephron, filtered FDG is poorly reabsorbed and a large proportion is excreted in the urine.

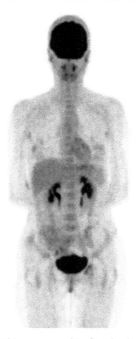

Fig. 2. The distribution of FDG within a normal individual

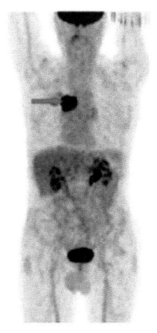

Fig. 3. A FDG +ve right hilar squamous cell carcinoma.

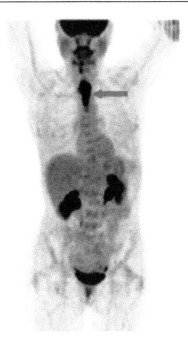

Fig. 4. An upper oesophageal squamous cell carcinoma.

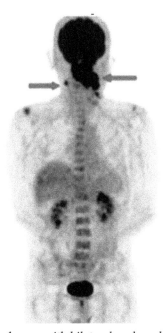

Fig. 5. A naso-pharyngeal lymphoma with bilateral neck node involvement.

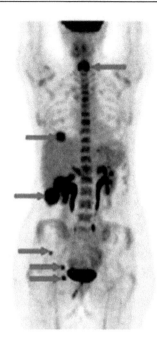

Fig. 6. Recurrent colorectal cancer with metabolically active deposits in the liver and right hemipelvis. The uptake in the neck is due to a coincidental thyroiditis.

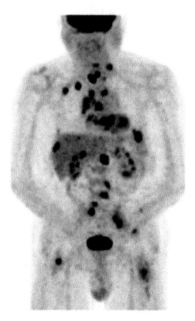

Fig. 7. Multiple bony metastatic deposits.

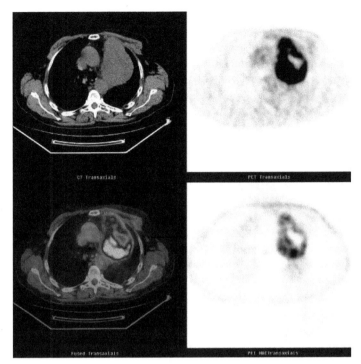

Fig. 8. Fused PET-CT image of a lung cancer.

Figure 3 to 7 is abnormal PET scans with the abnormality highlighted by arrows. Figure 8 is an example of a fused PET-CT image. The CT component is viewed in the top left hand corner and the attenuation-corrected PET in the top right hand corner. This image uses the CT data to correct for the effect of different positron absorption within different density tissues of the patient. The more intense the FDG (or glucose) uptake, the blacker it appears on the PET scan.

The fused PET-CT scan is seen in the bottom left hand corner of the image. This combines the anatomical data from the CT and the metabolic data from the PET, the colour scale chosen, shows the FDG uptake as increasingly orange to yellow, with increasing activity. The bottom right hand image is the non-attenuated PET image, which is effectively the raw PET data.

2.3 Scanning protocol and imaging sequence

Patients should arrive at the nuclear medicine department having fasted for at least four hours. This ensures most tissues are using free fatty acids as their energy source. Diabetic patients are advised to take their normal insulin or medication prior to arriving at the department.

After the staff has made all the necessary patient checks including correct patient identification and a check of blood glucose level, the injection of radioactive FDG can take place. The patient is advised to lie still for approximately 45 minutes to allow the FDG enough time to accumulate in metabolically active cells. Any unnecessary patient movement during this uptake period can result in muscular uptake than can cause confusion with later scan interpretation. Patients who are tense during this time often show physiological uptake within the muscles of the neck.

Following the uptake period, the patient is taken into the scanning room and lies supine on the table. A picture of a GE Discovery Lightspeed PET-CT scanner is shown in Figure 9.

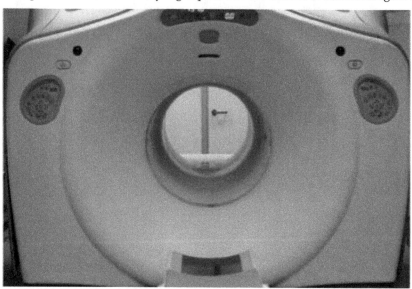

Fig. 9. GE Discovery Lightspeed PET-CT

Many centres now routinely use oral contrast enhancement to help visualise the bowel. Some centres also now recommend the use of intravenous contrast but this is presently not routine practice in the UK.

The CT scan is normally carried out from the base of skull to mid-thigh level. There are a number of reasons for performing this and not a whole body scan:

1. Brain metastases are difficult to detect using FDG as any brain lesion must have an intensity greater than or less than the surrounding brain tissue to be identified.
2. Only a few tumours have metastatic potential to disseminate to the distal lower limbs.
3. There is a decreased radiation burden to the patient from the CT.
4. There is a considerable amount of time saved which can be used to increase the patient throughput.

Whole body scans are carried out in some circumstances, for example patients with melanoma due to the widespread and unpredictable lymphatic dissemination that characterises this disease. A similar problem is encountered with the pattern of disease spread in non-Hodgkin's lymphoma, which often requires a larger scanning volume. Patients with head and neck disease often have scans that include the entire skull, and patients with soft tissue sarcomas may also require additional views.

After the CT images are acquired, which only takes a minute or so, when using a modern multislice scanner, the patient is then scanned again using the PET component of the machine. The detectors on the PET scanner can identify radioactive emissions from the FDG within the body. A ring of detectors surrounds the patient. This ring is approximately 15 cm long and images are therefore acquired in blocks of 15 cm from the base of the skull to mid thigh. In most individuals this area is covered in about five blocks (~75 cm), taller or shorter individuals will take more or less imaging time. The time required for each 15 cm image of the patient is between three and five minutes. This means that the PET component of the study can take at least 15-45 minutes to acquire. Any patient movement during this time will degrade the quality of the images obtained.

After the PET scan has been acquired the patient is free to go but is given warnings about exposure to individuals during the next few hours as the radioactivity decays and is excreted from the body.

2.4 Standard uptake value

A semi quantitative method is available to calculate the intensity of FDG uptake within a range of interest on the PET scan. This value is called the Standardised Uptake Value, SUV, and takes account of factors such as injected activity, patient weight and time from injection. Simply speaking, the SUV assumes that if there's an even distribution of radioactivity throughout the body the SUV would be measured as one. Obviously this is not the case but we can calculate the relative uptake within different parts of the body and relate them to each other. An area with an SUV of five means this area has five times the average uptake. Certain modifications can be made to the SUV calculation to take into account, for example, the patient's body fat, since FDG is not generally taken up into fatty tissue.

The SUV allows comparisons to be made between different parts of the body and between different scans on the same patient over a period of time. It must be emphasised that the SUV is only a semi-quantitative measurement and can vary considerably with changes in the patient's plasma glucose level and are dependent on the uptake time allowed prior to scanning. Therefore, is it important that PET facilities use a standard scanning and imaging protocol for all their patients.

It is the SUVmax that is usually quoted in PET reports and measured in research studies. However there is a growing interest in the measurement of SUVmean, as it is less susceptible to outliers. The maximum SUV represents only one single pixel (the pixel with the maximum SUV within the entire tumour), whereas, the mean SUV in a region of interest, represents the average SUV of the given number of pixels within the ROI. Some clinicians prefer to avoid numbers altogether, and simply use visual interpretation to compare the intensity of one area to another using the background blood pool as a guide to normality. There is evidence to suggest that both methods are equally accurate.

3. The prognostic potential of PET-CT in the clinical management of oesophageal cancer

3.1 Introduction

Oesophageal cancer is staged according to the current American Joint Committee on Cancer guidelines, which incorporate the T, N and M classification (9). The current staging modalities utilize an array of morphological imaging studies, and more recently, minimally invasive surgical techniques, to bridge the gap between clinical and pathological staging. The introduction of PET-CT has provided an incremental yield to the diagnostic accuracy in oesophageal cancer staging (10-11). PET-CT provides an increased sensitivity and specificity of metastatic disease compared to other morphological imaging techniques (PET-CT vs CT: sensitivity 71% vs 52% and specificity 93% vs 91%), changing the operability in up to 20% of patients (12-13).

PET-CT also provides a semi-quantitative value of biological aggressiveness of a malignancy by reporting the standard uptake value, which represents the amount of metabolic activity within the tumour. Like certain biochemical indices, this amount of metabolic activity has been shown to be related to the clinical behaviour for a specific type of tumour for a given patient (7, 14-19). Therefore, it has been suggested that the FDG SUV value, may have a role as a predictive tool for patient outcome in oesophageal cancer (7, 17-19). This has already been demonstrated in other types of malignancies such as lung cancer and head and neck cancer (20-21). However, to our knowledge, there are only limited data available with regards to oesophageal cancer (7, 17-19).

3.2 Methods and materials
3.2.1 Patient population
All patients diagnosed with oesophageal carcinoma that had undergone staging PET-CT imaging between the period of June 2002 and May 2008, were included in this study. The eligibility criteria included only patients diagnosed with adenocarcinoma or squamous carcinoma of the oesophagus, (specifically excluding lesions confined to the upper third of the oesophagus), including those who were suitable for curative surgery, either with or without neo-adjuvant chemotherapy.

Studies were performed at a single institution (Regional Thoracic Surgical Unit, Royal Victoria Hospital, Belfast) with a standardised procedure, a Total Thoracic Oesophagectomy with a cervical anastomosis and two field lymphadenectomy. All patients were discussed at a surgical cancer network multidisciplinary meeting that included a thoracic or upper gastrointestinal surgeon, a nuclear medicine radiologist, an oncologist and a pathologist.

The study protocol was approved by our local research ethics committee (08/NIR03/106). Only electronic patient files including cancer network meetings, pathology reports and nuclear medicine imaging were used to collect the clinical information.

3.2.2 Patient image acquisition of FGD PET-CT data
Patients were scanned after injection of 370MBq 18F-FDG and an uptake period of 45 minutes, on a GE Discovery Light Speed PET-CT scanner, using a standard diagnostic protocol.

3.2.3 Measurement of prognostic variables and clinical outcome
Standardised Uptake Value (SUVmean and SUVmax)

A region of interest (ROI) was created for every individual patient based on the diameter of the FDG avid oesophageal lesion, on the attenuated corrected PET image, with side by side comparison with the CT image. The ROI ranged from 1cm to 3cm in diameter accordingly. This was to prevent overestimation, if a large ROI was used from neighbouring structures especially the heart, or underestimation, if a small predetermined ROI was used. The SUVmean and SUVmax were calculated, with the SUVmean taken at the same corresponding level as the SUVmax for that particular patient.

Clinical Outcome

The outcome evaluated was overall survival, which was from the date of surgery to death, identified from the Hospital Episode Statistics Data. Follow-up was through March 2009, constituting our censoring date for survival.

3.2.4 Surgery and pathological staging

Only patients with middle, lower or OGJ tumours involved were included in this study, with a standard total thoracic oesophagectomy being performed in all patients. This consists of a left thorocolaparotomy incision, resection of all the thoracic and abdominal oesophagus with two field lymphadenectomy, mobilisation of the stomach on the right gastro-epiploic arcade, creating a neo-oesophagus that is then anastomosed in the neck via a left oblique cervical incison. The same experienced surgical team performed all procedures. A single pathologist reported all pathological specimens using the current TNM staging.

3.2.5 Statistical analysis

The associations between the SUVmax and SUVmean with clinical staging (T and N categories) were assessed using analysis of variance or t-test. Pearson's correlation was used to assess the association between the different prognostic variables. Log-Rank and Cox regression tests were performed for disease free survival analysis. A $p < 0.05$ was considered significant. All statistical analysis was performed using the SPSS Version 18 (SPSS, Chicago, IL).

3.3 Results

There were a total of 96 patients during this study period that underwent staging FDG PET-CT scans. Fifty-three patients proceeded to receive neo-adjuvant chemotherapy followed by surgery. A response scan was performed 3 weeks after completion of neo-adjuvant treatment. The remaining 43 patients proceeded directly to surgery following their staging PET-CT.

From the 96 patients, 68.7% had adenocarcinoma and 31.3% had squamous carcinoma. Tumours were located predominantly in the lower oesophagus, 59.4%, followed by OGJ and middle oesophageal lesions, with 25% and 15.6% respectively (Figure 10)

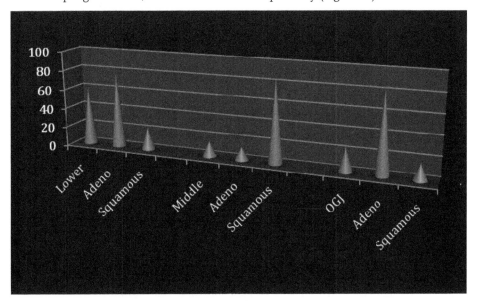

Fig. 10. Distribution of tissue type according to location.

The mean and median Staging SUV values were 10.3 and 9.3 for SUVmax, and, 6 and 5.8 for SUVmean, with a fairly normal distribution for SUVmean within the population studied (Figure 11 and 12).

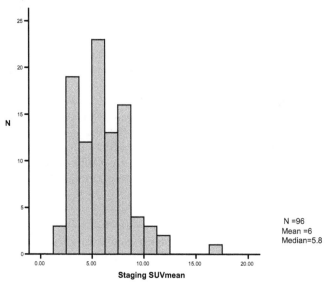

Fig. 11. Distribution of Staging SUVmean amongst study population.

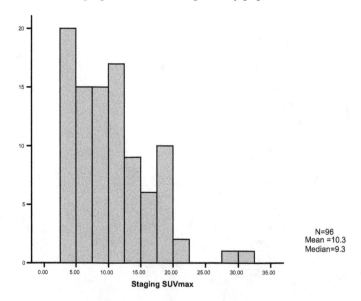

Fig. 12. Distribution of Staging SUVmax amongst the study population.

Both the Staging SUVmax and SUVmean correlated well, with a Pearson's correlation coefficient of 0.91 (p<0.01), Figure 13.

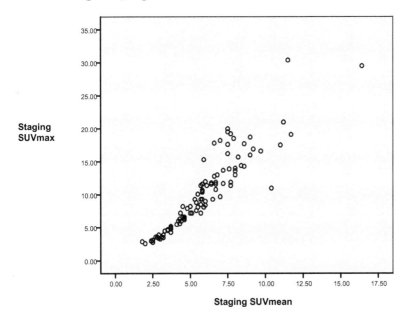

Fig. 13. Pearson's Correlation between SUVmax and SUVmean.

SUV_{max} and SUV_{mean} were both influenced by tissue type, with squamous carcinoma having a significantly higher uptake than adenocarcinoma, SUVmax 13.6 vs 8.8 (p<0.01) and SUVmean 7.3 vs 5.3 (p<0.01) respectively. SUVmax and SUVmean also varied according to locality, with tumours located in the middle oesophagus having the highest SUV uptake followed by the lower and then OGJ tumours. SUVmax varied from 13.4 to 10.5 to 8.0 (p=0.02) and for SUVmean from 6.7 to 6.1 to 5.2 (p=0.14) respectively. Logistic regression analysis demonstrated that the SUVmax dropped by 2.6 (p<0.01) and SUVmean by 0.8 (p=0.05) between tumour locations from proximal to distal oesophagus. However, the effect of tumour location on SUVmax (p=0.23) and SUVmean (p=0.37) lost its significance when corrected for tissue type.

Prognostically, staging SUVmean had a significant correlation with survival in patients with SUV values of less than 5 having a better survival than those above 5 (p=0.02), Figure 14. The risk of death was 2.4 times higher (95% CI 1.1, 5.0, p=0.02) in the latter group, after correcting for patients age, tumour type and tumour location. This survival advantage, however, wasn't demonstrated with a SUVmax of 10 and above (p=0.14), Figure 15. The effect of chemotherapy did not seem to influence survival in this cohort of patients (p=0.20).

Patients with advanced tumours, seemed to demonstrate an increase in metabolic activity, reflected by the increase in SUV uptake. The SUVmax for high-grade dysplasia, Stage I, II and III were 3.5, 5.1, 11.6 and 9.6 (p=0.02) and for SUVmean were 2.9, 3.9, 6.5 and 5.3 (p=0.03) respectively. Patients with nodal disease also demonstrated an increase in SUV uptake compared to N0 disease, with SUVmax of 11.4 versus 7.4 (p=0.02) and SUVmean of 6.1 versus 4.6 (p=0.03) respectively.

Survival

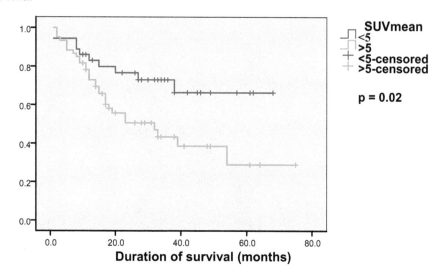

Fig. 14. Survival in operable oesophageal cancer patients around a SUVmean of 5.

Survival

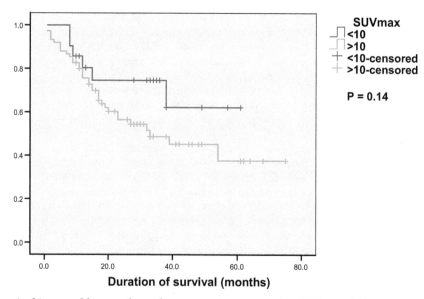

Fig. 15. Survival in operable oesophageal cancer patients around a SUVmax of 10.

3.4 Discussion

The treatment of oesophageal cancer, like any other solid organ tumour, is dependent of the stage of the cancer. However, the current TNM staging system is based only on anatomic and not on any biological factors. Interestingly, there is increasing evidence to suggest that biological factors influence prognosis just as much, if not more than, anatomical factors (22-24). FDG PET may aid in the detection of some of these biological factors that can't be identified with the current morphological imaging techniques. FDG PET has emerged as a useful metabolism-based whole body non-invasive imaging technique for the detection, characterization and staging of oesophageal cancer in recent years (25).

Van Westreenen et al. in a meta-analysis of the staging performance of FDG PET in oesophageal cancer, was able to demonstrate a moderate sensitivity and specificity for the detection of loco-regional metastases, but a reasonable sensitivity and specificity for the detection of distant metastases (26). The limited sensitivity and specificity for loco-regional metastases is due to the reduced spatial and contrast resolutions of PET-CT, and therefore limits visualization of the anatomic extent of the primary tumour as well as the ability to differentiate peri-oesophageal lymph nodes from the primary tumour (27). However, most morphological imaging scans as well as minimally invasive staging methods are able to compensate for this with a high accuracy for T and N staging. PET-CT, however, does have an excellent accuracy for the detection of M staging, accounting for up to 40% change in treatment strategies in patients as described by Chatterton et al. (28).

Recently, there is a growing body of evidence to suggest the prognostic potential of PET-CT in patients with oesophageal cancer, apart from its utility as a tool for radiotherapy planning or measuring tumour response in patients receiving neo-adjuvant treatment (7, 17-19). Its ability to identify metabolic activity within tumours reflects the biological aggressiveness of these cancers. This was first demonstrated by Fukunaga et al., who reported that patients with high SUV value within the primary tumour have a worse prognosis than those patients with a low SUV (29). A recent meta-analysis by Pan et al. demonstrated that patients with high SUV value not only have a worse survival prognosis, HR: 1.86, but also a reduced disease free survival with early recurrence, HR: 2.52 (30). The majority of these studies use SUVmax, to distinguish high from low SUV groups (30). Only one study utilized SUVmean (30).

From our data, we were able to demonstrate the independent predictor of survival using SUVmean and not SUVmax, both with univariate and multivariate analysis. SUVmean is less susceptible to outliers, but bear in mind, this study also showed both SUVmean and SUVmax to correlate well, with a correlation coefficient close to 1, and therefore it would be premature to disregard the prognostic potential of SUVmax. Hence, they should be used hand in hand to complement each other.

The metabolic activity is influenced by the biological properties of the tumour as we know. We demonstrated that squamous carcinomas have a higher SUVmax and SUVmean uptake compared to adenocarcinomas. Unfortunately, due to the small number in our series, we were unable to analyse the prognostic potential of the SUV values within the individual tumour types. Interestingly, both tumour types had a similar range distribution, with squamous carcinomas SUVmax and SUVmean ranging from 3.5 to 30.5 and 3.2 to 11.5 respectively, and, with adenocarcinomas SUVmax and SUVmean ranging from 2.6 to 29.5 and 2 to 16.4 respectively. Also, in the multivariate analysis, SUVmean was shown to be an independent predictor of survival after taking into account of tumour type.

The prognostic potential of SUV is strengthened by its relationship to the T and N staging. We found a linear increase in SUVmax and mean with the T staging apart for stage III, where there was a slight decrease. This could be attributed to the fact that there were more adenocarcinomas than squamous carcinomas (64% vs 36%). Also, the SUVmax and mean within the primary tumour also related significantly to nodal disease, with a higher incidence of nodal involvement when the SUVmean was greater than 5 (50% vs 23.5%). This relationship between metabolic activity and the current morphological staging has been correlated in only a handful number of papers (7, 17-18).

Finally, how do we translate the wealth of information we obtain from morphological, biological, biochemical and minimally invasive techniques to these patients diagnosed with oesophageal cancer? As we already now, the incidence of oesophageal cancer varies according to geographic location, as well as the treatment practices (31). Apart from the TNM staging which provides prognostic information to the clinician, it allows treatment based algorithms to be compared, with the idea of producing a uniform framework, enabling multi-disciplinary teams to tailor their treatment appropriately according to the disease stage. However, there are subgroups of patients where, surgery alone, even in early cancers (T2N0) will not provide cure, or cases, where surgery itself is prohibitive due to the significant co-morbidities of the patient. Here, the additional biological information provided by PET-CT can better inform the multi-disciplinary team and treat the patient accordingly.

For example patients who are currently staged as T2N0 oesophageal cancers, have no agreed consensus with regards to their optimal therapy. The risk-benefit analysis of proceeding directly to surgery, or being treated initially with neo-adjuvant treatment followed by surgery, fails to reach a clear consensus. When we analysed our data pertaining to this subgroup, it was interesting to find out that patients with a SUVmean < 5 (n=6), only 1 patient died, due to peri-operative complications. However, in patients with a SUVmean > 5 (n=11), 2 patients died due to recurrent disease, both of which were not treated with neo-adjuvant treatment. The remaining patients were alive, taking into account that nearly 90% of these patients had received neo-adjuvant treatment. Though these numbers seem small, the fact that these early tumours with an SUV > 5 demonstrate a greater malignant potential should alert the multi disciplinary team to adjust their treatment accordingly.

In conclusion, apart from PET-CT serving as a staging modality for oesophageal cancer, it provides important biological information that reflects the metabolic activity of the tumour. This pre-treatment or staging SUV, can provide important prognostic information that can supplement the current TNM staging to improve our decision making process, to ensure patients with oesophageal cancer receive the appropriate treatment care.

4. Future developments of PET-CT

As technology improvements parallel the increase utility of PET-CT, we anticipate further development prospects within the field of metabolic imaging. One such area is the development of new novel tracers that mimic cellular mechanisms, other than glucose uptake. Already tracers exist which can identify regions of hypoxia, examples include, Flourine and Copper labelled compounds, such as, (18F-fluoromisonidazole, 18F-fluoroazomycinarabinofuranoside, 64Cu-ATSM, and 18F-EF5). These tracers can modify chemotherapy and radiotherapy by highlighting areas of hypoxia. These regions can be particularly difficult to treat, and resistant clonal elements can survive, due to the delivery of sub toxic therapies. With this knowledge, dose modification can be carried out, for example using Intensity Modulated Radiotherapy (IMRT). Other potential areas for research include the development of tracers to assess the rate of tumour proliferation and the prospective clinical application of the integrated MRI-PET.

Another growing utility of PET-CT is the ability to predict tumour response to neo-adjuvant treatment by PET-CT (6, 32-35). Metabolic response is suggested when there was a certain relative decrease of the SUV between staging and response PET-CT scans, Figure 16.

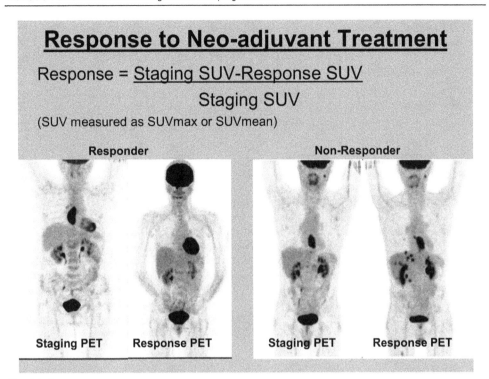

Response to Neo-adjuvant Treatment

Response = <u>Staging SUV-Response SUV</u>
                     Staging SUV

(SUV measured as SUVmax or SUVmean)

Fig. 16. Response measurement.

Several studies have concluded that FDG-PET is an effective modality for the non-invasive assessment of pathologic tumour response to neo-adjuvant treatment, but other investigations have seen no association between metabolic and histopathologic response (6, 32-35). The reason for these discrepancies between studies could be explained, at least in part, by various confounding factors that have an effect on SUV measurements; such as tissue activity factors, tissue state factors or normalisation factor; but also in part, by the definition of response in these respective studies (36). Simply using a specific cut-off value of SUV, to determine metabolic response from the response PET-CT scan, would be inappropriate, as we have demonstrated a wide distribution of SUV uptake amongst patients with oesophageal cancer, Figures 11 & 12 (34, 37). Additionally, the inflammatory response post neo-adjuvant treatment can complicate the interpretation of metabolic response, increasing the false positive rate of non-responders, as most of these patients have a background diffuse low FDG uptake, with an SUV value as high as 2.6 as demonstrated by Wieder et al (38).   More importantly, as we have demonstrated, the biology tissue type influences the SUV uptake, both max and mean, and therefore using a percentage drop of the SUV from the staging to response PET-CT scan would be more judicious.

Recent evidence would suggest an interval PET-CT at 14 days after commencing neo-adjuvant treatment, to judge treatment response and therefore determine further treatment course. Wieder et al was able to demonstrate this, predicting histopathologic response with a sensitivity and specificity of 93% and 88%, respectively, with treatment induced oesophagitis observed in less than 15% of the scans (38). Furthermore, the decrease in metabolic activity at 14 days was significantly associated with overall survival (38). This was also confirmed in the

MUNICON trial, confirming the usefulness of early response evaluation by PET, and therefore tailoring multimodal treatment in accordance with individual tumour biology (39). We anticipate that PET-CT will have a significant impact on patient management by allowing a new means to individualize neo-adjuvant treatment in patients with oesophageal cancer.

5. References

[1] Office of National Statistics, 2010 Mortality Statistics: Deaths Registered in England & Wales, 2008.

[2] Northern Ireland Statistics & Research Agency: Registrar General Annual Report 2010

[3] General Register Office for Scotland, 2010 Deaths Time Series Data, 1997-2008

[4] Jeganathan R, Kinnear H, Campbell J, Jordan S, Graham A, Gavin A, et al. A surgeon's case volume of oesophagectomy for cancer does not influence patient outcome in a high volume hospital. Interact.Cardiovasc.Thorac.Surg. 2009 Jul;9(1):66-69.

[5] Bruzzi JF, Munden RF, Truong MT, Marom EM, Sabloff BS, Gladish GW, et al. PET/CT of esophageal cancer: its role in clinical management. Radiographics 2007 Nov-Dec;27(6):1635-1652.

[6] Ott K, Weber WA, Lordick F, Becker K, Busch R, Herrmann K, et al. Metabolic imaging predicts response, survival, and recurrence in adenocarcinomas of the esophagogastric junction. J.Clin.Oncol. 2006 Oct 10;24(29):4692-4698.

[7] Cerfolio RJ, Bryant AS. Maximum standardized uptake values on positron emission tomography of esophageal cancer predicts stage, tumor biology, and survival. Ann.Thorac.Surg. 2006 Aug;82(2):391-4; discussion 394-5.

[8] Warburg O, Wind F, Negelein E. The Metabolism of Tumors in the Body. J.Gen.Physiol. 1927 Mar 7;8(6):519-530.

[9] Greene F, Fritz A, Balch C, et al. Esophagus. In: Greene F, Fritz A, Balch C, et al, eds. AJCC cancer staging handbook part III: digestive system-9 esophagus. 6th ed. New York, NY: Springer- Verlag, 2002.

[10] Kato H, Miyazaki T, Nakajima M, Takita J, Kimura H, Faried A, et al. The incremental effect of positron emission tomography on diagnostic accuracy in the initial staging of esophageal carcinoma. Cancer 2005 Jan 1;103(1):148-156.

[11] Kato H, Fukuchi M, Miyazaki T, et al. Positron emission tomography in esophageal cancer. Esophagus. 2005;2:111-121.

[12] van Vliet EP, Heijenbrok-Kal MH, Hunink MG, Kuipers EJ, Siersema PD. Staging investigations for oesophageal cancer: a meta-analysis. Br.J.Cancer 2008 Feb 12;98(3):547-557.

[13] Weber WA, Ott K. Imaging of esophageal and gastric cancer. Semin.Oncol. 2004 Aug;31(4):530-541.

[14] Wayman J, O'Hanlon D, Hayes N, Shaw I, Griffin SM. Fibrinogen levels correlate with stage of disease in patients with oesophageal cancer. Br.J.Surg. 1997 Feb;84(2):185-188.

[15] Shimada H, Oohira G, Okazumi S, Matsubara H, Nabeya Y, Hayashi H, et al. Thrombocytosis associated with poor prognosis in patients with esophageal carcinoma. J.Am.Coll.Surg. 2004 May;198(5):737-741.

[16] Guillem P, Triboulet JP. Elevated serum levels of C-reactive protein are indicative of a poor prognosis in patients with esophageal cancer. Dis.Esophagus 2005;18(3):146-150.

[17] Kato H, Nakajima M, Sohda M, Tanaka N, Inose T, Miyazaki T, et al. The clinical application of (18)F-fluorodeoxyglucose positron emission tomography to predict

survival in patients with operable esophageal cancer. Cancer 2009 Jul 15;115(14):3196-3203.

[18] Rizk N, Downey RJ, Akhurst T, Gonen M, Bains MS, Larson S, et al. Preoperative 18[F]-fluorodeoxyglucose positron emission tomography standardized uptake values predict survival after esophageal adenocarcinoma resection. Ann.Thorac.Surg. 2006 Mar;81(3):1076-1081.

[19] Choi JY, Jang HJ, Shim YM, Kim K, Lee KS, Lee KH, et al. 18F-FDG PET in patients with esophageal squamous cell carcinoma undergoing curative surgery: prognostic implications. J.Nucl.Med. 2004 Nov;45(11):1843-1850.

[20] Downey RJ, Akhurst T, Gonen M, Vincent A, Bains MS, Larson S, et al. Preoperative F-18 fluorodeoxyglucose-positron emission tomography maximal standardized uptake value predicts survival after lung cancer resection. J.Clin.Oncol. 2004 Aug 15;22(16):3255-3260.

[21] Sanghera B, Wong WL, Lodge MA, Hain S, Stott D, Lowe J, et al. Potential novel application of dual time point SUV measurements as a predictor of survival in head and neck cancer. Nucl.Med.Commun. 2005 Oct;26(10):861-867.

[22] Wijnhoven BP, Pignatelli M, Dinjens WN, Tilanus HW. Reduced p120ctn expression correlates with poor survival in patients with adenocarcinoma of the gastroesophageal junction. J.Surg.Oncol. 2005 Nov 1;92(2):116-123.

[23] Yamazaki K, Hasegawa M, Ohoka I, Hanami K, Asoh A, Nagao T, et al. Increased E2F-1 expression via tumour cell proliferation and decreased apoptosis are correlated with adverse prognosis in patients with squamous cell carcinoma of the oesophagus. J.Clin.Pathol. 2005 Sep;58(9):904-910.

[24] Kato H, Takita J, Miyazaki T, Nakajima M, Fukai Y, Masuda N, et al. Correlation of 18-F-fluorodeoxyglucose (FDG) accumulation with glucose transporter (Glut-1) expression in esophageal squamous cell carcinoma. Anticancer Res. 2003 Jul-Aug;23(4):3263-3272.

[25] Kuipers EJ, Haringsma J. Diagnostic and therapeutic endoscopy. J.Surg.Oncol. 2005 Dec 1;92(3):203-209.

[26] van Westreenen HL, Westerterp M, Bossuyt PM, Pruim J, Sloof GW, van Lanschot JJ, et al. Systematic review of the staging performance of 18F-fluorodeoxyglucose positron emission tomography in esophageal cancer. J.Clin.Oncol. 2004 Sep 15;22(18):3805-3812.

[27] Rice TW. Clinical staging of esophageal carcinoma. CT, EUS, and PET. Chest Surg.Clin.N.Am. 2000 Aug;10(3):471-485.

[28] Chatterton BE, Ho Shon I, Baldey A, Lenzo N, Patrikeos A, Kelley B, et al. Positron emission tomography changes management and prognostic stratification in patients with oesophageal cancer: results of a multicentre prospective study. Eur.J.Nucl.Med.Mol.Imaging 2009 Mar;36(3):354-361.

[29] Fukunaga T, Okazumi S, Koide Y, Isono K, Imazeki K. Evaluation of esophageal cancers using fluorine-18-fluorodeoxyglucose PET. J.Nucl.Med. 1998 Jun;39(6):1002-1007.

[30] Pan L, Gu P, Huang G, Xue H, Wu S. Prognostic significance of SUV on PET/CT in patients with esophageal cancer: a systematic review and meta-analysis. Eur.J.Gastroenterol.Hepatol. 2009 Sep;21(9):1008-1015.

[31] Parkin DM, Bray F, Ferlay J, Pisani P. Global cancer statistics, 2002. CA Cancer.J.Clin. 2005 Mar-Apr;55(2):74-108.

[32] Downey RJ, Akhurst T, Ilson D, Ginsberg R, Bains MS, Gonen M, et al. Whole body 18FDG-PET and the response of esophageal cancer to induction therapy: results of a prospective trial. J.Clin.Oncol. 2003 Feb 1;21(3):428-432.

[33] Kato H, Kuwano H, Nakajima M, Miyazaki T, Yoshikawa M, Masuda N, et al. Usefulness of positron emission tomography for assessing the response of neoadjuvant chemoradiotherapy in patients with esophageal cancer. Am.J.Surg. 2002 Sep;184(3):279-283.

[34] Song SY, Kim JH, Ryu JS, Lee GH, Kim SB, Park SI, et al. FDG-PET in the prediction of pathologic response after neoadjuvant chemoradiotherapy in locally advanced, resectable esophageal cancer. Int.J.Radiat.Oncol.Biol.Phys. 2005 Nov 15;63(4):1053-1059.

[35] Brink I, Hentschel M, Bley TA, Walch A, Mix M, Kleimaier M, et al. Effects of neoadjuvant radio-chemotherapy on 18F-FDG-PET in esophageal carcinoma. Eur.J.Surg.Oncol. 2004 Jun;30(5):544-550.

[36] van Baardwijk A, Baumert BG, Bosmans G, van Kroonenburgh M, Stroobants S, Gregoire V, et al. The current status of FDG-PET in tumour volume definition in radiotherapy treatment planning. Cancer Treat.Rev. 2006 Jun;32(4):245-260.

[37] Swisher SG, Maish M, Erasmus JJ, Correa AM, Ajani JA, Bresalier R, et al. Utility of PET, CT, and EUS to identify pathologic responders in esophageal cancer. Ann.Thorac.Surg. 2004 Oct;78(4):1152-60; discussion 1152-60.

[38] Wieder HA, Brucher BL, Zimmermann F, Becker K, Lordick F, Beer A, et al. Time course of tumor metabolic activity during chemoradiotherapy of esophageal squamous cell carcinoma and response to treatment. J.Clin.Oncol. 2004 Mar 1;22(5):900-908.

[39] Lordick F, Ott k, Krause BJ, Weber WA, Becker K, Stein HJ, et al. PET to assess early metabolic response and to guide treatment of adenocarcinoma of the oesophagogastric junction: the MUNICON phase II trial. Lancet Oncol. 2007 Sep;8(9):797-805.

12

Pathophysiology of Extravascular Water in the Pleural Cavity and in the Lung Interstitium After Lung Thoracic Surgery

Giuseppe Miserocchi and Egidio Beretta
University of Milano-Bicocca, Department of Experimental Medicine,
Italy

1. Introduction

Thoracic surgery implies a considerable imbalance of fluid dynamics in the pleural space and in the lung interstitium, and this is of relevance when considering that the volume of water in these compartments is physiologically very low thanks to very powerful mechanisms of control able to offset potential causes leading to an increase in this volume. There are reasons to believe that severe complications of lung fluid balance may occur after lung resection surgery and that the critical period is 24-48 hours after intervention. This paper wishes to present an updated review of pathophysiology of fluid balance in the respiratory system to be discussed within the specific frame of lung resection surgery. Some concept were only marginally considered in a paper previously published that was mostly dedicated to alterations in respiratory mechanics following lung resection surgery (Miserocchi et al, 2010).

2. Control of pleural liquid volume

Pleural fluid turnover occurs at parietal pleural level in physiological conditions: a pressure gradient causes fluid to filter from the capillaries of the parietal pleura into the cavity and is drained through the lymphatics stomata that connect the pleural space to the submesothelial lymphatic network of the parietal pleura itself (Miserocchi & Negrini, 1997).

Fig.1 highlights schematically that fluid filtration mostly occurs in less dependent regions and pleural fluid is drained towards preferential absorption sites at the bottom and in the mediastinal region. The absorption pressure of lymphatics (Fig. 2) sets a subatmospheric pressure of the pleural fluid that averages ~ -10 cmH$_2$O at mid heart level (it is more negative in the less dependent regions of the cavity and less negative at the bottom, where it reaches ~ 0 cmH$_2$O). This pressure acts to keep the lung in close apposition of the chest wall. Note that the lung and the chest wall develop an elastic recoil that would tend to pull them apart (red arrows in the insert in Fig. 2), however, the pressure generated by such recoil (about 4 cmH$_2$O at the functional residual capacity) is less subatmospheric than that generated by the lymphatic pump, therefore, lung and chest wall are actually pushing one against the other. This mechanical condition does not impair the reciprocal movements of the parietal and visceral pleura (about 25000 km in a life span) due to a very efficient lubrication system (see insert in Fig.2) based on reciprocal repulsive forces of negative charges carried by polar phospholipids adsorbed on the opposing pleural surfaces and assures a friction coefficient as low as 0.02 (comparable to that of ice on ice) (Hills, 1992).

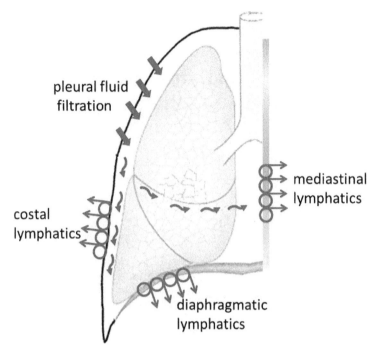

Fig. 1. Fluid turnover in the pleural cavity.

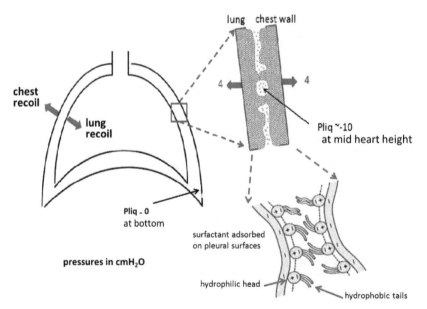

Fig. 2. Mechanical coupling between lung and chest wall.

2.1 Pathophysiology of pleural effusion

Pleural lymphatics act as efficient regulators of pleural liquid volume avoiding hydrothorax formation by increasing the draining flow (up to ~ 20 fold) in proportion to the increase in filtration rate (Miserocchi, 2009). As a matter of fact, for a tenfold increase in filtration rate, the volume of the pleural fluid would only be hardly doubled (Miserocchi, 2009). Any increase in pleural fluid filtration can in principle easily accumulate in the chest due to the opposite retraction of the lung and chest wall (Fig. 3).

When filtration exceeds the maximum lymphatic flow, pleural effusion results favoured by three conditions: an increase in systemic capillary pressure, an increase in permeability of the parietal/visceral pleura, a strong limitation to an increase in lymphatic flow. Pleural effusion are classified as exudates when the fluid/serum total protein ratio (indicated as TPR) exceeds 0.5 (Joseph et al, 2001; Joseph et al, 2002; Joseph et al, 2003). The degree of mesothelial lesion can be related to the concentration of lactic dehydrogenase (Joseph et al,2001) in the pleural fluid (indicated as FLDH); a cut off for FLDH at 163-200 U/L has been proposed for diagnostic.

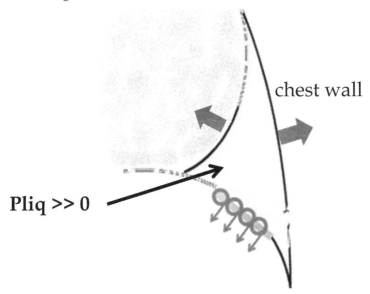

chest wall

Pliq >> 0

Fig. 3. Pleural lymphatics act as efficient regulators of pleural liquid volume.

3. Control of extravascular water volume

The thinness of the air-blood barrier (0.2-0.3 microns) reflects a functionally "dry" condition (Conforti et al, 2002), therefore, as much as for the pleural liquid, also for the extravascular space of the lung one can speak of a "minimum" volume of water. This ensures, in turn, a high efficiency of the gas diffusion. Similarly to the pleural fluid, also lung interstitial fluid is kept at a subatmospheric pressure (also ~ -10 cmH$_2$O, Fig.4) due to the powerful draining action of lymphatics in face of a very low microvascular permeability (Miserocchi, 2009). The latter feature allows to keep microvascular filtration as low as $1 \cdot 10^{-4}$ ml/cm^2 in 24h. Fig. 4 also presents important molecules, belonging to the proteoglycans (PGs) family, whose role appears crucial to control the extravascular water volume, as they act as highy hydroplhilic link proteins. Perlecan, an heparansulphate PG (MW 0.1-0.5 MDa) is placed in the basement membrane and controls the porosity to water and solutes; versican (MW 0.5 MDa), a large PG bound to hyaluronan (a random coiled molecule), provides rigidity to the tissue by establishing multiple non-covalent links with other molecules of the matrix and with cells (Roberts et al, 1997).

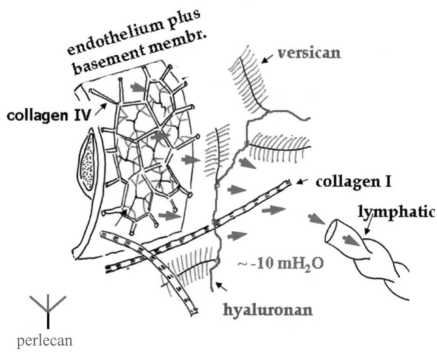

Fig. 4. Lung interstitial fluid dynamics and some macromolecular components of the interstitial matrix.

The volume of the extravascular water is strictly controlled so that the lung appears quite resistant to the development of edema. In fact, at least three mechanisms cooperate to allow only minimal variations in extravascular water volume relative to the steady state condition (Miserocchi, 2009). First, the glycosaminoglycan chains of PGs can bind excess water to form gel-like structures; this results in an increase in the steric hindrance of proteoglycans and corresponding decrease in the porosity of the basement membrane and thus also in microvascular permeability. Second, the assembly of large matrix PGs within the extracellular matrix provides low tissue compliance and this represents an important "tissue safety factor" against the development of edema. In fact, a minor increase in extravascular water in response to increased microvascular filtration, causes a marked increase in interstitial pressure (e.g., from ~ -10 to ~ 5 cmH_2O) (Miserocchi, 2009) that buffers further filtration. Third, arteriolar vasoconstriction represents an important reflex to avoid or actually decrease capillary pressure when filtration is increased due to an increase in microvascular permeability (Negrini, 1995, Rivolta et al, 2011).

4. Pathophysiology of lung edema

The development of severe edema is known as a tumultuous event taking place in minutes (Miserocchi et al, 2001a). Experimental models in animals allowed to attribute the sudden increase in extravascular lung water (Miserocchi et al, 2001a) to the loss of integrity of the proteoglycan components of the macromolecular structure of the lung interstitial space. Fragmentation/degradation of PGs of the basement membrane cause an increase in microvascular permeability of the paracellular pathway as pore size can reach 50-100 nm allowing easy leak of albumin. Finding of red blood cells in the alveolar fluid reflects major lesions of the air blood barrier. Fragmentation of matrix PGs removes the "tissue safety factor" by causing an increase in interstitial compliance. The loss of integrity of PGs reflects the sustained increase in parenchymal stresses, the weakening of the non-covalent bonds due to increased water binding, and the activation of tissue metalloproteases (Miserocchi et al, 2001a).

One shall consider interstitial edema as a sharp edge between tissue repair and severe disease: in fact, the transition from interstitial to severe lung edema occurs through an "accelerated" phase when the loss of integrity of the interstitial matrix proceeds beyond a critical threshold. Interestingly, the same pathophysiological mechanism can be extended to all forms of lung edema, the only difference being the time sequence of fragmentation of the families of PGs. The initial degradation process involves the large matrix PGs in cardiogenic edema, while in the lesional edema model, the initial process involves PGs of the basement membrane. In the hypoxia lung edema model, both PGs families are involved (Miserocchi et al, 2001a). Lung cellular activation for matrix remodelling and repair was documented as differential expression of signalling-transduction platforms on plasma membrane (Sabbadini et al, 2003; Palestini et al, 2002; Palestini et al, 2003; Daffara et al, 2004; Botto et al, 2006; Botto et al, 2008) and the hypothesis was put forward of differential activations of these platforms (lipid rafts or caveolae) to trigger redeposition of specific matrix components. A further peculiar feature of lung edema is that to develop in a patchy way, thus revealing regional differences in the efficiency of control of extravascular water volume. These differences have been recently documented in a hypoxic edema model (Rivolta et al, 2011) and the hypothesis was put forward that alterations in the geometry of the microvascular-alveolar design might favor an imbalance in interstitial fluid dynamics.

5. Specific conditions pertaining to thoracic surgery as potential causes of disturbance in extravascular water fluid dynamics

5.1 Pleural space

Evacuation of air from the cavity is the most immediate problem after thoracic surgery to allow re-expansion of the remaining lung. Air (and fluid) drainage are accomplished via a chest tube placement, and we address the reader to a recently published consensus definition (Brunelli et al, 2011). As a matter of fact, tube management is basically left to personal surgeon's evaluation despite the fact that such practice is a major factor affecting the length of recovery, the cost and the morbidity of patients undergoing lung resection surgery. Many surgeons use only a single drain, likely differently oriented, to drain both air and pleural fluid. The initial gas drainage is better performed by having the chest tube opening placed in the retrosternal region where air collects in the supine posture (see below). Conversely, pleural fluid is profitably drained by having the tube opening in the lowermost part of the pleural space (dorsal costodiaphragmatic sinus, both in supine and head up posture (Miserocchi et al, 1988; Haber et al, 2001) where fluid collects. Hydrothorax may develop due to surgical insult and/or to excessive subatmospehric pressure applied to the chest tube favouring fluid filtration. Note that pleural liquid pressure in the costodiaphragmatic sinus is close to 0 cmH$_2$O in physiological conditions and may become positive with increasing liquid pooling.

Thus, the recommended strategy is simply that of having the chest tube open to atmosphere (Fig. 5A): whenever pressure, in the hydrothorax will exceed atmospheric pressure fluid will drain into the tube. To avoid suction of liquid/air back into the pleural cavity when a subatmospheric pleural pressure is generated on inspiration, a one way valve should be placed on the tube outlet. In case fluid advances down the tube (by 10cm in Fig. 5B) a subatmospheric pressure (-10 cmH$_2$O) is generated at tip of chest tube in the pleural space, a condition speeding up the drainage.

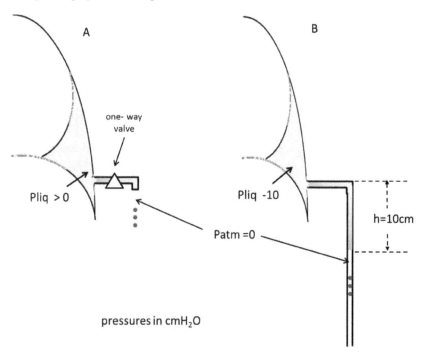

Fig. 5. Fluid mechanics of hydrothorax drainage from the costodiaphragmatic sinus.

For a pressure at tip of the order of about -60 cmH$_2$O (the case of a fluid column from patient bed down to the floor) the pressure gradient for fluid filtration into the cavity would be increased by about 10 times! No wonder that such pressure would contribute to increased fluid filtration and hydrothorax formation. Interestingly, the negative pressure generated at tip remains basically confined to the fluid pool and is not transmitted to the rest of the pleural space due to the extremely high flow resistance of the pleural space once the visceral pleura adheres to the parietal one (Miserocchi et al, 1992). Recovery from pleural effusion may be slow, ranging from weeks to months (Cohen & Sahn, 2001). Removal of chest tubes after fluid drainage of 400-450 cc /day or less appears reasonable (Cerfolio & Bryant, 2008; Cerfolio et al, 2010; Bertholet et al 2010) as it is in the range of physiological daily pleural fluid filtration (an estimated value of 350 ml/day (Miserocchi & Negrini, 1997).

5.2 Lung interstitium

The important point to be considered here is that the compliance ($\Delta V/\Delta P$) of the remaining lung is decreased in proportion to the amount of the resected portion: so, for example, a 50% reduction in lung volume, would entrain a similar reduction in lung compliance.

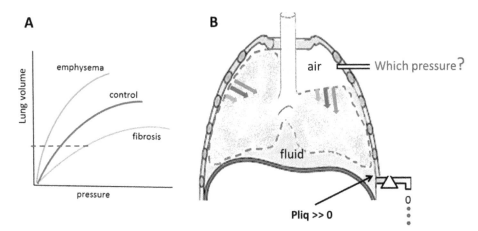

Fig. 6. Safe strategy to re-expand the lung after resection: gas pressure must generate the pre- operation lung distending pressure that depends upon the functional state of the lung.

Therefore re-expansion of the remaining lung to match the original chest volume would obviously require considerable greater distending pressure (over-distension) as well as a remarkable deformation of its natural shape. As thoroughly discussed in a previous paper (Miserocchi et al, 2010), to avoid lung over-distension re-expansion of the remaining lung should match the pre-operating distending pleural pressure that vary however as described by the volume-pressure relationship (Fig. 6A): fibrosis (blue) increases lung distending pressures on the abscissa and decreases compliance, while the opposite occurs in emphysema (green), relative to control (red). In practice, an air bubble ought to remain in the pleural cavity and the pressure generated by the suction line (Fig.6B) must be equal to that exerted by the lung before resection. The elastic properties of the lung can be described during a pneumological functional examination by relating lung volumes to the corresponding values of transpulmonary pressures as deduced from oesophageal pressure.

6. Lung over-distension: The risks of air leak and lung edema

6.1 Air leak

If no leaks are present, the gas bubble is reabsorbed (~1%/day), following the gradient in gas partial pressures in the blood and in the gas phase, until physical equilibration is reached. Reabsorption of the gas bubble is initially slow because the flow of O_2 to the blood is opposed by CO_2 flow to the bubble; furthermore, N_2 slows down the reabsorption process because of its low solubility in blood. Washing the cavity with oxygen would speed up the reabsorption process. The corresponding decrease in pleural pressure would increase fluid filtration so that, over time, liquid will replace gas.

Air leak after pulmonary resection may be due to bronchopleural or bronchoalveolar-pleural fistulas (Rice et al, 2002) due to failure to obtain a perfect surgical seal. An estimate of air leak would be useful to decide about chest drainage removal, however the methods of detecting air bubbles along the chest tube during forced expiratory maneuvers appears rather imprecise, while more refined methods are available (Varela et al, 2009). Measuring the change in pressure in the air bubble (ΔP) by a chest tube would allow an indirect estimate of the change in air volume (ΔV) considering that $\Delta V = Crs * \Delta P$, where Crs is the compliance of the respiratory system. Considering the mechanical arrangement of the lung and of the chest wall, one has:

$$\frac{1}{Crs} = \frac{1}{Cl} + \frac{1}{Cw}$$

where Cl and Cw are the compliance of lung and chest wall respectively. In physiological conditions, one has $Cl=Cw = 0.2$ L/cmH_2O, so that one has $Crs=0.1Cl$. As mentioned above, Cl reflects the functional state of the lung and furthermore is decreased in proportion of the decrease in lung volume. No such measurements are considered so far in the clinical practice: yet, we believe that a pneumological functional evaluation would provide important information concerning the trend of an air leak.

6.2 Lung edema

Severe complications representing the major cause of morbidity after lung resection ("idiopathic edema", ALI, atelectasis, ARDS) share a similar patho-physiological basis essentially represented by an acute increase in microvascular filtration, thus, simply, edema formation (Miserocchi et al, 2010). In post lung resection surgery, this can be due to:

- lung overinflation on re-expansion and/or prolonged mechanical ventilation with excessive tidal volume (Miserocchi et al, 1991). Stretching of lung parenchyma results indeed in a marked subatmospheric interstitial pressure, that, in turn, favours microvascular filtration potentially evolving towards matrix fragmentation and an "accelerated phase" (Miserocchi et al, 2001a);
- lack of clearance of the fragments, neutrophil and macrophage activation (Adair-Kirk & Senior, 2008), production of reactive oxygen species, leading to diffuse alveolar damage and inhibition of the active alveolar fluid reabsorption (Khimenko et al, 1994);
- large amounts of intraoperative fluid administration (Zeltin et al, 1984; Slinger, 2006), particularly when coupled to increased microvascular permeability, as clearly shown by experimental models of lung edema (Miserocchi et al, 2001a);
- the remaining lung is hosting a greater blood flow and this is accomplished by capillary recruitment and increased blood flow velocity and shear rate that lead to an increase in microvascular permeability (Min-Ho et al, 2005);
- local hypoxia, a known factor favouring edema formation (Miserocchi et al, 2001b), may develop due to edema itself as well as to ventilation/perfusion mismatch;

- finally, due to the decrease in vascular bed, pulmonary vascular resistances are likely to increase leading to pulmonary hypertension that is potentially correlated to the risk of developing pulmonary edema (Grünig et al, 2000; Rivolta et al, 2011).

7. The "postoperative residual pleural space"

The "postoperative residual pleural space" refers to the fate of the volume left free by lung resection (Misthos et al, 2007). As much as in physiological conditions, **the main variable setting the volume of the postoperative residual pleural space is the absorption pressure of the pleural lymphatics**. If their capacity to drain flow and generate a subatmospheric pressure have remained unchanged, they will still tend to reduce pleural liquid volume to a minimum. However, the new "minimum" will reflect a state equilibrium resulting from the modified lung-chest wall coupling and the actual filtration/absorption balance of pleural fluid. In practice, the volume left free by lung resection will be occupied (Fig. 7) in part by pleural fluid, in part by an increase in volume of the remaining lung, and in part by the displacement of the diaphragm and of the mediastinum.

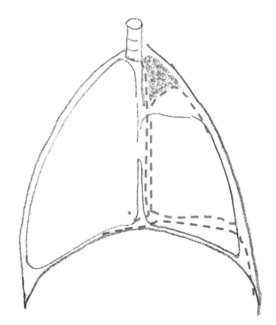

Fig. 7. The "postoperative residual pleural space"(blue area).

8. Cardiac output, lung fluid-balance and oxygen diffusion-transport

As delineated in section 2, control mechanisms are present in the lung to limit the increase in extravascular volume such as when lung capillary recruitment occurs in response to an increase in cardiac output. However the efficiency of these mechanisms, as from experimental models, varies among lung regions and among individuals, particularly when tissue hypoxia is also present (Rivolta et al, 2011).

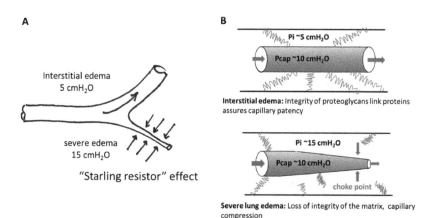

Fig. 8. A: lung capillary squeeze in relation to interstitial fluid pressure ("Starling resistor" effect). B: role of proteoglycans (in pink) fragmentation in favouring the squeeze of microvessels in severe edema.

Fig. 8A shows that in regions where severe edema develops, the increase in interstitial pressure is such as to squeeze the microcirculation ("Starling resistor" effect) thus impairing blood flow (Rivolta et al, 2011). In fact, the patency of microvessels is critically dependent upon the integrity of the proteoglycan molecules linking the matrix to the endothelial surface: as suggested in Fig. 8B, the integrity is preserved in interstitial edema, while massive fragmentation occurs when severe edema develops. The decrease in vascular bed causes a rise in pulmonary vascular resistances leading to an increase in pulmonary artery pressure, whose entity reflects the extension of severe edema (Rivolta et al, 2011). The variability concerning the proneness to develop lung edema and associated pulmonary hypertension in response to an increase in cardiac output, particularly when associated with alveolar hypoxia, is documented not only in animals but also in humans (Grünig et al, 2000). One can now remark that after resection surgery, the remaining lung, as described in section 4.2, is also exposed to increased blood flow and, owing to potential ventilation/perfusion mismatch, also to local hypoxia. Therefore, the risk of developing post-lung resection surgery pulmonary edema may depend upon the extension of the resection as well as on the individual proneness to develop lung edema. It appears therefore justified to assess the latter point by performing a pre-operation cardio-pulmonary exercise test and gather data on cardiac output, pulmonary artery pressure, pulmonary vascular resistance as well as indirect evidence of increase in lung water (see paragraph 7 below). These data may be compared to post-resection surgery condition.

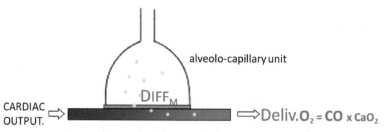

Fig. 9. Lung water balance related mechanisms limiting oxygen delivery

Fig. 9 summarizes the lung-water balance related mechanisms that may limit oxygen delivery defined as $DelivO_2$ = Cardiac Output x CaO_2, where CaO_2 is the oxygen concentration at the lung capillary outlet. A membrane "diffusion limitation" ($DIFF_M$) may result from the reduction in alveolar surface available for diffusion and/or from the presence of edema fluid. "Perfusion limitation" in oxygen transport has also to be envisaged because $DelivO_2$ is critically dependent upon regional lung blood flow and this, in turn, depends upon the local patency-compression condition of microvessels (see Fig. 8). Finally, the increase in blood flow velocity slows down the alveolo-capillary oxygen equilibration. All together, these alterations result in an alveolo-capillary oxygen pressure difference.

9. Indexes to assess alteration in pleural and lung interstitial fluid balance

Most of the complications of post-thoracic surgery relate to a severe disturbance in lung extravascular water and occur in the early postoperative period (Alvarez et al, 2007; Khan et al, 1999), similarly to what is observed after lung transplant (Khan et al, 1999).

Pre-operative:
-   lung compliance: needs measurement of transpulmonary pressure by using an esophageal balloon (more easily performed once the patient is anesthetized)
-   lung diffusion DLCO, Krogh factor (DLCO/alveolar volume). After lung resection DLCO will be reduced in proportion of resected volume, however, if the remaining lung works as an efficient diffusor, the Krogh factor will be normal.
-   respiratory impedance (in particular reactance at low oscillation frequency , 1 Hz). A recent paper highlights that reactance significantly decreases for an increase in extravascular water of about 10% (Dellacà et al, 2008).
-   lung comets determined by echocardiography, as a sign of interstitial lung edema (Picano et al, 2006).
-   cardio-pulmonary exercise test to evaluate the efficiency of the oxygen diffusion-transport system and the proneness to develop pulmonary edema

Immediate Post-operative:
-   measure lung compliance at the end of operation while the patient is still under anaesthesia
-   sensitive methods to assess a disturbance in lung fluid (respiratory impedance, comets)
-   time course of pressure in the pleural air bubble to monitor the trend of a potential air leak
-   lung diffusion: DLCO, Krogh factor (DLCO/alveolar volume)

Later on:
-   cardio-pulmonary exercise test to evaluate the efficiency of the oxygen diffusion-transport system

10. References

Adair-Kirk T.L. & Senior R.M. (2008). Fragments of extracellular matrix as mediators of inflammation. *Int J Bioch. Cell Biol*, Vol.40, pp. 1101–1110.

Alvarez JM, Tan J, Kejriwal N, Ghanim, K., Newman, M.A., Segal, A., Sterret, G. & Bulsara, M.K. (2007). Idiopathic postpneumonectomy pulmonary edema: Hyperinflation of the remaining lung is a potential etiologic factor, but the condition can be averted by balanced pleural drainage. *J Thorac Cardiovasc Surg*, Vol. 133, pp. 1439-4147.

Bertholet, J.W., Joosten J.J., Keemers-Gels M.E., van den Wildenberg F.J. & Barendregt W.B. (2010) Chest tube management following pulmonary lobectomy: change in protocol results in fewer air leaks. *Interact Cardiovasc Thorac Surg*, Vol. 12, No. 1, pp. 28-31.

Botto, L., Beretta, E., Bulbarelli, A., Rivolta I., Lettiero, B., Leone, B.E., Miserocchi, G. & Palestini, P. (2008). Hypoxia-induced modifications in plasma membranes and lipid microdomains in A549 cells and primary human alveolar cells. *J Cell Biochem*, Vol. 105, No 2, pp. 503-513.

Botto, L., Beretta, E., Daffara, R., Miserocchi, G. & Palestini P. (2006) Biochemical and morphological changes in endothelial cells in response to hypoxic interstitial edema. *Respir Res*, Vol. 7, No. 1, pp. 7.

Brunelli, A., Beretta, E., Cassivi, S.D., Cerfolio, R.J., Detterbeck, F., Kiefer, T., Miserocchi, G., Shrager, J., Singhal, S., Van Raemdonck, D. & Varela, G. (2011). Consensus definitions to promote an evidence-based approach to management of the pleural space. A collaborative proposal by ESTS, AATS, STS, and GTSC. *Eur J Cardiothorac Surg.* Vol. 40(2), pp.291-297.

Cerfolio, R.J. & Bryant, A.S. (2008). Results of a prospective algorithm to remove chest tubes after Pulmonary resection with high output. *J Thorac Cardiovasc Surg*, Vol. 135 pp. 269-273.

Cerfolio, R.J., Varela, G, & Brunelli, A. (2010). Digital and smart chest drainage systems to monitor air leaks: the birth of a new era? *Thorac Surg Clin*, Vol. 20, pp. 413-420.

Cohen, M. & Sahn, S.A. (2001). Resolution of Pleural Effusions. *Chest*, Vol. 119, pp. 1547-1562.

Conforti, E., Fenoglio, C., Bernocchi, G., Bruschi, O. & Miserocchi, G. (2002). Morpho-functional analysis of lung tissue in mild interstitial edema. *Am J Physiol (Lung Cell Mol Physiol)*, Vol. 282, pp. L766-L774.

Daffara, R., Botto, L., Beretta, E., Conforti, E., Faini, A., Palestini, P. & Miserocchi, G. (2004). Endothelial cells as early sensors of pulmonary interstitial edema. *J Appl Physiol*, Vol. 97, No 4, pp. 1575-1583.

Dellacà, R.L., Zannin, E., Sancini, G., Rivolta, I., Leone, B,E,, Pedotti, A. & Miserocchi, G. (2008). Changes in the mechanical properties of the respiratory system during the development of interstitial lung edema. *Respir Res*, Vol. 12, No. 9, pp. 51-60.

Grünig E., Mereles D., Hildebrandt W., Swenson E.R., Kübler W., Kuecherer H. & Bärtsch P. (2000). Stress Doppler echocardiography for identification of susceptibility to high altitude pulmonary edema. *J Am Coll Cardiol*. Vol. 35, No. 4, pp. 980-987.

Haber, R., Grotberg, J.B., Glucksberg, M.R., Miserocchi, G., Venturoli, D., Del Fabbro, M. & Waters CM. (2001). Steady-state pleural fluid flow and pressure and the effects of lung buoyancy. *J Biomech Engineering*, Vol. 124, pp. 485-492T

Hills, B.A. (1992). Graphite-like lubrication of mesothelium by oligolamellar pleural surfactant. *J Appl Physiol*, Vol. 73, pp. 1034-1039.

Joseph, J., Badrinath, P., Basran, G.S. & Sahn, S.A. (2001). Is the pleural fluid transudate or exudate? A revisit of the diagnostic criteria. *Thorax*, Vol.56, pp. 867-870.

Joseph, J., Badrinath, P., Basran, G.S. & Sahn, S.A. (2003). Do we need all three criteria for the diagnostic separation of pleural fluid into transudates and exudates? An appraisal of the traditional criteria. *Med Sci Monit*, Vol. 9, No. 11, pp. CR474-476.

Joseph, J., Badrinath, P., Basran, G.S. & Sahn, S.A. (2002). Is albumin gradient or fluid to serum albumin ratio better than the pleural fluid lactate dehydroginase in the diagnostic of separation of pleural effusion? *BMC Pulmonary Medicine*, Vol. 22, No. 2, pp. 1.

Khan, S.U., Salloum, J., O'Donovan, P.B., Mascha, E.J., Mehta, A.C., Matthay, M.A. & Arroliga, A.C. (1999). Acute Pulmonary Edema After Lung transplantation. *Chest*, Vol.116, pp. 187-194.

Khimenko, P.L., Barnard, J.W., Moore, T.M., Wilson, P.S., Ballard, S.T. & Taylor, A.E. (1994). Vascular permeability and epithelial transport effects on lung edema formation in ischemia and reperfusion. *J Appl Physiol*, Vol. 77, No. 3, pp. 1116-1121.

Min-Ho, K., Harris, N.R. & Tarbell, J.M. (2005). Regulation of capillary hydraulic conductivity in response to an acute change in shear. *Am J Physiol Heart Circ Physiol*, Vol. 289, pp. H2126–H2135.

Miserocchi, G., Negrini, D., Pistolesi, M., Bellina, C.R., Gilardi, M.C., Bettinardi, V. & Rossitto F. Intrapleural liquid flow down a gravity dependent hydraulic pressure gradient. *J Appl Physiol*, Vol. 1988, No. 64, pp. 577-584.

Miserocchi, G., Negrini, D. & Gonano, C. (1991). Parenchymal stress affects interstitial and pleural pressures in in situ lung. *J Appl Physiol*, Vol. 71, No. 5, pp. 1967-1972.

Miserocchi, G., Venturoli, D., Negrini, D., Gilardi, M.C. & Bellina, R. (1992). Intrapleural fluid movements described by a porous flow model. *J Appl Physiol*, Vol. 73, pp. 2511-2516.

Miserocchi, G. & Negrini, D. (1997). Pleural space: pressure and fluid dynamics, In: *THE LUNG, Scientific Foundations*, Crystal, R.G. West, J.B., Weibel, E.R. & Barnes, P.J., pp. 1217-1225, Lippincott-Raven Pub, New York..

Miserocchi, G., Negrini, D., Passi, A. & De Luca, G. (2001a). Development of lung edema: interstitial fluid dynamics and molecular structure. *News Physiol Sci*, Vol. 16, pp. 66-71.

Miserocchi, G., Passi, A., Negrini, D., Del Fabbro, M. & De Luca. (2001b). Pulmonary interstitial pressure and tissue matrix structure in acute hypoxia. *Am J Physiol (Lung Cell Mol Physiol)*, Vol. 280, pp. L881-L887.

Miserocchi, G. (2009). Mechanisms controlling the volume of pleural liquid and extravascular lung water. *Eur Respir Rev*, Vol. 18, pp. 244–52.

Miserocchi, G., Beretta, E. & Rivolta, I. (2010). Respiratory mechanics and fluid dynamics after lung resection surgery. *Thorac Surg Clin*, Vol. 20, pp. 345-357.

Misthos, P., Kokotsakis, J., Konstantinou, M., Skottis, I. & Lioulias, A. (2007). Postoperative Residual Pleural Spaces: Characteristics and Natural History. *Asian Cardiovasc Thorac Ann*, Vol. 15, pp. 54–58.

Negrini, D. (1995). Pulmonary microvascular pressure profile during development of hydrostatic edema. *Microcirculation*, Vol. 2, pp. 173-180.

Palestini, P., Calvi, C., Conforti, E., Botto, L., Fenoglio, C. & Miserocchi, G. (2002). Composition, biophysical properties and morphometry of plasma membranes in pulmonary interstitial edema. *Am J Physiol Lung Cell Mol Physiol*, Vol. 282, pp. L1382-L1390.

Palestini, P., Calvi ,C., Conforti, E., Daffara, R., Botto, L. & Miserocchi, G. (2003). Compositional changes in lipid microdomains of air-blood barrier plasma membranes in pulmonary interstitial edema. *J Appl Physiol*, Vol. 95, pp. 1446-1452.

Picano, E., Frassi, F., Agricola, E., Gligorova, S., Gargani, L. & Mottola, G. (2006). Ultrasound lung comets: a clinically useful sign of extravascular lung water. *J Am Soc Echocardiogr*, Vol. 19, No. 3, pp. 356-363.

Rice, T.W., Okereke, I.C. & Blackstone, E.H. (2002). Persistent air-leak following pulmonary resection. *Chest Surg Clin N Am*, Vol. 12, pp. 529-539.

Rivolta, I., Lucchini, V., Rocchetti, M., Kolar, F., Palazzo, F., Zaza, A. & Miserocchi, G. (2011). Interstitial pressure and lung oedema in chronic hypoxia. *Eur Respir J*, Vol. 37, pp. 943-949.

Roberts, C.R., Wight, T.N. & Hascall, V.C. (1997). Proteoglycans. In: *The LUNG scientific foundtaions.*, Crystal, R.G. West, J.B., Weibel, E.R. & Barnes, P.J. pp. 757-767, Lippincott-Raven Pub, New York.

Sabbadini, M., Barisani, D., Conforti, E., Marozzi, A., Ginelli, E., Miserocchi, G. & Meneveri, R. (2003). Gene expression analysis in interstitial lung edema induced by saline infusion. *Bioch Bioph Acta-Mol Basis of Dis*, Vol. 1638, pp. 149-156.

Slinger, P.D. (2006). Postpneumonectomy pulmonary edema. *Anesthesiology*, Vol. 105, pp. 2-5.

Varela, G., Jimenez, M.F., Novoa, N.M. & Aranda, J.L. (2009). Postoperative chest tube management: measuring air leak using an electronic device decreases variability in the clinical practice. *Eur J Cardiothorac Surg*, Vol. 35, pp. 28–31.

Zeldin, R.A., Normadin, D., Landwing, B.S. & Peters, R.M. (1984). Postpenumonectomy pulmonary edema. *J Thoracic Cardiovasc Surg*, Vol. 87, pp. 359-365.

13

Extracorporeal Membrane Oxygenation in the Transition of Emergent Thoracic Surgery

Shao-Jung Hsu and Kuang-Yao Yang
Department of Chest Medicine, Taipei Veterans General Hospital,
School of Medicine, National Yang-Ming University,
Taiwan, Republic of China

1. Introduction

Extracorporeal membrane oxygenation (ECMO) has been used more extensively since it became known as a potential bridge therapy, in patients with severe respiratory failure even under optimum conventional mechanical ventilator support, for further definite therapy. In the area of thoracic surgery, ECMO may have already become a useful life-saving tool but studies on this treatment method remain scarce. Currently available reports and case series reveal that patients with massive hemoptysis or critical tracheal stenosis may be benefit from temporary ECMO therapy during the transition of emergent thoracic surgery.

2. ECMO

ECMO, also called extracorporeal life support, is a type of cardiopulmonary bypass. In May 1953, Gibbon (Gibbon, 1954) used artificial oxygenation and perfusion support for the first successful open heart surgery. Then it was first also effectively used in an adult patient with acute post-traumatic respiratory failure in 1972 (Hill et al., 1972). The following preliminary studies in 1970s suggested that ECMO could support oxygenation in patients with profound respiratory failure. Recently, the CESAR trial demonstrated that ECMO-based management can improve survival in patients with severe acute respiratory failure (Peek et al., 2009). As technological continues to advance, increasing indications and reports suggest that ECMO has a role to play in the transition of emergent thoracic surgery (Hsu et al., 2011).

There are two types of ECMO: venous-arterial (VA) and venous-venous (VV) ECMO. VV ECMO supports isolated oxygenation failure, whereas VA ECMO provides hemodynamic and respiratory support. Although VA ECMO applies cardiopulmonary bypass, it has more complications due to the alteration of hemodynamic system. As a result, VV ECMO is typically used for respiratory failure while VA ECMO is used for cardiac failure.

2.1 Initiation of ECMO

ECMO is composed of a pump, an oxygenator and a heat exchanger. Once cannulation established, a large volume of blood is extracted from vessels by the mechanical pump. It passes through the oxygenator and heat exchanger. The oxygenated blood is then finally re-infused into the vessels. A complete circuit can be established in 40 minutes by an experience team. In VV ECMO, blood is drawn distally into the right atrium and returned into right atrium in an attempt to minimize recirculation. To achieve this, a drainage cannula is inserted in the right common femoral vein and the other infusion cannula is inserted in the right internal jugular vein. The tip of each cannula should be placed near the junction of the vena cava and the right atrium (fig. 1A). Alternatively, a double lumen cannula can be placed in one major vein (fig. 1B).

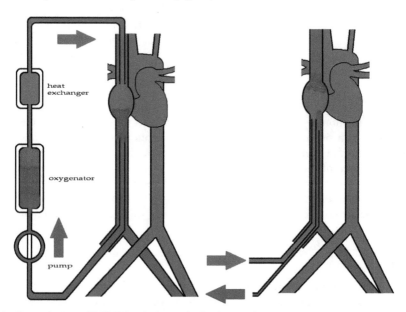

Fig. 1. A: Cannulation of VV ECMO through the femoral vein and jugular vein.
B: Alternative cannulation with a double lumen cannula through one major vein.

In VA ECMO, blood is drawn from the common femoral vein and returned into the femoral artery (fig. 2A). Venous blood is oxygenated and pumped back into arterial circulation. As a result, both the heart and lungs are bypassed. The main concern in femoral artery cannulation is hypoxia of the ipsilateral leg. On the other hand, if native heart function was presence, the oxygenated blood may not reach the proximal aorta and this would result in hypoxia of the heart and upper body. Alternatively, carotid artery cannulation could be performed (fig. 2B). But the risk of watershed cerebral infarction increases when utilizing this method. Because ECMO draw a large volume of blood from vessels, the circuit should be primed with fluid. In most cases, the circuit is re-circulated with normal saline, heparin and crystalloid first. A typical regimen is normal saline 2000ml with heparin 2000units/liter. Once ECMO activated, packed red blood cells are transfused to compensate for the diluting effects of the priming fluid. There is no consensus about the total amount of units that should be transfused. This depends on the volume of the circuit, the perfusion status of patients and the underlying disease. Typically, the goal is to make the hematocrit more than 30% and the mean arterial pressure more than 65mmHg.

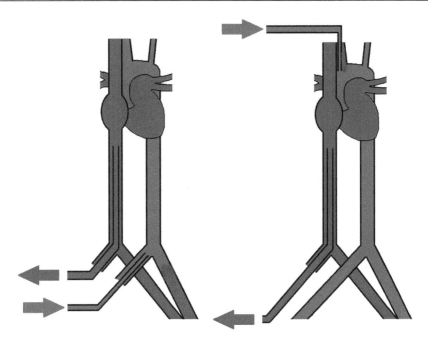

Fig. 2. A: Cannulation of VA ECMO through the femoral vein and artery. B: Cannulation through the femoral vein and carotid artery. Each path has its own unique risks with regards to complications.

2.2 Maintenance of ECMO
During the extracorporeal circulation, thrombosis may occur in the circuit and induce an embolism because of blood surface interaction. As a result, anticoagulation with a continuous infusion of unfractionated heparin is mandatory. The anticoagulant is monitored by activated clotting time (ACT). In general, ACT should be titrated to 210 to 230 seconds. The target should be decreased if the patients have a tendency towards bleeding. Platelets are continuously consumed because of the exposure to the foreign surface and the sheer force. As a result, platelet counts should also be monitored frequently. Sedation is definitely needed during ECMO. Adequate sedation can decrease the anxiety and suffering of patients and put the cardiopulmonary system at rest. The common agents for sedation in ICU are a continuous infusion of midazolam or propofol. Muscle relaxants could be added as well if the patients cannot tolerate use of mechanical ventilators well. Regardless, ECMO should only be utilized when patients are adequately sedated.

2.3 Complications
ECMO alters hemodynamic stability and induces a large amount of blood run in a device out of body. As a result, complications including localized tissues ischemia and hemostastic instability may occur. The VA ECMO also changes the direction of blood flow which may cause more complications than VV ECMO.

2.3.1 Complications in VV and VA ECMO

Bleeding tendency is usually increased and profound bleeding may even become life-threatening. The occurrence rate of bleeding ranges from 7-34%. The contributing factors are due to the mandatory continuous infusion of unfractionated heparin, platelet consumption and sometimes the underline diseases such as massive hemoptysis and sepsis-related DIC. Effective management depends upon the sites and the causes of bleeding. For example, if the bleeding source is mucosa or gastrointestinal tract, medical management including correcting thrombocytopenia and transfusing with fresh frozen plasma may be necessary. If the bleeding persists or develops into profound bleeding, unfractionated heparin infusion must be withheld temporarily. After the bleeding stops, heparin should be added once again but the target ACT could be adjusted. On the other hand, bleeding from the surgical or device-insertion wounds, including ECMO cannulation site, often requires surgical intervention. This ranges from bedside electrocautery to surgical exploration to achieve bleeding stoppage.

Thrombosis occurs at a rate of 8-17% and heparinization may help to reduce the incidence rate, but could also increase the potential for bleeding events. The balance between homeostasis and thrombosis require frequent clinical and laboratory monitoring. The pressure gradient across the oxygenator is a useful tool to be monitored, and a sudden change in the gradient may suggest a thrombus formation.

Bleeding from a cannulated site is not uncommon. Vascular perforation and arterial dissection may occur during the placement of the cannula. Thus, the utilization of an experienced surgeon is quite important to avoid such complications.

2.3.2 Complications only in VA ECMO

In VA ECMO, oxygenated blood is infused into carotid artery or femoral artery, which forms a countercurrent to native blood flow from the left ventricle. As a result, the increased afterload may worsen the cardiac output of the left ventricle. This results in left ventricle distension, acute pulmonary hypertension and then even pulmonary hemorrhage.

If the infusion cannula is placed in the femoral artery, not only the direction of blood flow of left ventricle, but also the blood flow of aorta is changed. Blood stasis in the aorta is induced if we are not able to maintain left ventricle output. Consequently, aorta thrombosis may develop.

In this type of situation, blood flow from ECMO supplies lower extremities and visceral organs, where as the brain, heart and upper extremities are supplied by the heart itself. It is obvious that the oxygen saturation from the blood vessels supplied by ECMO is much higher than that by heart. Under this type of condition, cerebral and cardiac hypoxia may occur without being recognized if saturation is only monitored by blood sampling from the lower extremities. As a result, monitoring blood saturation during VA ECMO only by digital oxymetry or single arterial line should be avoided.

2.4 Pumpless extracorporeal lung-assisted (pECLA) device

Pumpless extracorporeal lung-assisted device, a novel type of ECMO, had been developed in recent 10 years. In 1967, Rashkind and colleagues first proposed the concept of pECLA (Rashkind et al. 1967). In recent years, the commercialized devices are available and become more and more popular in intensive care unit (Walles, 2007).

During setting up, the blood was drawn from the common femoral artery and sent back to the femoral vein. The pressure gradient driving blood flow in the device was supplied by heart pumping. As a result, pECLA dose not need a centrifugal or roller pump. In this way, it could be set more easily with lower cost and lower dose of heparin than conventional ECMO. However, the device was built to remove carbon dioxide in patient with acute respiratory distress syndrome under lung protective ventilation strategy. Since the blood was drawn from the artery, the oxygenated ability of pECLA was not superior to conventional ECMO. In the management of massive hemoptysis or critical tracheal stenosis, the main problem encountered was hypoxemic respiratory failure, but not hypercapnia. As a result, the application of pECLA in these patients may need more strictly selection.

in summary, ECMO is a powerful therapeutic tool since it can replace the function of the heart and lungs. However, it has several potential complications and their risks increase as the duration of ECMO is prolonged. As a result, it can only serve as a salvage tool in life-threatening conditions and as a bridge to the definite therapy. There are two types of ECMO, the VA type and the VV type. Although VA type can supply perfusion pressure, it obviously has more complications than the VV type. In the field of emergent thoracic surgery, which we will introduce in the following sections, the cardiac function is usually preservative. As a result, VV type ECMO is the first choice in emergent thoracic surgery.

In thoracic surgery, there are 2 conditions, massive hemoptysis and major airway obstruction, where oxygenation is difficult to maintain. Under these conditions, if oxygenation could not be maintained by optimized mechanical ventilation or if the risk of life-threatening hypoxemia is very high, ECMO should be considered.

3. Massive hemoptysis

Massive hemoptysis is an important and potentially fatal event. It has been variably defined as an expectoration of blood amount ranging from 100-1000 ml in 24 hours (Dweik & Stoller, 1999). Since 200 ml of blood could fulfill the anatomical dead space of a major airway and 400 ml of blood might impede the oxygen exchange of alveolar space, massive hemoptysis can be defined as the expectorated blood volume that induces a life-threatening condition by virtue of airway obstruction or severe blood loss (Garzon et al., 1982).

3.1 Conventional management of massive hemoptysis

In the management of massive hemoptysis, protection of the non-bleeding lung and maintenance of adequate oxygen saturation are the major priorities. Then, the second step is to identify the source of the bleeding. The final step is the definite and specific treatment to prevent recurrent bleeding. Among the 3 steps, lung protection and maintenance of oxygenation are the most critical and could determine the outcome of patients. There are five methods for lung protection if the patient has continuous bleeding: decubitus position, selective intubation, double lumen intubation, Fogarty catheter placement and bronchoscope balloon tamponade (Lordan et al., 2003).

At first, an attempt should be made to identify the bleeding side of the lung. After that, the patient should be laid with the bleeding side down to isolate the bleeding lung and ventilate the normal lung. Single lung intubation could be performed if the amount of blood is too great (Gourin & Garzon, 1975). For right side bleeding, the bronchoscope could be placed in the left main bronchus and the endotracheal tube could be inserted in the left lung under the guidance of bronchoscope. For left side bleeding, the endotracheal tube could be placed in the right main bronchus simply by "pushing deeper"; however, this procedure has the risk of occluding the right upper lobe bronchus.

Double lumen endotracheal tube is an alternative method for lung isolation. However, it has four major disadvantages and is not routinely performed in ICU. First, it is difficult for a physician to decide whether double lumen tube should be inserted if the patient only has mild hemoptysis at presentation. Second, it is difficult for an operator to insert a double lumen catheter if the patient was under a hypoxemic status with large amount of blood in the trachea and pharynx. Third, an experienced operator is mandated to avoid the serious result of mal positioning, especially during the transference of patients from ICU to an angiography room. The last disadvantage is that there are still not enough trials to definitively demonstrate whether the double lumen catheter procedure is effective.

Fogarty catheter and bronchoscope balloon tamponade can be applied for lung isolation. A Fogarty catheter (14Fr/100cm length) can be placed over the bleeding bronchus under the guidance of bronchoscope. After inflated, the blood could be restricted in the bleeding side. Bronchoscope balloon tamponade may be more selective in restricting the blood. A 4-7 Fr balloon catheter is passed through the working channel of the bronchoscope and inflated to isolate the lung. However, both interventions need the guidance of bronchoscope. If the patient has massive bleeding, the large amount of blood in the trachea will impede the placement of a balloon catheter.

3.2 ECMO in massive hemoptysis

Several methods for lung isolation have been developed. Their aim is basically the same: to ventilate the good lung and to maintain adequate oxygenation. As a result, if a physician is able to establish a route for oxygenation without depending on inadequate ventilation support, the definite therapy could be applied more safely, even if we fail to protect the good lung. ECMO has such characteristics and might be useful in certain circumstances.

If the patient had "abrupt desaturation", ECMO can be implemented in 40 minutes by an experienced team. VV ECMO is the first choice, since most patients with massive hemoptysis are threatened by desaturation, rather than hypotension and shock. ECMO can be used as a bridge therapy for the definite treatment, such as angiography embolization and surgery.

Comprehensive review for ECMO use in life-threatening hemoptysis is lacking, and there are still no studies in the related literature on this topic. Since no original study has been published, the experience in application of ECMO in certain patients is largely based on case reports and case series. As early as in 1974, Hanson and colleague reported the first case with pulmonary hemorrhage rescued by ECMO (Hanson et al., 1974). However, not until the 1990s was there was a study or report about the use of ECMO in certain situations. There may be two reasons for this lack of reporting. The first, there is still the argument about the benefit of ECMO in an adult population at that era. And the second, heparinization during

Author, year (list in reference)	Underlie disease	Duration (days)	ACT (seconds)	Note
Hernandez et al., 2002	Wegener's granuloma	9	150	Pediatric
Kolovos et al., 2002	Autoimmune disease or sepsis	4.9	160-180	Pediatric, Case No. 8
Ahmed et al., 2004	ANCA vasculitis	12	Full anticoagulation since day 3	
Fujita et al., 2005	Fulminant hepatitis s/p liver transplant	4	N/A	
Agarwal et al., 2005	Microscopic polyangitis	7	160-180	
Arokianathana et al., 2005	Leptospirosis	7	N/A	
Sun et al., 2006	Idiopathic Pulmonary Hemosiderosis	5	170-200	
Zhong et al., 2008	Microscopic polyangitis	12	120-200	

Table 1. The application of ECMO in the 8 reported cases of diffuse alveolar hemorrhage.

ECMO may precipitate further lung hemorrhage. In 2002, Kolovos and colleague reported the largest series and again raised the profile of reconsidering the role of ECMO in severe hemoptysis and pulmonary hemorrhage (Kolovos et al., 2002). They reported 8 children, aged 2 months to 18 years, with pulmonary hemorrhage due to sepsis or autoimmune disease received ECMO as the final therapeutic method because of severe respiratory failure. The eight children exhibited varying degrees of coagulopathy but still received heparinization. The ACT was controlled between 160 to 180 seconds. There was no profound hemorrhage after they received ECMO and all of them were weaned from ECMO successfully after pulmonary hemorrhage was controlled. After that report, although bleeding tendency was still thought to be a relative contraindication for ECMO, it seems that some patients with severe pulmonary hemorrhage could be rescued by ECMO use.

As mentioned above, studies and reports in the related literature in this field are still scarce. To the best of our knowledge, there are only 13 reports about the application of ECMO in massive hemoptysis; 8 of them had diffused alveolar hemorrhage (DAH) (Table 1). In DAH, the use of ECMO has a stronger indication because there is no effective lung protective strategy. The patients in these reports were on ECMO support for 4 to 12 days. Heparin was used at a lower dosage to keep ACT around 120 to 200 seconds, instead of 210 to 230 seconds. Alternatively, delaying the application of heparin seems to be a safe method. All of the patients in these case reports were successfully weaned from ECMO after the underlying causes of severe hemoptysis were under control.

There are 5 reports about the use of ECMO in localized lung hemorrhage (Table 2). In 2 of them, the patients encountered abrupt desaturation during the procedure (bronchial artery embolization and operation), and lung protective therapy was difficult under that condition. Yuan et al. reported a patient with massive hemoptysis due to trauma and a double lumen endotracheal tube was intubated at the ER. However, the patient's clinical condition deteriorated and ECMO was used as a rescue method. In our experience, we have reported a case with bronchiectasis and massive hemoptysis (Hsu et al. 2011). The patient presented with acute respiratory failure due to a rapid progression of severe hemoptysis. A total of 4000 ml of packed red blood cells was transfused within 24 h to keep the hemoglobin level at around 10 mg/dl. The ventilator setting was in the volume control mode, at a positive end-expiratory pressure of 15 cm H2O, and a FiO2 of 100%; however, these setting only could maintain the arterial blood gas at a PaO2 of 62 mmHg. ECMO was applied due to high risk of transferring the patient from the intensive care unit to the angiography room and in-procedure mortality. After bronchial artery embolization successfully, ECMO was weaned 1 day later. No heparinization was performed because of the short term application of ECMO. The patient received left lower lobe lobectomy 2 weeks later due to intermittent small amount of hemoptysis. After the surgery, hemoptysis did not recur. He was discharged in ambulatory condition without any oxygen therapy.

Author, year (list in reference)	Underlie disease	Duration (days)	ACT (seconds)	Note
Fukui et al., 2006	Pulmonary hypertension	12	40-50 since day 3	
Bianchini et al., 2007	Swan-Ganz related trauma	2.5	N/A	During operation
Bedard et al., 2008	Aorto-pulmonary fistula	N/A	N/A	During bronchial arterial embolization
Yuan et al., 2008	Double lumen related trauma	10	60-80	
Hsu et al., 2011	Bronchiectasis	1	No heparin	

Table 2. The application of ECMO in the 4 reported cases of localized lung hemorrhage.

The use of ECMO in massive hemoptysis may be beneficial for certain populations. However, there are still a number of debates about the use of ECMO, since available data is not sufficient in this field. First, setting up ECMO is an invasive procedure, and physicians may not maximize the "conventional therapy" before initiating ECMO. Second, heparinization is usually necessary in ECMO, but it may produce a more severe hemorrhage. Third, ECMO itself may bring about some complications, such as platelet consumption, bleeding and/or thromboembolism.

In summary, maintenance of oxygenation is the most important object in the management of massive hemoptysis. ECMO should be used if all other methods fail or cannot be performed to maintain adequate oxygenation. However, there is still some uncertainty that needs to be addressed, such as the selection criteria of patients and the method of heparinization. Based on currently available evidence, the use of ECMO as a bridge tool for life-threatening hemoptysis can allow a patient to undergo definite therapy more safely.

4. Critical tracheal stenosis

Critical tracheal stenosis can be caused by either malignant or benign lesion. The symptoms may develop abruptly or slowly. In a chronic disease, such as malignancy, chronic inflammatory disease or collagen vascular disease, patients present with progressive dyspnea and stridor. While in acute conditions, such as blunt or penetrating neck trauma, patients may suffer from life-threatening asphyxia. The nature and severity of symptoms depends on the location and the magnitude of the lesion.

4.1 Conventional management of critical tracheal stenosis

Most patients with tracheal stenosis present with chronic symptoms. However, a 50% reduction in the cross-sectional area of the trachea usually results in dyspnea on exertion, whereas a 75% reduction in the cross-sectional area produces dyspnea and stridor at rest. This means that when these symptoms develop, the airway has been severely compromised with impending life-threatening obstruction (Wood, 2002). The patient may be compensated for airway obstruction, but even a small amount of secretion can be lethal. As a result, the strategies of management are different according to the time point of diagnosis.

If the tracheal stenosis is diagnosed early, physicians have enough time to make a complete study. The treatment options include surgical resection, reconstruction, therapeutic bronchoscopy with ablation and airway-stent placement. Before the management takes place, a secure airway could be performed utilizing an efficient method. The fiberoptic bronchoscope (FOB) provides a safe and effective way for airway control (Ovassapian, 2001). With FOB, the lesion could be evaluated vividly and the residual lumen of airway could be estimated. After that, the largest endotracheal tube (ETT) that can pass the lumen should be chosen, since the airway pressure is inversely proportional to the inner diameter of the ETT. To avoid trauma to the airway or the trachea lesion, the ideal size of FOB is 1mm smaller than the internal diameter of ETT. The ideal-sized FOB should be used if available. After determining the size of ETT and FOB, intubation could be performed by experienced anaesthesiologist.

If critical airway stenosis has developed, management will then become more difficult. The position of stenosis is important in this circumstance. For upper airway stenosis, FOB - assisted intubation or emergent tracheotomy can stabilize the airway. For severe mid-level tracheal stenosis, intubation above the stenotic portion can be performed first. After positive pressure ventilation, the residual lumen will be mildly dilated. Then a smaller tracheal tube is placed under the assistance of FOB through trachea or directly placed into main bronchus by the surgeon during surgery.

However, sometimes endotracheal intubation may be impossible, and even dangerous, possibly leading to complete airway obstruction. For most patients, emergent tracheotomy is ineffective because it cannot bypass the obstructive lesion. FOB may precipitate cough, bleeding or further mucosal edema and worsen the obstruction. There are only few choices for patients with this type of life-threatening major airway obstruction. One way is place the patient in a quiet room with very mild sedation and cool humidified oxygen. Nebulized epinephrine and dexamethasone help decrease the contraction and edema of the airway. It may temporary attenuate the symptoms and facilitate subsequent procedure, and FOB - assisted intubation.

4.2 ECMO in critical tracheal stenosis

In patients with critical tracheal stenosis, the key to saving their lives is to maintain safe and efficient gas exchange. However, conventional anesthetic technique has a high risk of causing airway total occlusion, and the risk is inversely proportional to the residual lumen of the airway. As a result, if intubation is performed under a "back up" system, that can maintain adequate oxygenation even under total airway occlusion, it becomes safer for patients and less challenging to anaesthesiologists. Thus, ECMO serves as an ideal tool in this situation.

In paediatric surgery, an increasing number of reports and small-scale patient studies have pointed out that ECMO, either elective or emergent, serves as a good-bridge tool for trachea reconstruction. In neonates with congenital trachea anomalies, ECMO reduces the risk of surgery to allow more precise and unrushed airway reconstruction (Huang et al., 2007)(Kunisaki et al., 2008). Elective ECMO uses in postoperative period also contribute to improve patients' outcome (Connonlly & McGuirt, 2001).

However, in the field of adults with critical trachea stenosis, we remain in the "case report era." In 1999, Onozawa and colleagues first reported a case with critical airway obstruction due to thyroid cancer. The diameter of residual lumen of trachea was only 5mm. VA ECMO was applied before induction and the surgery was performed smoothly. After the partial resection of the thyroid tumor and the insertion of tracheostomy, ECMO was decannulated successfully. Following that, there are total 7 case reports with 9 adult patients involving the application of ECMO during critical tracheal stenosis surgery (table 3). These physicians attempted to intubate the patients reported but failed in two of them. One of them even experienced hypoxia cardiac arrest. Emergent ECMO was activated and this saved the patient's life. Among them, the variable etiologies ranged from benign to malignant origin. The residual lumens of trachea are between 1mm to 5mm. The locations of trachea lesion distribute from 1.5cm above carina to upper level of trachea. VA ECMO was first used and more recently VV ECMO has been applied in cases of critical tracheal stenosis. Both types of ECMO can supply adequate oxygenation for performing the definite therapy.

Author, year (list in reference)	Underlie disease	Diameter & position of residual lumen	Ecmo type	Note
Onozawa et al., 1999	thyroid tumor	5mm	VA ECMO	
Kurokawa et al., 2000	tracheolysis	3mm	VV ECMO	
Chen et al., 2004	neurofibroma	more than 5.5mm, 5cm above carina	N/A	ETT, ECMO stand by only
Zhou et al., 2007	Post intubation trachea stenosis	2-3mm, 1.5cm above carina	VA ECMO	ETT but failure, emergent ECMO
	Leiomyoma	1mm, 6cm below vocal cords	VA ECMO	
Jeon et al., 2009	Thyroid tumor	N/A (3x4 cm)	VV ECMO	
Smith et al., 2009	Papilloma	N/A (2.5x2.8 cm), 2.5cm above carina	VV ECMO	
	Papilloma	N/A, extend 2 cm below vocal cords to just above carina	VV ECMO	Bronchoscope ETT related hypoxic cardiac arrest
Shao et al., 2009	Bilateral nodular goiter	5mm,	VA ECMO	

Table 3. The application of ECMO in critical airway stenosis during surgery

In summary, although there is still no original study published in this field, the related case reports have provided useful information. If the residual lumen of trachea is less than 5mm or the ETT cannot pass the lesion, a "stand by" ECMO should be considered before anaesthesia induction. VV ECMO is preferred since it can maintain adequate oxygenation with fewer complications.

And finally, it is worth noting that the criteria for patient selection still needs further investigation to demonstrate the benefits of ECMO as a bridge therapy in critical trachea stenosis. The cost-effectiveness of this method is also worthy of further investigation. Before a definitive conclusion can be made, ECMO should be kept in mind as one option for clinical physicians when handling a patient with critical tracheal stenosis.

5. Conclusion

During the transition of emergent thoracic surgery, the most important objective is to maintain vital signs, ensuring that they are stable. However, in cases of massive hemoptysis and critical airway stenosis, it remains difficult for physicians to achieve adequate oxygenation since these conditions share the same challenge: difficult airway maintenance. In this field, ECMO serves as the rationale option if conventional therapy cannot achieve adequate oxygenation. Due to the lack of an original study, the role of ECMO in the transition of emergent thoracic surgery still deserves further investigation regarding its utilization and cost-effectiveness. Based on the current evidence available, ECMO could make the transition of emergent thoracic surgery safer.

6. References

Ahmed, SH. et al. (2004). Use of extracorporeal membrane oxygenation in a patient with diffuse alveolar hemorrhage. *CHEST*, No.126, Vol.1, (July 2004), pp. 305–309, ISSN 0012-3692.

Arokianathana, D. et al. (2005). Leptospirosis: a case report of a patient with pulmonary haemorrhage successfully managed with extra corporeal membrane oxygenation. *The Journal of Infection*, Vol.50, No.2, (February 2005), pp. 158-162, ISSN 0163-4453.

Agarwal, HS. et al. (2005). Extra corporeal membrane oxygenation and plasmapheresis for pulmonary hemorrhage in microscopic polyangiitis. *Pediatric Nephrology*, Vol. 20, No.4, (April 2005), pp. 526-528, ISSN 0931-041X.

Bedard, E. et al. (2008). Life-threatening hemoptysis following the Fontan procedure. *The Canadian Journal of Cardiology*, Vol.24, No.2, (February 2008), pp. 145-147, ISSN 0828-282X.

Bianchini, R. et al. (2007). Extracorporeal membrane oxygenation for Swan-Ganz induced intraoperative hemorrhage. *Ann Annals of Thorac Surgery*, Vol.83, No.6, (Jun 2007), pp. 2213– 2214, ISSN 0003-4975.

Chen, PT. et al. (2004). Anesthetic management of a patient undergoing segmental resection of trachea with an endotracheal neurofibroma and nearly total occlusion of trachea. *Acta Anaesthesiology Taiwanica*, Vol.42, No.4, (December 2004), pp. 233-236, ISSN 1875-4597.

Connonlly, KM. & McGuirt, WF Jr. (2001). Elective extracorporeal membrane oxygenation: an improved perioperative technique in the treatment of tracheal obstruction. *The Annals of Otology, Rhinology and Laryngology*, Vol.110, No.3, (March 2001), pp. 205-209, ISSN 0003-4894.

Dweik, RA. & Stoller, JK. (1999). Role of bronchoscopy in massive hemoptysis. *Clinics in Chest Medicine*, Vol.20, No.1, (March 1999), pp. 89–105, ISSN 0272-5231

Fujita, S. et al. (2005). Expanded efficacy and indication of extracorporeal membrane oxygenation for preoperative pulmonary bleeding on pediatric cadaveric orthotopic liver transplantation. *Transplantation*, Vol.79, No.11, (June 2005), pp. 1637, ISSN 0041-1337.

Fukui, S. et al. (2006). Recovery from hemorrhagic pulmonary damage by combined use of a left ventricular assist system and right ventricular assist system and extracorporeal membrane oxygenation. *The Journal of Heart and Lung Transplantation*, Vol.25, No.2, (February 2006), pp. 248–250, ISSN 1053-2498.

Garzon AA.; Cerruti MM. & Golding ME. (1982). Exsanguinating hemoptysis. *The journal of Thoracic and Cardiovascular Surgery*, Vol.84, No.6, (December 1982), pp. 829–833, ISSN 0022-5223.

Gibbon, JH. Jr. (1954). Application of a mechanical heart and lung apparatus to cardiac surgery. *Minnesota Medicine*, Vol.37, No.3, (March 1954), pp. 171-178, ISSN 0026-556X.

Gourin, A. & Garzon, AA. (1975). Control of hemorrhage in emergency pulmonaryresection for massive hemoptysis. *Chest*, Vol.68, No.1, (July 1975), pp. 120–121, ISSN 0012-3692.

Hanson, EL. et al. (1974). Venoarterial bypass with a membrane oxygenator: Successful respiratory support in a woman following pulmonary hemorrhage secondary to renal failure. *Surgery*, Vol.75, No.4 (April 1974), pp. 557–565, ISSN 0039-6060.

Hernandez, ME. et al. (2002). Acute onset of Wegener's granulomatosis and diffuse alveolar hemorrhage treated successfully by extracorporeal membrane oxygenation. *Pediatric Critical Care Medicine*, Vol.3, No.1, (January 2002), pp. 63–66, ISSN 1529-7535.

Hill, JD. et al. (1972). Prolonged extracorporeal oxygenation for acute post-traumatic respiratory failure (shock-lung syndrome). Use of the Bramson membrane lung. *The New England Journal of Medicine*, Vol.286, No.12, (March 1972), pp. 629-634, ISSN 0028-4793.

Hsu, SJ. et al. (2011). Life-threatening hemoptysis due to left inferior phrenic artery to pulmonary artery fistula rescued by extracorporeal membrane oxygenation therapy. *Interactive Cardiovascular and Thoracic Surgery*, Vol.12, No.2, (February 2011), pp. 337-338, ISSN 1569-9293.

Huang, SC. et al. (2007). Perioperative extracorporeal membrane oxygenation support for critical pediatric airway surgery. *European Journals of Pediatrics*, Vol.166, No.11, (November 2007), pp. 1129-1133, ISSN 0340-6199.

Jeon, HK. et al. (2009). Extracorporeal oxygenation support for curative surgery in a patient with papillary thyroid carcinoma invading the trachea. *The Journal of Laryngology and Otology*, Vol.123, No.7, (July 2009), pp. 807-810, ISSN 0022-2151.

Kolovos, NS. et al. (2002). Extracorporal life support for pulmonary hemorrhage in children: A case series. *Critical Care Medicine*, Vol.30, No.3, (March 2002), pp. 577–580, ISSN 0090-3493.

Kunisaki, SM. et al. (2008). Extracorporeal membrane oxygenation as a bridge to definitive tracheal reconstruction in neonates. *Journal of Pediatric Surgery*, Vol.43, No. 5, (May 2008), pp. 800-804, ISSN 0022-3468.

Kurokawa, S. et al. (2000). Anesthetic management using extracorporeal circulation of a patient with severe tracheal stenosis by thyroid cancer. *The Japenese journal of anesthesiology*, Vol.49, No.11, (November 2000), pp. 1242-1246, ISSN 0021-4892.

Lordan, JL.; Gascoigne, A. & Corris, PA. (2003). The pulmonary physician in critical care * Illustrative case 7: Assessment and management of massive haemoptysis. *Thorax*, Vol. 58, No.9, (September 2003), pp. 814-819, ISSN 0040-6376.

Onozawa, H. et al. (1999). Anesthetic management using extracorporeal circulation of a patient with severe tracheal stenosis by thyroid cancer. *The Japenese journal of anesthesiology*, Vol.48, No.6, (June 1999), pp. 658-661, ISSN 0021-4892

Ovassapian, A. (2001). The flexible bronchoscope. A tool for anesthesiologists. Clinics in Chest Medicine, Vol.22, No.2, (June 2001), pp. 281-299, ISSN 0272-5231.

Peek, GJ. et al. (2009). Efficacy and economic assessment of conventional ventilatory support versus extracorporeal membrane oxygenation for severe adult respiratory failure (CESAR): a multicentre randomised controlled trial. *Lancet*, Vol.374, No.9698, (October 2009), pp. 1351–1363, ISSN 0140-6736.

Rashkind, WJ. et al. (1967). Hemodynamic effects of arteriovenous oxygenation with a small-volume artificial extracorporeal lung. *The Journal of Pediatrics*, Vol.70, No.2, (March 1967), pp. 425-429, ISSN 0022-3476

Shao, Y. et al. (2009). Extracorporeal membrane oxygenation-assisted resection of goiter causing severe extrinsic airway compression. *The Annals of Thoracic Surgery*, Vol.88, No.2, (August 2009), pp. 659-661, ISSN 0003-4975.

Smith, IJ. et al. (2009). Use of extracorporeal membrane oxygenation during resection of tracheal papillomatosis. *Anesthesiology*, Vol.110, No.2, (February 2009), pp.427-429, ISSN 0003-3022.

Sun, LC. et al. (2006). Extracorporeal membrane oxygenation to rescue profound pulmonary hemorrhage due to idiopathic pulmonary hemosiderosis in a child. *Pediatric Pulmonology*, Vol.41, No.9, (September 2006), pp.900–903, ISSN 8755-6863.

Walles, T. (2007). Clinical experience with the iLA Membrane Ventilator pumpless extracorporeal lung-assist device. *Expert Review of Medical Device*, Vol.4, No.3, (May 2007), pp. 297-305, ISSN 1743-4440

Wood, DE. (2002). Management of malignant tracheobronchial obstruction. *The Surgical Clinics of North America*, Vol.82, No.3, (June 2002), pp. 621–642, ISSN 0039-6109.

Yuan, KC. et al. (2008). Treatment of endobronchial hemorrhage after blunt chest trauma with extracorporeal membrane oxygenation. *The Journal of Trauma*, Vol.65, No.5, (November 2008), pp. 1151–1154, ISSN 0022-5282.

Zhong, H. et al. (2008). Extracorporeal membrane oxygenation for pulmonary hemorrhage in microscopic polyangiitis. *Chinese Medical Journal*, Vol.121, No.24, (December 2008) ,pp. 2622-2623, ISSN 0366-6999.

Zhou, YF. Et al. (2007). Anesthetic management of emergent critical tracheal stenosis. *Journal of Zhejiang University. Science. B.*, Vol.8, No.7, (July 2007), pp. 522-525, ISSN 1673-1581.

Permissions

The contributors of this book come from diverse backgrounds, making this book a truly international effort. This book will bring forth new frontiers with its revolutionizing research information and detailed analysis of the nascent developments around the world.

We would like to thank Paulo F. Guerreiro Cardoso MD, Ph.D., for lending his expertise to make the book truly unique. He has played a crucial role in the development of this book. Without his invaluable contribution this book wouldn't have been possible. He has made vital efforts to compile up to date information on the varied aspects of this subject to make this book a valuable addition to the collection of many professionals and students.

This book was conceptualized with the vision of imparting up-to-date information and advanced data in this field. To ensure the same, a matchless editorial board was set up. Every individual on the board went through rigorous rounds of assessment to prove their worth. After which they invested a large part of their time researching and compiling the most relevant data for our readers. Conferences and sessions were held from time to time between the editorial board and the contributing authors to present the data in the most comprehensible form. The editorial team has worked tirelessly to provide valuable and valid information to help people across the globe.

Every chapter published in this book has been scrutinized by our experts. Their significance has been extensively debated. The topics covered herein carry significant findings which will fuel the growth of the discipline. They may even be implemented as practical applications or may be referred to as a beginning point for another development. Chapters in this book were first published by InTech; hereby published with permission under the Creative Commons Attribution License or equivalent.

The editorial board has been involved in producing this book since its inception. They have spent rigorous hours researching and exploring the diverse topics which have resulted in the successful publishing of this book. They have passed on their knowledge of decades through this book. To expedite this challenging task, the publisher supported the team at every step. A small team of assistant editors was also appointed to further simplify the editing procedure and attain best results for the readers.

Our editorial team has been hand-picked from every corner of the world. Their multi-ethnicity adds dynamic inputs to the discussions which result in innovative outcomes. These outcomes are then further discussed with the researchers and contributors who give their valuable feedback and opinion regarding the same. The feedback is then collaborated with the researches and they are edited in a comprehensive manner to aid the understanding of the subject.

Apart from the editorial board, the designing team has also invested a significant amount of their time in understanding the subject and creating the most relevant covers. They scrutinized every image to scout for the most suitable representation of the subject and create an appropriate cover for the book.

The publishing team has been involved in this book since its early stages. They were actively engaged in every process, be it collecting the data, connecting with the contributors or procuring relevant information. The team has been an ardent support to the editorial, designing and production team. Their endless efforts to recruit the best for this project, has resulted in the accomplishment of this book. They are a veteran in the field of academics and their pool of knowledge is as vast as their experience in printing. Their expertise and guidance has proved useful at every step. Their uncompromising quality standards have made this book an exceptional effort. Their encouragement from time to time has been an inspiration for everyone.

The publisher and the editorial board hope that this book will prove to be a valuable piece of knowledge for researchers, students, practitioners and scholars across the globe.

List of Contributors

N. Barbetakis
Consultant Thoracic Surgeon, Thoracic Surgery Department, The agenio Cancer Hospital, Greece

Hidir Esme and Sevval Eren
Konya Education and Research Hospital, Dicle University, School of Medicine, Turkey

Jung-Jyh Hung and Yu-Chung Wu
Division of Thoracic Surgery, Department of Surgery, Taipei Veterans General Hospital and School of Medicine, National Yang-Ming University, Taipei, Taiwan

James D. Maloney, Nicole K. Strieter and Joshua L. Hermsen
University of Wisconsin School of Medicine and Public Health, William S. Middleton Memorial VA, USA

Petre Vlah-Horea Botianu and Alexandru Mihail Botianu
Surgical Clinic 4, University of Medicine and Pharmacy from Targu-Mures, Romania

Paulo F. Guerreiro Cardoso
Department of Cardio-Pneumology, Division of Thoracic Surgery, Heart Institute (InCor)-Hospital das Clínicas, Faculdade de Medicina, Universidade de São Paulo, Brazil

Dariusz Sagan
Department of Thoracic Surgery, Poland

Jerzy S. Tarach and Andrzej Nowakowski
Department of Endocrinology, Poland

Maria Klatka
Department of Pediatric Endocrinology and Neurology, Poland

Elżbieta Czekajska-Chehab and Andrzej Drop
1st Department of Radiology, Poland

Beata Chrapko
Department of Nuclear Medicine, Poland

Janusz Klatka
Department of Otolaryngology and Laryngeal Oncology, Medical University of Lublin, Poland

Ashish K. Sharma, Matthew L. Stone, Christine L. Lau and Victor E. Laubach
University of Virginia Health System, Charlottesville, VA, USA

Lucas G. Fernández, James M. Isbell and David R. Jones
University of Virginia Health System, Charlottesville, VA, USA

Francesco Puma and Jacopo Vannucci
University of Perugia Medical School, Thoracic Surgery Unit, Italy

Reubendra Jeganathan, Jim McGuigan and Tom Lynch
Royal Victoria Hospital, Belfast, United Kingdom

Giuseppe Miserocchi and Egidio Beretta
University of Milano-Bicocca, Department of Experimental Medicine, Italy

Shao-Jung Hsu and Kuang-Yao Yang
Department of Chest Medicine, Taipei Veterans General Hospital, School of Medicine, National Yang-Ming University, Taiwan, Republic of China

Printed in the USA
CPSIA information can be obtained
at www.ICGtesting.com
JSHW011811301024
72690JS00002B/41